Continuing care: the management of chronic disease

Oxford General Practice Series 7

Edited by

JOHN HASLER

*Regional Postgraduate Adviser
and Clinical Lecturer in General Practice,
University of Oxford*

and

THEO SCHOFIELD

*Associate Regional Postgraduate
Adviser in General Practice, Oxford*

OXFORD
OXFORD UNIVERSITY PRESS
NEW YORK TORONTO MELBOURNE
1984

Oxford University Press, Walton Street, Oxford OX2 6DP

London Glasgow New York Toronto
Delhi Bombay Calcutta Madras Karachi
Kuala Lumpur Singapore Hong Kong Tokyo
Nairobi Dar es Salaam Cape Town
Melbourne Auckland

and associates in
Beirut Berlin Ibadan Mexico City Nicosia

Oxford is a trade mark of Oxford University Press

British Library Cataloguing in Publication Data
Hasler, John
Continuing care: the management of chronic
disease.—(Oxford general practice series; 7)
1. Chronic diseases
I. Title   II. Schofield, Theo
615.5   RC108
ISBN 0-19-261364-2

Library of Congress Cataloging in Publication Data
Main entry under title:
Continuing care.
(Oxford general practice series; 7)
Bibliography: p.
Includes index.
1. Chronic diseases—Addresses, essays, lectures.
I. Hasler, John.   II. Schofield, Theo.   III. Series:
Oxford general practice series; no. 7. [DNLM:
1. Chronic disease—Therapy. 2. Long term care. W1
OX55 no. 7/WT 500 C762]
RC108.C65 1984   616   83-19473
ISBN 0-19-261364-2 (pbk.)

Typeset by Cotswold Typesetting Ltd, Cheltenham
Printed in Great Britain by Wm. Clowes Ltd, Beccles, Suffolk

Foreword

David Metcalfe
Professor of General Practice, University of Manchester

The populations of economically developed countries survive the perils of being born, the vulnerability to infectious diseases, and the dangers of giving birth, only to live into an old age beset by the disability and debility of chronic disease! This sad fact reflects a shortfall in prevention which has proved singularly difficult to correct because such prevention would require behaviour change (and that in the areas of gratification). The failure of primary prevention of these diseases, however, is compounded by a failure in tertiary prevention: that is the prevention of avoidable disability and suffering in people with established chronic diseases.

This is gravely disappointing in a country whose primary care service, based on general practitioners, boasts of providing continuity of care which should be comprehensive and free at the point of contact for the whole population. Yet there is much evidence, some of it meticulously researched and a lot anecdotal, including clinical audits done by both general practitioners and their trainees, which gives much cause for concern. It is easy, of course, to put down such failures of surveillance and control to lack of skill or motivation among general practitioners, but this is a simplistic and largely unrewarding approach. It neglects the fact that patients are autonomous and make their own complex and sophisticated decisions about the way in which they enter care, continue in care, and adhere to management plans made for them by general practitioners. Elegant management plans aimed at correcting and controlling biochemical anomalies may appeal to doctors but ignore the fact that many chronically ill people have a rooted dislike of being seen as chronically ill, of occupying the sick role, or accepting the 'invasion of their space' implicit in the plan in question. Just as we are unlikely to be effective at primary prevention unless we understand the dynamics of behaviour change we are unlikely to be effective at tertiary prevention.

This welcome book goes far to achieving a balance between the biological and behavioural components of care of patients with chronic diseases. The first section should give the reader real insights into what it feels like to have chronic disease, and what the world looks like from that position. Only with an understanding like this can care be properly planned. But planning care also includes looking at practice organization not in terms of practicability for the doctor, but practicability for the patient. This too is well covered. When these basic considerations have been laid before the reader, the second section goes on to applying them to those chronic diseases which are common and serious and which are becoming the very stuff of general practice.

Acknowledgements

When we started to plan this book, we decided that not only should all the clinical contributors be general practitioners, but, if possible, they should come from training practices in the Oxford Region. In the event, that wish became a reality and all the chapters in Part II have been written by course organizers, trainers, or partners of trainers. We thank them and hope that they are as pleased as we are in the demonstration of the high standard of clinical medicine that we have come to expect of our training practices.

The two non-medical contributors in Part I are of course well known for their contributions in their fields and it is a particular pleasure to thank them.

Finally, Mrs Barbara Vaughan and Mrs Ruth Warren, our charming, efficient, and long-suffering secretaries, deserve our earnest gratitude.

Contents

Contributors

Martyn Agass, MA, MRCP, MRCGP
General Practitioner, Berinsfield and
Clinical Assistant in Venereology, Royal Berkshire Hospital

Robert Gilchrist, FRCGP, D. Obst.RCOG
General Practitioner and Vocational Training Scheme Course Organizer, Banbury and
Clinical Assistant in Chest Diseases, Horton General Hospital

John Hasler, MD, FRCGP, DA, DCH
General Practitioner, Sonning Common and
Regional Adviser and Clinical Lecturer in General Practice, University of Oxford

Marie Johnston, B.Sc., Ph.D., Dip.Clin.Psych.
Senior Lecturer in Clinical Psychology, Royal Free Hospital School of Medicine

Michael Kenworthy-Browne, MA, MRCP, FRCGP
General Practitioner and Vocational Training Scheme Course Organizer, Oxford

Martin Lawrence, BA, MRCP, FRCGP
General Practitioner, Chipping Norton and
Clinical Assistant in Ophthalmology, Horton General Hospital

Gordon Lennox, FRCGP, MRC.Psych., D.Obst.RCOG, DPM
General Practitioner, Didcot; Tutor in General Practice, University of Oxford; and
Hospital Practitioner in Psychiatry, Fairmile Hospital

Ian Lister Cheese, Ph.D., MRCP
General Practitioner, Wantage

Andrew Markus, MA, MRCP, FRCGP
General Practitioner, Thame and
Tutor in General Practice, University of Oxford

David Millard, MA, FRC.Psych.
University Lecturer in Applied Social Studies, University of Oxford

Theo Schofield, MA, MRCP, FRCGP, D.Obst.RCOG
General Practitioner, Shipston-on-Stour and
Associate Regional Adviser in General Practice, Oxford

Tom Stewart, FRCGP, DCH
General Practitioner, Sonning Common and
Clinical Assistant in Rheumatology, Royal Berkshire Hospital

John Toby, MRCP, FRCGP
General Practitioner and Vocational Training Scheme Course Organizer, Northampton
and Clinical Assistant in Rheumatology, Northampton General Hospital

Part I

1 The size and nature of the problem

John Hasler

By any account, the number of people in the United Kingdom requiring some kind of continuing medical support is staggering. The original concept of a national health, or perhaps sickness, service, gradually producing a population of healthier individuals became a myth long ago. Every day, patients with chronic problems attend their doctor's surgery or hospital outpatient department at inconvenience and cost to themselves, making large demands on medical and supporting services. The problems are likely to get larger with an increasing elderly population. So could we in general practice provide this care more effectively for more people, with greater benefit to the patient? And what are the implications for us and the National Health Service?

THE SIZE OF THE PROBLEM

General practice

The most comprehensive analysis of the work done in general practice in the United Kingdom is the second National Morbidity Survey (Office of Population Censuses and Surveys 1974) analysing workload over a 12-month period at the beginning of the seventies. Amongst other things, the number of consultations and the number of patients consulting per 1000 population are analysed. Table 1.1 shows the rates for some of the common chronic diseases. Fry (1979) has also produced figures for events occurring annually in a typical general practice of 2500 and some of his figures for chronic disease are shown in Table 1.2. These figures are of course only means, affected considerably by such things as the age and sex structure of the practice population, the number attending outpatients, and the number of times the doctor asks the patient to reattend. General practitioners with a high proportion of old people on their lists, for example, will know that their elderly arthritics may create much more work than the figures quoted above. It is also important to emphasis that the data obtained for the National Morbidity survey were from selected practices and not a random sample.

In another analysis of the general practitioner's work at the beginning of the seventies by the Royal College of General Practitioners (1970), the number of patients consulting the average general practitioner was itemized. In addition to looking at chronic disease in the conventional sense, the authors also examined

Table 1.1. *Consultation rates and number of patients consulting per 1000 population for certain long-term problems. (Source: derived from Office of Population Censuses and Surveys Second National Morbidity Statistics from General Practice)*

Disease	Consultations (all ages)	Patients consulting (all ages)
Diabetes mellitus	17.2	4.5
Anxiety neurosis	73.1	34.0
Depressive neurosis	89.9	31.4
Epilepsy	8.0	2.9
Benign hypertension	77.3	18.7
Congestive heart failure	25.9	5.9
Chronic bronchitis	38.4	11.5
Asthma	34.3	10.2
Osteoarthritis and allied conditions	43.5	18.2
Rheumatoid arthritis and allied conditions	18.9	5.0

social pathology and estimated there might be 100 people receiving supplementary social security benfits, 50 people living on their own, and 60 one-parent families. General practitioners are only too well aware of the problems, both potential and real, that such patients may present. Also estimated were the number of undiagnosed conditions such as hypertension (250 persons) and chronic bronchitis (150 persons).

Has the workload of general practitioners changed in recent years? An analysis carried out by Billsborough (1981) showed that visiting rates have decreased substantially in the last 30 years but no significant trend has been identified in attendance rates. Since 1971 general practitioners have referred a constant number of patients on to hospitals as outpatients. There is, however, no evidence that workload in terms of consultations in general practice is increasing. On the other hand, it may be that the service that the general practitioner is offering is more comprehensive and the time he is taking per consultation is getting longer.

More information from the patients themselves is available from the General Household Survey in 1978 (Office of Population Censuses and Surveys 1980).

Table 1.2. *Annual prevalence of certain long-term diseases in a general practice with a population of 2500. (Source: derived from Fry (1979))*

Disease	Persons per year
Chronic rheumatism	100
High blood pressure	100
Chronic mental illness	460
Coronary artery disease	50
Chronic bronchitis	35
Asthma	30
Diabetes	20
Epilepsy	10

Questions were included which were designed to examine the extent to which people considered they had health problems, the effect of these problems on their lives, and how they coped with ill-health. Overall, 56 per cent of men and 70 per cent of women reported that they had a health problem all the time, or one that kept recurring, and for both sexes the proportion increased with age. There was an association between chronic ill-health and socio-economic group. Nine per cent of men and 12 per cent of women had seen a general practitioner in the preceding 14 days about their reported chronic or short-term ill-health.

Thus, using these figures, general practitioners having populations with a large proportion of elderly patients, or with a large proportion of patients from a low socio-economic group, will have an increase proportion of patients who are likely to report chronic health problems.

During 1981 the Royal College of General Practitioners published three reports of subcommittees of a Working Party on prevention (Royal College of General Practitioners 1981a–c). In all these reports a more positive approach to prevention was rightly urged on general practitioners. For arterial disease, the authors argued the case for bringing the routine management of hypertension and non-insulin-dependent diabetes back to general practice from hospital outpatients, and for handling smoking and obesity as clinical problems in their own right. About 4 per cent of the adult population have arterial pressures at or over levels requiring intervention and life-long follow-up. If lower levels of blood pressure are shown to need intervention, this figure could rise to 18 per cent. Two per cent of adults are diabetics, 40 per cent are cigarette smokers, and 20 per cent are above ideal weight for height. The resource implications are serious.

Psychological problems are reputed to be prominent in about a quarter of adult general practice attenders and there is strong evidence that particular life-events produce psychological reactions and disorders for which the general practitioner is consulted. The authors of the Report on the Prevention of Psychiatric Disorders (1981) believed that, unlike for arterial disease, the work involving more anticipatory care would not represent a large increase, but rather a change of skills and attitudes on the part of the doctor.

In 1978 approximately 2 200 000 women received contraceptive advice from their family doctors. Yet there is evidence that 44 per cent of all known conceptions to married women with two or more children are regretted (Cartwright 1978). During 1977 over 72 000 women under the age of 20 became pregnant outside marriage and over 30 000 women in this age group had the pregnancy terminated.

Whenever we look, the potential for continuing care in general practice is large, and to some, alarming.

The hospital service

If the problems of numbers seems large to our general practitioner service, it is no less so to the hospital service.

An analysis of outpatients statistics for England in 1977 (Department of Health and Social Security 1980) showed 140.5 new outpatients per 1000 population for acute specialties excluding obstetrics and accident and emergency, and 4.2 for psychiatric specialties. Each new outpatient generated 4.2 outpatient attendances for acute specialties and 8.5 attendances for psychiatry.

There have been varying changes in new outpatients according to specialty (Office of Health Economics 1981). For rheumatology and rehabilitation for example, a specialty much concerned with long-term problems, the number rose only by 2 per cent between 1969 and 1978 and is just below 200000 for England. Cardiology, on the other hand, whilst having a smaller number overall, rose from around 26000 by 55 per cent to 40000. New outpatients in geriatrics rose from 21000 to 36000.

The total numbers of new outpatients in England rose from 6.3 million in 1952 to 7.9 million in 1971. After that, however, there was a slight decline in the numbers of new outpatients seen in hospitals with the figure fluctuating between 7.5 million and 7.7 million between 1976 and 1979. Total numbers of outpatients attendances have also remained constant. Some of the outpatient referrals of course are for short-term problems but many are not.

It is clear from these figures that there is no evidence that general practitioners are passing more cases to hospital outpatients. It should be noted in passing that the numbers of doctors in the hospital service has increased steadily and at a faster rate than the numbers of general practitioners (Office of Health Economics 1981).

The ambulance service statistics also reflect some of the size of the problem. In the year ending 31 December 1978 the ambulance service for England carried over 16 million patients, excluding emergencies and the hospital car service over three million. The mileage involved was in excess of 130 million for these non-emergency cases. Most of this load would be for outpatients or day-ward attendances and many of the patients would be infirm with long-term problems.

Figures of this size seem almost meaningless. But it is clear that our hospital services are coping with a problem of major significance.

What does it cost?

The cost for outpatients has been steadily rising even though the number of outpatient referrals was static during the seventies. The cost per outpatient attendance at acute hospitals outside London was £2.87 in 1970/71 and had risen to £9.99 by 1976/77 (Department of Health and Social Security 1980). The actual cost per outpatient case outside London at an acute hospital was £41.61 in 1976/77. The total cost of the ambulance service for England in 1979/80 was in excess of £150 million although naturally some of this cost is for emergency services.

General practitioner, nursing, health visitor, and social services time is difficult to quantify. Suffice it to say that a very large proportion of time is spent in dealing with patients with long-term problems.

Cost has to be measured also in terms other than of NHS resources. The cost to the patient in relation to his time, work and domestic arrangements, and lifestyle may be considerable.

HOW WELL DO WE COPE?

Hospital care

It is clear that in any system of health care embodying a primary (general practice) and a secondary (specialist) service, the work of caring for people with long-term problems will be shared between the two. In theory most of the routine care should be given in general practice using the specialist as a consultant if there is a problem of diagnosis or management. In practice, however, in the United Kingdom much of the routine supervision has been taken over by the specialist services.

Does it matter?

On balance it probably does. In the first place, many of the chronic diseases are intimately related to the patients' domestic environment. The hospital doctor is not to know automatically whether the widow with heart failure or the unemployed man with chronic bronchitis have to climb two flights of stairs to reach their front doors. He will not have seen the empty chocolate box in the diabetic's drawing room, or the three cats which always set off the young girl's asthma. The physical and psychological difficulties of looking after an elderly grandmother may have to be witnessed at first hand to be fully grasped.

Second, the doctor who sees the patient for repeat outpatient attendances is often not the consultant, but maybe the registrar or sometimes the senior house officer – himself possibly a general practice trainee. Thus, the medical supervision by the specialist service may not be carried out by the specialist himself and the doctor may change from one outpatient attendance to the next.

Third, much of the care of long-term problems involves prescribing drugs or a different way of life. It is known that many patients fail to take their pills either according to instructions, or at all, and there is evidence which shows that certain factors influence compliance. In an editorial in the *Journal of the Royal College of General Practitioners* (1979) some of these factors were identified. The fewer the number of doctors prescribing for each patient, the better. The more the patient is involved in decisions about treatment, and the more he has the opportunity to discuss his treatment, the more likely he is to take it. Charney and Colleagues (1967) showed that the taking of penicillin by children was improved when the prescription was issued by the personal doctor rather than a partner. As the above Editorial stated 'the prescription symbolically represents the doctor himself and may well be treated in the same way'. It would be discourteous to our hospital colleagues to suggest that they do not take these matters into consideration or that they do not form effective personal relationships with patients. The fact remains, however, that it is more difficult for them to do so than for the general practitioner, especially if the doctor concerned changes at intervals.

Shaw (1981) outlined some of the problems of hospital outpatient visits to the hospital. For the individual patient, the cost will depend upon a number of factors, including the distance travelled, type of transport, time spent, and investigation or treatment given. If this expense is to be justified he argued there must be some clinical advantage which the patient could not have obtained from a visit to his general practitioner. Busy clinics sometimes become a vicious circle, giving little opportunity to revew all patients adequately or for the consultant to be consulted. Shaw also pointed out that the decision to recycle outpatients lies largely within the hospital. Inexperienced junior staff may lack the confidence to discharge chronic patients, interesting cases may be brought back for research or teaching, or the hospital staff may not be confident that the GP will adequately follow-up or inform the patient of the results of investigation. Ironically, in the short term, discharging a patient from the clinic involves the doctor in more work than asking the patient to come back.

On the other hand, are there advantages in the hospital consultant following-up chronic problems? It can be argued that the patient is more certain of benefiting from the latest advances in the specialty and that the consultant is more likely to be knowledgeable about the problem than the general practitioner. Furthermore, seeing the patient for only one condition means that the notes are not congested with notes for other problems.

What would seem most appropriate for the specialist service is for the consultant to be consulted for the more difficult problems of diagnosis or management leaving the routine management to the family doctor who should relieve some of the pressure on hospital outpatient clinics leaving the consultant more time for a smaller number of patients, who need expertise that the general practitioner does not possess.

General practice

Moving the care of long-term problems from the hospital service to general practice, as argued in the previous section has big implications for general practitioners. Could we cope, and do we want to?

The difficulties in general practice are of a different kind. First, because the general practitioner sees the patient for a number of different complaints at different times, monitoring one particular condition may be difficult. This is largely an organizational problem and can be overcome by a special flow sheet in the medical record or, as some general practitioners have done, by instituting a special follow-up clinic.

Second, the standards of medical records in many practices are still poor and it is sometimes difficult, without a special sheet, to see when, for example, a blood pressure or blood sugar was last measured.

Third, the introduction of repeat prescription systems into many practices has made it easy for patients to receive drugs over long periods without any direct contact with the doctor or the nurse.

These difficulties are, however, largely organizational and there are reasons why they should be overcome, not only for the patient but for the doctor as well. The patient, as we have seen, benefits from being more likely to comply and from not having the cost, in every sense of the word, of repeated visits to the hospital. If the communication and consultation between the patient and his family doctor is good, if the patient is involved in the decision making, and if the doctor carefully supervises the patient by appropriate examination and investigation, then there should be no better care for routine follow-up purposes.

The main advantage is to do with professional standards and expertise. If a general practitioner prefers to have many of his patients supervised by specialists, then inevitably his confidence and expertise will diminish. If he attempts to deal only with acute and self-limiting problems then his range of clinical skills will inevitably be narrower and less interesting than if he attempts to provide comprehensive care. It is evident from a number of publications that many doctors have welcomed the chance to expand their role and responsibility.

The obvious implication and difficulty is to do with time and resources. Do busy general practitioners have the time?

The question of time is a difficult one. It is quite clear that many doctors and their patients believe they are short of time and in many instances this is undoubtedly true. Practitioners such as Marsh (1980), however, argue that doctors could look after more patients and still provide a comprehensive and effective service. We probably do not know the complete answer. Many doctors are extremely busy, but their workload is more under their control than many of them imagine.

High prescribing of antibiotics, cough medicines, and tranquillizers condition the patient to believe that a prescription from the doctor is the appropriate remedy for many self-limiting ills. But ironically, like discharging hospital out-patients, it takes longer to tell a patient so, than to write another prescription. The ability to communicate effectively is not something that comes naturally to every doctor and from looking at video recordings of a large number of consultations, we have learnt that what is most frequently lacking is establishing what the patient really believes is wrong with him and sharing the decisions about his management with him. Both these features of a consultation are vital for the management of a long-term problem, and will save time in the long run. For example, an asthmatic patient who is angry about her dependence on doctors and drugs, and feels unable to share in her own management, may present with frequent acute attacks of asthma because of failure to heed warning signs.

Much follow-up does not need a doctor at all and can easily be delegated to a nurse. Blood pressure readings, blood sugar estimations, visual acuity measurements, weighing and measuring, peak flow readings are all examples of activities that nurses usually enjoy carrying out. Counsellors are starting to be used in practices for some patients with long-term emotional problems. Family planning nurses can easily deal with the routine follow-up of patients on oral contraceptives and secretaries can take care of ensuring that patients attend for regular assessment. And yet, although the Government refunds 70 per cent of staff salaries up to a maximum of two whole-time equivalents per doctor, many practices do not claim for as many staff as they could and still receive reimbursement for all of them. In short, most general practitioners should be able to manage the majority of their patients with chronic illness without an unbearable burden of work and with an added clinical interest.

COMMUNICATION BETWEEN HOSPITAL AND GENERAL PRACTITIONER

But whatever the skill of the general practitioner in managing his patients with long-term problems, there will be some patients who, because of the complexity of the problem, will need to be managed by both consultant and general practitioner. Equally, there may be other general practitioners who are happy to manage the majority of problems, provided that they feel that they have some kind of intermittent support from the hospital services.

Most of the publications describing innovations in this field relate to diabetes. Malins and Stuart (1971) described the setting up of a diabetic clinic in a general practice of four doctors with 9500 patients of which 50 were known diabetics. The clinic was held annually and involved not only the four general practitioners but also two consultants, a senior registrar, secretary, and technician who all visited the practice. In Poole a community care service for diabetics was established in 1972 (because of an increasing workload for the hospital) and has been described by Hill (1976). The patients attending the hospital clinic were surveyed and subsequently each general practitioner was supplied with the list of his patients and invited to meet the hospital staff to agree the future management. A co-ordinated service was then established with agreed guidelines and this included a community care co-operation booklet which was carried by the patient and was a means of communication between all concerned as well as a source of information for the patient himself.

Tulloch (1979) has reviewed the care of long-term disorders and points out that although much of this activity has to be done jointly by general practitioner and consultant, little attempt is made to co-ordinate it. Hospital and family doctors have rarely met to identify the objectives of management and to develop a clear programme of care. Nor are regular communications the rule. After the first referral letter from the general practitioner and the initial reply from the consultant, subsequent letters from the consultant may be sporadic and from the general practitioner usually non-existent. Co-operation cards, similar to those used for maternity care, could be used to advantage for a number of disorders.

THE VIEWS OF CONSUMERS

Cartwright and Anderson (1981) carried out a survey of patients' views about general practice in 1964 and compared the results with those from a similar survey in 1977. They found an increase in the number of people who said they had attended a hospital outpatient or casualty department in the previous 12 months, but this figure almost certainly included those attending diagnostic departments, and it is known that there has been a 25 per cent increase in those attending accident and emergency departments.

All the patients who had consulted a general practitioner at all in the previous 12 months were asked if there was any occasion when they felt the general practitioner might have examined them more fully: 11 per cent said yes. This proportion was higher among those who had been to outpatients, than among those who had not. The former were less likely to feel their doctor had a well-equipped, up-to-date surgery. But there was no indication that attendance at outpatients weakened ties between patients and their general practitioners.

Whether or not the patients had been to outpatients or casualty was unrelated to the procedures the doctors carried out, the number of patients they looked after, the number of doctors they worked with whether a nurse worked at the surgery, or their training. But those who had certain equipment such as peak-flow meters had a lower proportion of patients attending outpatients in the second survey. The authors commented that some hospital attendances would probably be reduced if general practitioners were prepared to arrange for more procedures and examinations to be carried out at the surgery and if they could spend more time with some patients. In both surveys the majority preference was for a general practitioner who did a number of tests himself rather than one who sent patients to hospital if they needed any investigation.

MEDICAL EDUCATION

If then we detect problems in the way we manage our patients with their long-term problems, are there clues to be found in the education we receive as medical students and young doctors?

Undergraduate education

Many of the facets of continuing care are to do with our clinical skills in history-taking, examination, investigation, and management especially in the field of therapeutics. No one would disagree with the necessity to be competent in these fields. In this respect our undergraduate medical education serves us reasonably well. Only in the field of probabilities is there likely to be cause for concern. The medical student largely learns in a hospital environment where a mere 10 per cent of the patients present: his enthusiasm for some of the more exotic investigations has to be tempered when he reaches general practice. But, as McCormick (1979) argues in his book, *The doctor—father figure or plumber,* which all aspiring general practitioners should read, medical schools, by emphasizing with good reason the scientific aspects of practice, have unwittingly diminished concern for patients as people. He points out that the strength of academic departments in clinical subjects has been the rigorous application of scientific method to the diagnosis and management of disease. This has encouraged a mechanistic approach and has tended to undervalue other areas that are less easily measured. Yet some of the most fundamental aspects of caring for patients with long-term problems are to do with the relationship between the doctor and patient, particularly in the field of therapy. The scientific physician if concerned mainly with diagnosis and investigation tends to see his role within relatively narrow confines. Those fields where no cure is possible, but only support, tend to become comparatively neglected. Is this then why we seem to be better at coping with acute problems, whether major or self-limiting, rather than the longer-term ones where much of the care is not to do primarily with science but more with support?

Vocational training for general practice

If there are deficits in undergraduate training for those young doctors who choose general practice as a career, can they be remedied during their period of vocational training for general practice? Unfortunately attitudes die hard, and a value system which puts scientific aspects of disease in a more important category than helping people is remarkably difficult to alter quickly. The fact that two-thirds of vocational training takes place in the hospital environment is a positive hindrance. There is little doubt that in the future we shall have to be much more explicit early in vocational training about the need for each doctor to examine his own values and attitudes.

We have already seen that both compliance and support are heavily dependent on the quality of consultation and communication between doctor and patient. This is a largely neglected area of undergraduate education for the reason described previously. Yet we now have some considerable experience in teaching communication skills to trainees in the Oxford Region (Pendleton and Hasler 1983; Pendleton *et al.* 1983). We are convinced of the necessity for all trainers and trainees to be aware of how they consult with patients, preferably by means of videotape, and to know how they can improve.

In spite of advances in teaching techniques in vocational training there is strong anecdotal evidence that both trainers and trainees prefer to learn experientially. Many trainers and trainees still base their tutorials on the patients that the trainee has managed or one the areas that the trainee asks to discuss. We now have evidence suggesting that the pattern of clinical care that the trainee deals with is not the same as that for a principal general practitioner.

In a study involving nearly 60 trainees in the Oxford Region between 1976 and 1979, Hasler (1982) examined their contact with 16 conditions requiring long-term supervision. Data collected included not only the number of patients in each category but the number of subsequent consultations with the trainee for the condition in question.

There was little difference between numbers of patients consulting per 1000 population for trainees and numbers derived from the second National Morbidity Study (Office of Population Censuses and Surveys 1974) except for depression, osteoarthritis, and rheumatoid arthritis where the figures for trainees were less than 50 per cent of the National Morbidity Study. But for consultations per 1000 population there were more discrepancies. Analysis of some individual diseases demonstrates some of the problems, and asthma, diabetes, epilepsy, and osteoarthritis are good examples.

Table 1.3 shows the total number of patients recruited by 36 trainees on 11- or 12-month attachments to training practices and what happened to them subsequently.

Table 1.3. *Total number of patients with four chronic diseases recruited by 36 trainees during 11 or 12 months in a training practice and subsequent numbers of consultations*

Condition	Total no. all patients	Percentage of patients seen			
		Once only for condition	Twice only for condition	Twice or more *after* first consultation For condition	For anything
Asthma	619	50	22	28	34
Diabetes	259	52.5	22	25.5	33
Epilepsy	103	72	18	10	17.5
Osteoarthritis	353	46	22	32	42

It can be clearly seen that approximately half the patients (72 per cent of the epileptics) were never seen again by the trainee after the initial consultation. Roughly another 22 per cent were only seen twice for the condition. This left less than a third (10 per cent of the epileptics) who were seen twice or more after the initial consultation for the condition in question. A slightly higher number came to see the trainee again but for something else. It must be borne in mind that the actual numbers of patients were in some cases quite small and some trainees were getting a very thin experience indeed. It would appear from analysing trainee prescribing that trainees see a larger proportion of self-limiting illness than do their trainers.

CONCLUSION

In a National Health Service where every patient has access to a personal general practitioner, every general practitioner access to a hospital consultant, and where every patient has a personal medical record following him or her from cradle to grave, could we not look afresh at the management of those patients with long-term problems? A modern, well-organized general practice should be able to provide routine care that is both of a high clinical standard and based on a close and effective personal relationship between patient and doctor. The practice team should be used to the full where appropriate, and both clinical medical records and practice registers should provide the support the general practitioner needs. The majority of patients should be under the full care of their own doctor. Where patients need the expertise of the consultant we should be looking at better systems of shared care. As Tulloch (1979) wrote 'the time has come for the haphazard methods of current shared care to give way to well planned integrated care of chronic disorders. Ignorance of, or indifference to, current problems by doctors (and not least general practitioners) represents the main obstacle to such progress.' Finally, we need to look again at the medical education of our young doctors and the continuing education of the older ones.

REFERENCES

Billsborough, J. S. (1981). Do patients consult the doctor less often than they used to? *Jl R. Coll. Gen. Practrs* **31**, 99–105.

Brown, G. W. and Harris, T. O. (1978). *The social origins of depression*. Tavistock, London.

Cartwright, A. (1978). *Recent trends in family building and contraception*. Office of Population Censuses and Surveys. Studies on Medical Population Subjects No. 34. HMSO, London.

—— and Anderson, R. (1981). *General practice revisited*. Tavistock, London.

Charney, E., Bynum, R., Eldredge, D. *et al.* (1967). How well do patients take oral penicillin? A collaborative study in private practice. *Pediatrics* **40**, 188–95.

Department of Health and Social Security (1980). *Health and personal social services statistics for England 1978*. HMSO, London.

Fry, J. (1979). *Common diseases*, 2nd edn. MTP, Lancaster.

Hasler, J. C. (1982). Clinical experience of trainees in general practice. MD thesis, University of London.

Hill, R. D. (1976). Community care service for diabetics in the Poole area. *Br. med. J.* **i**, 1137–9.

Journal of the Royal College of General Practitioners (1979). Editorial. *Jl R. Coll. gen. Practrs* **29**, 387.

McCormick, J. S. (1979). *The doctor—father figure or plumber*. Croom Helm, London.

Malins, J. M. and Stuart, J. M. (1971). Diabetic clinic in general practice. *Br. med. J* **iv**, 161.

Marsh, G. N. (1980). Cutting the cost of the National Health Service – a personal view. *Br. med. J.* **i**, 1140–1.

Office of Health Economics (1981). Briefing No. 18. *Doctors, nurses and midwives in the National Health Service*. London.

Office of Population Censuses and Surveys (1974). *Morbidity statistics from general practice. Second National Study 1970–71*. OPCS, RCGP and DHSS. HMSO, London.

—— (1980). *General Household Survey, 1978*. HMSO, London.

Pendleton, D.A. and Hasler, J.C. (eds.) (1983). *Doctor–patient communication*. Academic Press, London.

——, Schofield, T. P. C., Tate, P. H. L., and Havelock, P. B. (1984). *The consultation: an approach to learning and teaching*. Oxford University Press.

Royal College of General Practitioners (1970). *Present state and future needs of general practice,* 2nd edn. Reports from General Practice, 13. London.

—— (1981*a*). *Prevention of arterial disease in general practice.* Report from General Practice, 19. London.

—— (1981*b*). *Prevention of psychiatric disorders in general practice.* Report from General Practice, 20. London.

—— (1981). *Family planning. An exercise in preventive medicine.* Report from General Practice, 21. London.

Shaw, C. D. (1981). The problems of outpatient visits. *Health Trends,* No. 4, Vol. 13, pp. 107–8. DHSS and Welsh Office.

Tulloch, A. J. (1979). Integrated patient care. *Update,* Nov. 1105–10.

2 Psychological aspects of chronic disease

Marie Johnston

We often describe a patient's problem as psychological, but this description has a wide variety of meanings. Sometimes we refer to the aetiology of an illness such as peptic ulcer, whereas on other occasions we refer to the symptoms or even to the patient's response to the symptoms.

In lay use, when a problem is described as psychological it may have derogatory implications which may offend and confuse the patient. Thus it may be taken to imply that the symptoms do not exist and that the patient is imagining the symptoms or is malingering, i.e. is pretending to have symptoms in order to avoid some unpleasant tasks; a patient suffering severe pain may be insulted or angered if he makes this interpretation of a doctor's suggestion that his symptoms have a psychological element. Alternatively, it may be taken to imply that the illness is the patient's own fault or within his or her own control; a patient who is suffering severe asthmatic attacks may feel frightened and helpless given this interpretation. The other common interpretation is that the patient is suffering from a psychiatric illness which must be dealt with before the symptoms can be alleviated; the habitual cigarette smoker may be alarmed if this is how he interprets a suggestion that his problem is psychological.

In a psychological analysis one examines how the individual thinks, feels, and acts, and in this chapter we shall consider how these factors impinge on patients with chronic disease. The chapter is organized to follow the career of the patient with chronic disease, starting at the premorbid state when he or she may show signs that predict later disease and where early detection of psychological predictors may give opportunities for prevention. The second section deals with the ill patient, the thoughts, feelings, and actions that may be symptoms of disease or that may influence their presentation. The third section examines the response by the patient and other people. Given a diagnosed disease, how do the patients and others in their environments including their doctors respond to the illness, what do they think, how do they feel, and what do they do? Finally we consider the psychological aspects of treatment in the fourth section in terms of the compliance with all kinds of treatment regimes and in the fifth section the opportunity for treatments that intervene by changing the psychological factors.

PREDICTION AND PREVENTION

If the antecedents of disease are known then the opportunity for prevention exists, as the population at risk and possible causal agents have been identified. Before proceding to the psychological aspects of caring for patients with chronic disease, it is appropriate to examine the psychological antecedents of disease, i.e. the psychological factors which might alert the general practitioner to engage in 'anticipatory care'. Is there any evidence that particular ways of thinking, feeling, or behaving predict or even cause chronic disease? It is commonly accepted that some diseases may be psychosomatic, i.e. the pathological processes result from psychological causes, and textbooks of medicine will commonly include asthma, duodenal ulcer, essential hypertension, and ulcerative colitis amongst the psychosomatic diseases. Sometimes an illness is attributed to psychological factors because no physical cause can be identified, a dangerous procedure both because it distracts attention from a continuing search for physical causes, and because the psychological aetiology is often poorly specified and therefore cannot be reversed or modified. It should be possible to be more precise about the nature of the causes than simply to say 'it's psychological'.

The most commonly suggested psychological factors are stress, personality, and habits, i.e. the disease may be seen as the result of excessive stress on the individual, due to having a personality that predisposes the person to develop such a disease or due to habitual levels of drinking, smoking, eating, etc.

Stress

It is commonly accepted that stress can cause disease and we are not surprised if, 'pressure at work' or the strain of caring for an elderly relative begins to tell on the individual's health. Some occupations are seen as being more stressful and there is indeed evidence that the workers may be more susceptible to disease. For example, air-traffic controllers whose jobs require intense concentration and where errors are serious clearly have stressful work and they show a high incidence of essential hypertension. While some people may have stressful jobs, others endure the stress of becoming unemployed and there is now a growing body of evidence showing that redundancy and unemployment can also lead to elevated blood pressure which may persist if no work is found.

In the early studies relating stressful life-events and disease, patients were asked about stressful events occurring prior to the onset of their current illness and these reports were compared with those of healthy individuals. While the patients did indeed report more stresses, such studies are unable to establish a causal role as patients might be more likely to remember and identify such stresses in looking for a cause for their illness and some of the stresses identified might be associated with early symptoms of the illness rather than being causal.

In later studies, the stresses have been more clearly specified. For example,

Parkes (1975) studied men whose wives had died and compared them with men of a similar age, examining the prevalence of morbidity and mortality in the subsequent six months, and showed that the widowers were much more likely to become ill and even to die, usually of cardiovascular disease. An alternative strategy has been to use standard questionnaires to measure both the number of stresses experienced and the amount of adaptation they would require. The earliest questionnaire of this kind, the Social Readjustment Rating Scale (Holmes and Rahe 1967) is illustrated in Table 2.1. The individual checks the items he has experienced in the previous 6 or 12 months and gets a score in life change units (LCU) by adding up the values of the items checked; a high score is obtained either by having many events or by experiencing events which have high values. People with high scores are more likely to become ill than those with low scores. Using similar life-events assessments, it has been shown that those having more life-events are more likely to develop leukaemia, colds and fevers, fractures, heart attacks, etc. than those with lower scores. Thus life events predict morbidity but do not predict which disease the individual will develop.

While the studies on human beings show that stressful psychological conditions may predate disease, their true causal nature is best demonstrated in the animal studies (see Henry and Stephens 1977). In these, the animals are subjected to stressful living conditions over long periods and the resulting pathological changes studied both while the animal is alive and at post mortem. In a situation somewhat comparable to a stressful work environment, monkeys were required to press a lever to avoid shock whenever a light flashed; over a period of months the animals showed increases in blood pressure. Various social stresses have also been used. For example, tree shrews were given a daily experience of being defeated by a more dominant tree shrew and spent the rest of the day separated from their opponents only by a wire screen. The subordinated animals remained in a state of sustained sympathetic arousal for more than 90 per cent of their waking time and many of the animals died in less than two weeks, not because of injuries or starvation, but because they developed fatal uraemia.

Thus animal and human studies confirm that psychological stress can cause disease. Current research is attempting to define more precisely what is meant by psychological stress, as well as investigating whether there may be individual ways of dealing with stress that make one less susceptible. There is also some interest in identifying particular stresses or particular methods of coping which make some diseases more likely than others. For example, it has been hypothesized that stresses which elicit active coping are more predictive of cardiovascular disorders while more passive coping is associated with neoplastic changes.

Personality

In clinical practice, one hears reference to the 'asthmatic personality' or the 'rheumatoid personality' suggesting that particular personality types go with

Table 2.1. *Social readjustment rating scale*

	LCU values
Family	
Death of spouse	100
Divorce	73
Marital separation	65
Death of close family member	63
Marriage	50
Marital reconciliation	45
Major change in health of family	44
Pregnancy	40
Addition of new family member	39
Major change in arguments with wife	35
Son or daughter leaving home	29
In-law troubles	29
Wife starting or ending work	26
Major change in family get-togethers	15
Personal	
Detention in jail	63
Major personal injury or illness	53
Sexual difficulties	39
Death of a close friend	37
Outstanding personal achievement	28
Start or end of formal schooling	26
Major change in living conditions	25
Major revision of personal habits	24
Changing to a new school	20
Change in residence	20
Major change in recreation	19
Major change in church activities	19
Major change in sleeping habits	16
Major change in eating habits	15
Vacation	13
Christmas	12
Minor violations of the law	11
Work	
Being fired from work	47
Retirement from work	45
Major business adjustment	39
Changing to different line of work	36
Major change in work responsibilities	29
Trouble with boss	23
Major change in working conditions	20
Financial	
Major change in financial state	38
Mortgage or loan over $10 000	31
Mortgage foreclosure	30
Mortgage or loan less than $10 000	17

particular diseases. While there is no evidence that particular disease are associated with particular personality types, there is some evidence of an association between neuroticism and chronic disease. However, there is little support for the notion that this personality made the individual more susceptible to the disease.

Neuroticism

Using tests such as the Eysenck Personality Questionnaire (EPQ) and the Minnesota Multiphasic Personality Inventory (MMPI) it has been shown that physically impaired or chronically ill patients are more neurotic than comparable, healthy subjects. The 'neurotic triad' of high hypochrondriasis (Hs), depression (D), and hysteria (Hy) has been found in patients with as diverse chronic disabling conditions as rheumatoid arthritis, multiple sclerosis, spinal cord injuries, intestinal cancer, coronary heart disease, and various back and limb injuries. Thus patients with chronic disease have been shown to have different personality patterns from a normal population.

However, it would be wrong to conclude that the personality is a predictive or a causal factor in the disease. It seems equally plausible that the disease leads to personality change, patients experiencing painful and distressing symptoms and becoming more neurotic as a result. If this were the case then cured patients should show normal personality patterns and such evidence as exists confirms this hypothesis; patients attending a chronic pain clinic who showed the neurotic personality pattern were found to be less neurotic as their pain was successfully treated. One might also expect that asymptomatic undiagnosed patients would show normal personality patterns and Robinson (1969) has shown that undiagnosed hypertensives were no more neurotic than normal healthy individuals; his work, and work with other diagnostic groups, shows that it is the neurotic individual who is more likely to consult a doctor and be referred to specialist clinics so that research on clinical samples will have a higher proponderance of neurotic patients, not because neuroticism is associated with disease, but because it is associated with consultation and referral. Other research on hypertensives selected in a factory rather than a clinic has in fact suggested that they are *less* neurotic than normal samples.

Thus although an association has been found between neuroticism and chronic illness it is unlikely that the neurotic personality makes the individual more susceptible to disease. Rather more probable is that being chronically ill is likely to lead to emotional disturbances and, in addition, that doctors and research workers may get a biassed view of those with chronic disease if they look at clinic populations.

Type A personality

There is one clearly demonstrated association between personality and disease that allows the possibility of a causal role for personality, namely the role of Type A personality in coronary heart disease. Friedman and Rosenman (1974) have described Type A behaviour, a behaviour pattern 'primarily characterized by intense ambition, competitive "drive", constant preoccupation with occupational "deadlines", and a sense of time urgency'. In a longitudial study of 3524 men over an eight-year period they found that men who exhibited the Type A behaviour pattern at the outset had twice the rate of fatal heart attacks of the Type B men, i.e. those lacking the Type A features. Subsequent studies have confirmed this relationship between Type A behaviour and coronary heart disease and have shown that Type A is an independent and important risk factor. The measures of Type A behaviour encompass a complex and multi-faceted pattern and it is not yet clear which aspects of this coronary-prone style is most closely associated with coronary risk. Thus interventions aimed at reducing the risk either attempt to alter the global pattern of Type A behaviour, or they make some guess at the critical features and try to change them. Preliminary results suggest that such interventions are not only feasible but can also reduce the risk of myocardial infarction. The high incidence of coronary heart disease makes the research into Type A behaviour and its modification an important field of study.

Habits

Many of the other risk factors for coronary heart disease as well as for lung cancer, chronic bronchitis, cardiovascular disorders, etc. are behavioural. Habits of smoking, over-eating, consuming excess salt or saturated fats are well established risk factors for various diseases. The analysis of the causal chain often stops at the level of the toxic substance, e.g. the tar from cigarettes causes lung cancer, but it is important to go one step back in the causal chain and look at the behaviour that lead to the introduction of the toxic substance into the body. There is a considerable amount of research on smoking and obesity reflecting the complex psychological and physiological components. Many attempts have been made, using many different theoretical models to reduce the frequency of these risk behaviours. A detailed review of this work is outside the scope of this chapter, but recent reviews of treatments for smoking and obesity can be found in Prokop and Bradley (1981). While there is some optimism about the effectiveness of programmes designed to reduce smoking, there is less success in reducing obesity, even in the most obese, most at risk subjects.

Thus there are psychological antecedents of chronic disease some of which have been illustrated. General practitioners are already aware of the risks of obesity and cigarette smoking, but they might additionally wish to consider whether their Type A patients are at risk of heart disease or whether patients who have frequent severe like events are at risk of becoming ill in a variety of ways. The general practitioner is often well-placed to notice life-events such as illness in the family or bereavement or to detect the presence of many life-change units in patients presenting with mild complaints. These may be exciting opportunities for 'anticipatory care'.

SYMPTOMS AND THEIR PRESENTATION

Psychological symptoms

For some chronic illnesses the presenting symptoms are psychological. This is obviously the case for psychiatric illnesses, and is also common in neurological disease. For example, changes in cognitive functioning may be the first symptoms of a brain tumour or Alzheimer's disease and in either case the patient may complain of memory difficulties. A precise evaluation of the patients intellectual abilities, often involving psychometric assessment, can indicate whether deterioration is occurring and if so whether it is limited to certain abilities which would indicate a localized organic lesion or more wide-spread, suggesting general cerebral atrophy.

Other patients may present with changes in mood or motivation, the presentation sometimes being a complaint from the family that the patient has become irritable or aggressive, or that they no longer participate in the chores or the leisure activities of the family. Such symptoms may indicate organic brain disease or temporary functional impairment, perhaps associated with depressive illness. The observation of changes in patients' behaviour, thinking style, and emotional state are clearly important in the diagnostic process.

They may also be important in assessing prognosis. It has been shown that changes in the level of intellectual functioning are predictive of the patient's future ability to look after himself and may predict the amount of care (e.g. hospital, sheltered accommodation, home care) that will be required (Pattie and Gilleard 1979). Some measures of intellectual functioning may even predict when the patient will die.

Symptom presentation

When a patient presents a symptom to a doctor, a number of interpretations of the symptom are possible. Most obviously, the symptom may be indicative of organic disease. However, it is worth remembering that surveys have shown a similar prevalence of symptomatology in patients not attending their general practitioner and presentation at the general practitioner may reflect some additional feature such as a high incidence of life-events, an anxious individual, or the presence of more severe symptoms.

There are indications that patients who present with multiple symptoms of physical disfunction are likely to be suffering from a psychological disorder. Indeed attempts to develop survey methods of assessing morbidity have faltered on the poor validity of reports of widely varied symptoms. The Cornell Medical Index was developed to measure the incidence of various symptoms in numerous body systems is indicative of psychiatric disorder.

The doctor's behaviour may also influence the presentation of symptoms, an assumption that is fundamental to the Balint approach of dealing with patients' problems in general practice. The doctor's response to patients' complaints may affect the rate of symptoms according to the principles of operant conditioning; a positive reinforcing response should increase the frequency of complaints whereas if complaints are ignored but healthy behaviour is given ample attention then one should expect fewer symptoms. Support for this notion was found in a study by Hallauer (1972) in which patients were given a list of symptoms and asked to say how frequently they experienced each one. After an initial, baseline, of 20 symptoms, the interviewing 'doctor' reinforced the response 'often' in half of the patients and 'never' in the remainder, the reinforcements being the ordinary social responses of agreement or support such as 'good', 'yes', 'uh-huh'. Patients increased the frequency of the reinforced response, i.e. the first group reported having many symptoms 'often' while the second group had relatively few symptoms 'often' and many symptoms 'never'.

While these studies do not deal specifically with patients with chronic disease, these patients are likely to visit their general practitioners quite frequently and are therefore particularly susceptible to any misinterpretation of symptoms or to selective reinforcement of symptoms. The role of Byrne and Long's (1976) 'miscellaneous professional noises' in maintaining patients symptoms remain to be clarified. It would be unfortunate if the chronically ill patient's reports of, and perhaps their experience of or attention to, uncomfortable symptoms was exacerbated by the doctors encouragement or excessive attention to those symptoms.

Pain

One of the most frequently reported symptoms is pain. Since pain is a private experience, one can only know of someone else's pain by how they behave and what they report and these behaviours and reports may be susceptible to numerous influences other than simply tissue damage and neural inputs (see Melsack and Wall 1982). The classical examples of religious rituals (such as walking on hot coals or hanging from hooks inserted in the muscles of the back) which would under other circumstances result in pain and injury illustrate the role of psychological factors.

The amount of pain experienced is clearly affected by the circumstances in which it occurs. Each of us has experienced the disappearance of headache, toothache, etc. when something suitably distracting or pleasant occurs with its reappearance during boring or unpleasant tasks. The meaning of the pain may also be important and one might expect that angina pain might be experienced as more painful because of the threat involved.

Social and cultural factors also influence pain reports and various studies indicate that some cultural groups, especially Jews and Italians, express more pain than others. It has been suggested that pain behaviour is a learned response, learned by observing how others around us respond to painful stimuli. For example, in one study two people were subjected to the same painful stimulus. One person was the experimenter's confederate and he was programmed either to report high or low levels of pain. It was found that the real subject imitated the confederate's behaviour – in other words he decided how much pain to report by observing the other's behaviour. Further investigations suggested that the subjects not only *report* more or less pain when they observe the stooge, they also *experience* different levels of pain.

Thus when faced with a patient whose pain and suffering seem greater than expected from the organic pathology, one might wonder whether the patient was unduly fearful of the pain, or if there was little to distract attention from it, or if he came from a family or culture which was particularly expressive of pain. At least some of these factors can be reversed, allowing the patient to be less restricted by pain.

RESPONSE TO CHRONIC DISEASE: I   BY THE PATIENTS

Some psychological changes following onset of disease are symptomatic of the disease while others reflect the individual's response to the disease. For example, emotional behaviour in a brain-damaged patient may be directly symptomatic and diagnostic of the location of damage, or it may be part of the patient's response to loss of function and disability caused by the organic damage. Similarly such a patient may be unable to walk due to failure of neural ennervation or due to depression and lack of motivation in response to his or her condition.

Developmental stage

The response to the disease will obviously vary with the nature of the disease. It seems likely that the adaptation to a condition present from birth will be different from those having a later onset, even where the symptomatology may be similar. Even acquired diseases may have different implications for the subsequent life-style depending on whether they were acquired prior to adolescence, prior to adult independence, or following the establishment of an independent social, marital, occupational, and domestic existence. If the disease or disability is congenital or begins early in the child's life, certain changes in the normal infant care pattern may contribute to poor cognitive, social, and personality development. In the early stages the infant may be hospitalized, perhaps experiencing social or maternal deprivation or even sensory deprivation where the condition requires a very restrictive environment or where the child has sensory loss, especially deafness or blindness; such deprivations are known to be associated with poor intellectual development due to lack of stimulation and poor social development due to failure to establish satisfactory early relationships, even in healthy children. The school-aged child with chronic disease may be unable to attend school and may be restricted to home or hospital either permanently or intermittently. It hardly seems surprising if they are educationally backward or immature in their relationships with their peer groups. As adolescents, physique and appearance become more important attributes and the child with deficits is likely to be less highly regarded by his or her peers and may develop poor self-esteem as a result. Children and adults who are physically impaired are likely to be subject to the stigmatizing attitudes of others especially if the impairment is visible or restricts communication and this may affect their view of themselves and lead the individual to avoid social contacts. Such influences on the development of the child or adult with a chronic disorder have been shown in several surveys. They are also apparent in clinical work with individual patients where an awareness of such detrimental influences may help to minimize their effects on the development of the individual. The presence of multidisciplinary teams working with handicapped children may also have beneficial effects.

Different illnesses have different likely ages of onset and may therefore have different developmental implications. Thus congenital disorders such as cerebral palsy have implications for the development of the child, while later-onset conditions such as multiple sclerosis may influence the young adult's role as wage earner, spouse and parent, whereas cerebrovascular accidents tend to occur in more elderly victims and have their main impact on the individual's ability to function independently.

Predictability

The adjustment to a particular disorder of disability may be quite different when it results from a static condition such as injury due to a road traffic accident and when it is due to a progressive disease such as rheumatoid arthritis or multiple sclerosis. Many psychological theories hypothesize that individual adjustment will be better when events, even distressing events, are predictable and others suggest that the important factor is a degree of personal control over events. One of the most popular theories, Seligman's 'learned helplessness' theory, predicts that animals or human beings who have repeated experience of unavoidable failure or punishment acquire 'learned helplessness', a state in which they no longer try to succeed or influence their environment and in which people describe themselves as feeling depressed. The theory has been used to explain depressive disorders in individuals who have experienced failure or loss. It would also appear to be relevant to the helplessness experiences associated with illness, especially progressive illnesses with unpredictable, uncontrollable progression, and might lead one to expect depressed mood and poor motivation to succeed.

Three aspects of the response to illness by patients will be considered in more detail. The emotional response i.e. how it affects the patient's mood, the cognitive response, i.e. how the individual thinks about his or her disorder, and the behavioural response, i.e. how the disorder changes the patient's activities.

Emotional response

The association between chronic illness and neurotic personality has already been mentioned and it seems likely that chronic illness may lead to emotional problems and problems in personal adjustment. Chronic illness may bring problems of pain and discomfort; unpleasant medical procedures and treatments; admission to hospitals and the associated separation from home, family, and friends; restrictions in the individual's choices of occupation, hobbies, leisure activities, social contacts, etc.; changes in the appearance and functioning of the body; changes in the reactions of others; threats of future loss of functioning or even life, all of which demands some degree of adjustment and may evoke anxiety, depression, irritability, anger, etc.

Depressive reactions are more common in all types of physically disabled groups when compared with healthy individuals and they are particularly likely at acute stages such as the onset of the illness, the time of a relapse or sudden deterioration or of an acute episode requiring hospitalization or extra care. These reactions can be considered in terms of 'learned helplessness'. Others have described this as a 'mourning' process, the functions of the body or parts of the body which may be lost at that stage being mourned in a pattern comparable to that of dying or bereavement. The notion that such mourning may be a healthy process allowing better later adjustment and recovery is still controversial.

The clinical manifestations of the depressive reactions include not only the mood of sadness, hopelessness, and self-deprecation but also reduced activity and social interaction, insomnia, changes in appetite and weight, lack of libido, increased somatic complaints, etc. There is some evidence of increased suicide rates and increased incidence of self-destructive behaviours in patients with various orthopaedic difficulties, diabetes, heart disease, etc. compared with the rates for the general population.

The development of depressive symptoms is not necessarily related to the severity of the condition. For example, patients with both mild and severe heart disease are likely to become depressed. However, if the heart disease is mild, the depression is likely to be of shorter duration than if it is severe.

An alternative type of emotional reaction is a *phobic reaction*, where the patient become unduly fearful of symptoms or situations associated with symptoms and learns to avoid any situation which might elicit symptoms, at the same time developing protective behaviours. Such cases are a familiar part of clinical practice, e.g. a middle-aged woman with angina who became too fearful of the pain to leave her house, an elderly woman with a cerebellar tumour who became excessively fearful of falling and unable to walk unaccompanied, a middle-aged man with mild diabetes which was controlled by diet whose life became dominated by fears of cardiac complications, restricting his activities, ceasing to take exercise, taking his pulse 20–25 times per day, etc., and a woman who had had a breast removed due to cancer some seven years previously who sought treatment for numerous aches and pains experienced due to her fearfulness of recurrence and undue attention to somatic changes. Some success was achieved in treating these phobic reactions in a similar manner to other phobic reactions using behavioural treatments.

The probability, nature, and severity of emotional reaction to chronic disease are likely to be affected not so much by the presence of the disease, but by the individual's perception of his or her disease, and the ways in which patients think of their illness will be discussed in the next section. Further discussion of emotional factors in illness and disability is presented in McDaniel (1976).

Cognitive response

In this section we consider how the individual thinks about his disease. It is commonly observed that two individuals with the same disorder and similar levels of disability may see their conditions in very different ways. For example, one stroke patient with weakness in the left hand described herself as perfectly well and healthy but with a useless left hand, whereas another with a similar disability saw her health as totally ruined and her future as that of an invalid who would slowly deteriorate and die.

The style of thinking adopted can be seen not simply as a response to the disease but as a way of dealing with the disease, it can be seen as a defence mechanism or a coping strategy.

Defence mechanisms and coping strategies

The concept of defence mechanisms derives from Freudian psycho-analytic theory. Defence mechanisms are said to prevent unconscious material from intruding into consciousness where it would cause unmanageable anxiety. Denial is the defence mechanism most often attributed to ill or disabled people. They may deny that they are ill or disabled, they may describe their illness as trivial, denying the more major or threatening aspects or their disorder, or they may recognize the illness but attribute it to some benign cause. In each case the anxiety-evoking aspects are denied, allowing the patient to cope with some less threatening, more manageable condition. Denial has been reported in a wide variety of conditions and there are many published examples of blatant denial in the face of obvious contradiction, e.g. a wheelchair patient describing herself as having been dancing the previous week. A less blatant form of denial can be seen in patients with a static or deteriorating condition who describe a rosy future such as the terminally ill patient with a life expectancy of weeks talking about the holiday he will take next year.

While some patients do talk and act as if they believed their illness did not exist or was not serious in the face of clear evidence to the contrary, this does not necessarily prove that an unconscious defence mechanism is at work. The alternative approach has been to view denial as one of a series of possible 'coping strategies' available to the patient. Many systems have been evolved which try to classify patients' coping strategies, or more general coping strategies for dealing with a wide range of stresses. A recent paper by Ray *et al.* (1982) describes a scheme for classifying patients' coping themes in response to breast cancer and to surgery. Two main dimensions are defined: the degree to which the patient recognizes the threat, i.e. a dimension similar to denial: and the degree to which the patient sees herself to be helpless or to have some control. A patient who was high on helplessness but low on denial of threat is described as coping with 'resignation', saying things like 'well, you can't do anything about it, just go on with life'. By contrast, a patient high on control but also high on denial would show 'minimization', saying, 'He said the lump was terribly small. That's what I wanted to hear'.

Adaptive and maladaptive coping

Without discussing the theoretical literature on coping in any more detail, we can turn to the important question of whether one form of coping is better than another. Are there adaptive and maladaptive forms of coping? Discussions of denial often suggest that this is a maladaptive style of coping, largely because it denies reality. On the other hand an effective denial strategy should reduce the distress experienced by the patient. There are two main criteria of what constitutes adaptive/maladaptive styles of coping, emotional criteria and disease criteria. It is possible that one style of coping might be adaptive on emotional criteria but maladaptive on disease criteria or vice versa. For example a patient who 'minimized' her breast cancer might cope well emotionally but fail to see the need for radiotherapy and therefore be unco-operative in treatment. The notion that different strategies may be helpful in controlling fear and in controlling danger has been useful in studies of individual's facing a wide variety of treats, including health threats and some unrelated to health.

Considering just the emotional criteria, it seems plausible, although not well documented, that those who deny or minimize the presence of a threatening condition will be less depressed and anxious and exhibit more stable mood. It also seems plausible, however, that such individuals are more vulnerable to new information. Studies of surgical patients have shown that patients who avoid collecting information about what is going on cope better emotionally than those who seek out as much information as they can get. However, if these patients are subjected to a preoperative information session, it is possible that the avoidant patients may experience more distress, perhaps because they are considering the real threats for the first time, whereas the information-seeking patient can be helped by such a session. In chronic disease, one might expect a denial strategy to be effective until some additional input of information from doctors, other patients, friends, family, etc., or some new experience of symptoms makes the strategy untenable. Some form of minimization or denial strategy is probably quite common, making the patient more vulnerable to distress when the condition is exacerbated leading to the increased incidence of depression associated with acute episodes of illness and treatment.

Turning to the disease implications, two conflicting pieces of evidence are of interest here. In a study of asthmatic patients, those patients showing either very high or very low levels of fearfulness were more likely to require inpatient hospital care than those with moderate fearfulness. The authors suggest that the low-fear patients ignore their symptomatology and therefore do not take protective steps when mild symptoms occur, resulting in more extreme episodes due to neglect. The high-fear patients pay undue attention to symptomatology, thereby exacerbate the condition and are more likely to present at the clinic. On the other hand, the moderately fearful patients neither neglect nor exaggerate their condition and achieve the minimal need for hospital care. In the second study coronary care patients who showed moderate levels of awareness of physical symptoms had the worst outcome in terms of rehospitalization and death. These authors suggest that the low-awareness patients, those expressing a form of denial may be experiencing a healing endorphin response which simultaneously makes the patient less aware of symptoms and reduces future risk. The high-awareness patient on the other hand is aware of his condition and is motivated to act to reduce risk; they produce evidence to show that these patients are more compliant with medical advice to change diet, alcohol, and exercise habits and suggest that these changes mediate the successful outcomes. The moderate-awareness patient is most at risk because he is neither protected by this highly speculative form of the endorphin response, nor by behaviour change leading to reduced risk.

While these studies appear to be in conflict, note that both describe a level of awareness or fearfulness that is necessary to behave in such a way as to minimize dangers. Perhaps it requires a greater degree of fearfulness to achieve the motivation required to change risky habits in coronary heart disease than to respond appropriately to onset of symptoms in asthma. These studies are consistent with a wide literature that suggests that there is an optimal level of recognition of threat for taking successful avoiding action; too little we fear will fail to motivate the individual; too much will lead to inefficient, confused behaviour.

The doctor is thus placed in the unenviable position of giving the patient information about the condition, its prognosis, and treatment in such a way as to allow the patient to develop a coping style which makes the patient able to cope emotionally and at the same time evokes a sufficient level of fearfulness to motivate the patient to take the actions required to control the particular disease. In a wide range of studies doctors have more often been criticized for giving too little information than for giving too much.

Behavioural response

Chronic disease can lead to many changes in the individual's behaviour. Some of these are associated with treatment of the condition, e.g. taking medication, attending clinics, taking exercise or resting, and factors influencing patient's compliance with prescribed medical regimes is discussed in the next section. Other changes result from the disease either directly or indirectly and can be seen as disabilities, often resulting in loss of independence or loss of valued hobbies and activities.

The relationship between disease, physical impairments, disability and social handicap is a complex one (World Health Organization 1980), and it is impossible to make simple predictions of the degree of disability or handicap from knowledge of the impairment alone. The patient's personality, skills, occupation, social and physical environment all play a part. For example, facial scarring may lead to no changes in the behaviour of one individual while another may become housebound for fear of other people's reactions; minor injuries such as loss of teeth or loss of a fingertip may have no implications for the majority of people but may render a flautist or violinist unemployed.

The possibility of secondary gain is frequently discussed, the loss of some function actually leading to some net gain. For example an injured lorry driver became wheelchair bound, received a disability pension and became able to study for a university degree as he had always wished. There is ample evidence of patients who are currently seeking financial compensation showing lower rates of success in rehabilitation programmes than those with no legal cases pending.

The patients attitudes and expectations may also be important. For example, Rutter (1979) has shown that the best predictors of return to work in a group of chronic bronchitics were not the measures of lung function but the patients' attitudes towards their illness and work. The placebo response is also a good example of the role of expectations; the size of the analgesic effect varies with the patient's expectations of the effect, less pain reduction being achieved by inert compounds when administered as aspirin than when administered as morphine.

Sexual functioning

The complex interaction of psychological factors and disease processes in determining disability is well illustrated in the area of sexual functioning. Many chronic diseases may affect the mechanical aspects of sexual functioning directly, as in impotence due to failure of neural mechanisms in demyelinating disease or lack of vascular supply to the pelvis in cardiovascular disease, or indirectly, e.g. due to inability to meet the extra oxygen demand in patients with chronic obstructive lung disease, or due to limits in movements or position in chronic arthritis, or due to fatigue and weakness associated with many disorders. There is now evidence that psychosexual problems often accompany physical disease of many types. Such problems may also be due to medically prescribed drugs such as hypotensives, psychotropics, and cytotoxics. But in addition many psychological factors may affect sexual adjustment.

The patients may anticipate failure in a sexual role either because they have a stereotyped view of the invalid as a sexless individual or because some transient physical effects of the disease have led to experience of failure. Recent research has shown that many diabetic men who report erectile impotence do have morning erections and the authors suggest that the problems may result in part from a progressive physical disorder such as peripheral neuropathy but with a superimposed psychological reaction of the patient and his partner which may worsen the problem. Sexual adjustment may be disturbed because of anticipation of pain or harm and this may be an important factor in patients with recent myocardial infarction or patients having recent surgical procedures especially colostomy or ileostomy. In addition they may worry about being rejected, perhaps seeing themselves as less sexually attractive, e.g. after mastectomy or amputation. Their partners may have similar anxieties about failure or harm, they may find the patients less attractive or they may feel guilty about their own continuing sexual desires. Any anxieties in patient or partner concerning sexual functioning are likely to interfere with performance and lead to the common psychosexual dysfunctions of general unresponsiveness, vaginismus, or orgasmic dysfunction in women and erectile impotence, premature ejaculation, and ejaculatory failure in men. There may be problems in the nature of the relationship perhaps due to changing roles following the onset of disease and disability, or due to poor previous sexual adjustment, and the unattached individual may have difficulties in establishing satisfactory sexual relationships.

Problems of sexual dysfunction in patients with physical illness are reviewed by Hawton (1982) who also points to the role of the medical profession in causing or maintaining problems. The doctor may exacerbate the problem by being inadequately informed about the nature of sexual dysfunction and its relationship to the patient's disease and treatment, or by offering cursory discussion which may serve to raise patients anxieties, or even by total avoidance of discussion due to his or her own embarrassment, ignorance, or assessment of the problem as not important enough to spend the required time. Hawton gives guidelines about the assessment of the patient's sexual problems including the nature of the problems, its relationship to organic factors, and to previous sexual adjustment, the patient and the partner's understanding of the problem, and their expectations. Treatment may involve clarification of the problem, reassurance, education, and advice, including advice about alternative sources of sexual satisfaction if coitus is impossible, and may be given by the patient's general practitiner, specialist in their disease and its rehabilitation, or specialist in psychosexual counselling. Such counselling should ideally form part of the patient's general rehabilitation and may have a preventive function if problems are anticipated, for example in myocardial infarction patients. The level of guidance should be adapted to the patient's requirements, and restricted to what is acceptable to the patient. As with other aspects in rehabilitation, sexual adjustment should be re-assessed at follow-up appointments.

The complex interplay of organic and psychological sources of disability and the potential role of the doctor has been discussed in some detail concerning sexual disability but clearly parallels can be drawn in other aspects of disability. If the clinician does not anticipate a problem and does not present an adequate opportunity for the patient to report it, he or she will be unable to help the patient to overcome the problem by simple information, advice or reassurance, by provision of mechanical aids, by referral to specialist rehabilitation therapists, by referral to clinical psychologists offering behavioural learning programmes, or by giving some form of psychotherapeutic intervention.

RESPONSE TO CHRONIC DISEASE: II   BY OTHER PEOPLE

An important part of the response to chronic illness, which may determine many of the outcomes, are the responses of other people than the patient. The patients' responses will be influenced by the emotional reactions, beliefs, and behaviours of those around. An overprotective family may prevent a disabled patient achieving independence simply by doing everything for him. In a ward or at home physical arrangements achieved by his helpers, such as placing his cup, books, and spectacles within or beyond his reach or siting his chair near to or far from the toilet, may determine whether the patient is independent and even whether he is incontinent. While there is much speculation about the possible motivation of these helpers and what needs the patients' invalidism might serve, such behaviours may simply reflect the knowledge and under-standing of the helper and problems may be remedied by quite simple advice. Including family and helpers in the educational and counselling aspects of treat-ment may often be useful.

Recently, behavioural psychologists have noted the role of social reinforce-ment in maintaining disability. Social attention interest and help is likely to be given when patients are unable to do something for themselves, independent behaviour being largely ignored. Where such social consequences are important for the patient and the effort involved in behaving independently is great, the disability may be unnecessarily maintained. For example, some nursing home residents were found to be using wheelchairs when they could walk indepen-dently, because of social contingencies; observers noted that staff and other residents were more likely to chat to the patients and offer assistance when they used their wheelchairs than when they walked to the dining room. During one experimental period, these contingencies were reversed so that the residents received little attention when using their wheelchairs but social conversation and encouragement when walking; within a short period these same residents chose to walk rather than ride to the dining room. There are many similar demonstrations of the role of apparently casual social interchanges in main-taining disability. Clearly the social and financial consequences may play a part in determining the degree of disability exhibited by a patient with a given severity of disease.

Prejudice

Family, friends, neighbours, employers, and even the general public may have stigmatizing attitudes towards particular diseases which prevent the sufferer from participating fully in the normal range of activities. Employers do discriminate against disabled applicants and it would appear that they are relatively more prejudiced against employing epileptics, former psychiatric patients, and the deaf, than candidates in wheelchairs. Such attitudes are often associated with fear or embarrassment in meeting the sufferer, especially if there are communication difficulties and familiarity probably serves to reduce these problems. Thus employers with experience of having disabled people say they are more willing to hire people with disabilities again and such attitude change may be a spin off from the quota system requiring all large employers to take on a minimum percentage of disabled people.

Not all prejudices are negative. While chronically sick or disabled people are often seen as inferior or unhappy, they may also be seen as more conscientious, more even-tempered, better friends, more understanding, etc. Perhaps the most difficult aspect of these attitudes is their stereotyped nature, the assumption that certain attributes will be shared by all people with a particular disorder. Similarly, patients may be stereotyped because of a temporary state such as incontinence during treatment with diuretics. In one study 18 patients in a psychiatric ward were selected by staff as bed-wetters suitable for a treatment programme. During the baseline period of two months, five of those patients did not wet their beds even once, and were thus given a inappropriate, stigmatizing label associated with earlier problems. Immediately we characterize the sufferers primarily by their condition, e.g. 'the disabled' or 'asthmatics' or 'enuretics' or 'epileptics', we run the risk of making stereotyped statements.

Finally, the reactions of the health-care staff, the doctors, nurses, physiotherapists, occupational therapists, etc., can be important. They may inadvertently encourage invalidism or lead the patient to seek and expect an active future. They may provide the information that patient requires about the illness, its prognosis, possible treatments, available mechanical aids, ways of overcoming common difficulties, etc., or they may be too diffident, embarrassed, ignorant, or uncaring to recognize or let the patient express a difficulty they are experiencing.

The reactions of others will frequently determine whether the individual with an impairment or a disability also becomes socially handicapped, i.e. whether he or she becomes a disadvantaged member of our society.

COMPLIANCE WITH TREATMENT

Failure of patients to comply with medical advice is well-documented (Sackett and Haynes 1976) and such problems may be exacerbated in patients with chronic illness. The usual reports are of failure to take medication or to take it as prescribed, or of failure to follow advice about exercise, resting, eating, working, etc. A detailed study in the United States showed that not only are large numbers of patients not taking the medication their doctors think they are taking, but large numbers also take medication which their doctors are unaware of. For chronic patients, the advice may apply to long periods or even a lifetime and may involve major changes of habits such as smoking or eating and such changes are notoriously difficult to achieve. The advice may concern a disorder which is symptomless and if this is compounded by disagreeable side-effects associated with medication, as in hypotensive medication, failures of compliance frequently occur. Advice may be aimed at the reduction of risk factors such as essential hypertension or smoking, rather than diseases per se and whereas healthy patients frequently fail to stop smoking as advised, patients on a coronary care unit having experienced one myocardial infarction were much more likely to give up smoking to avoid a second. As suggested earlier, a minimal level of fear may be necessary to motivate behaviour change.

Basic research demonstrating failures of compliance has been complemented by the development of explanatory theories the best known being Ley's cognitive hypothesis and Becker and Maiman's health belief model (Ley 1977; Becker and Maiman 1975).

The *cognitive hypothesis* states that patients may fail to comply with medical advice because they do not understand or remember it. Ley has collected evidence to show that much of the advice presented by doctors is not understood by patients either because it assumes knowledge and vocabulary which patients do not have or because the material is presented in a grammatical style that is too difficult for patients to follow. Names of parts of the body may mean different things to doctors and patients, e.g. in a multiple choice test the stomach was located accurately by 100 per cent of doctors but only 59 per cent of laymen. Even where doctors make efforts to be understood they may fail; for example, some leaflets designed to improve patients understanding were intelligible to only 24 per cent of the population. Difficult information is poorly remembered, but in addition too much information or poorly presented information is also forgotten. In a clever series of experiments Ley has shown that simple techniques lead to increases in understanding and memory of medical advice. General practitioners following Ley's guidelines managed to increase the amount of information remembered by their patients from an average of 56 per cent to 71 per cent. Obviously patients cannot comply with advice they do not understand or remember and he found that simple advice could lead to significant increases in patient compliance both in taking prescribed medication and in following diet instructions; patients taking psychotropic medication were more likely to take the correct number of tablets when given a simple explanatory leaflet and obese subjects lost nearly twice as much weight when given a simplified diet sheet than when given the original, more difficult to comprehend version of the diet.

The *health belief model* on the other hand suggests that compliance depends on the context in which the advice is given. Becker and Maiman propose the following three determinants of patients' compliance – the perceived seriousness of the condition, the perceived outcome of following the advice and the costs of following the advice. If patients do not think their illness is serious then they are less likely to follow the advice. Doctors and laymen do not necessarily agree about the seriousness of conditions and some research in the 1960s illustrates that dangerous discrepancies can occur. Amongst people questioned about lung cancer a considerable number thought it was an unpleasant, but not life-threatening, condition that could be cured by spending some months in a hospital or sanatorium; one could hardly expect people to give up smoking to avoid such a disease. Patients must also believe that following the advice is likely to be effective and that the benefits are related to their compliance. Several studies have shown that believing the illness to be serious and the advocated treatment to be effective is associated with higher compliance rates. But is it not clear how one would use these ideas as a basis for remedial action. One might suggest that the doctor's role is to persuade the patient of the seriousness of their condition and to 'sell' the proposed treatment so that the patient expects it to be effective. Perhaps more appropriately, this model suggests that the doctor should try to ensure that the patient has a realistic view of both the condition and the treatment, on which the patient can base her or his own decision about compliance.

The other factor in the patient's decision to comply are the costs involved. The costs may be psychological – he or she may feel tense and nervy without the usual quota of alcohol: or physical – it may be very painful or tiring to do the recommended exercises: or financial – the visits to the clinic may mean expensive bus fares and loss of wages. Anything which makes it easier for the patient is likely to improve compliance. In one study, subjects who had agreed to attend a clinic were more likely to attend if given a map directing them to the nearest clinic.

The cognitive hypothesis and the health belief model present the patient as a rational human being who decides to comply with doctor's recommendations when there is enough evidence in favour of compliance and when the recommendations are stated in a way that can be understood and remembered. And there is plenty of evidence in support. On the other hand, there is no support for the notion that patients fail to comply because they are irrational, aggressive, difficult, or unpleasant people. What we know about compliance, suggests that it depends not on the patient and his or her personality, but on the beliefs and knowledge that the patient has and, most importantly, on what takes place in the consultation between doctor and patient.

SYMPTOM CONTROL

Psychological techniques may be used to reduce risk behaviours such as smoking or alcohol abuse, or to alter the patient's response to illness, the emotional response, the coping-strategies used, or the level of disability adopted. They may also influence symptom presentation and compliance with treatment, but in this section we consider if and how psychological treatment may influence the disease process and its symptoms.

Recently there have been major advances in the field of behavioural medicine and books such as Katz and Zlutnick (1975) or Williams and Gentry (1977) describe examples of psychological treatments as applied to genitourinary, gastrointestinal, cardiovascular, musculoskeletal, respiratory, and nervous system complaints. These treatments are most likely to be applied as a course of treatment by specialists in behavioural medicine, usually clinical psychologists, unlike some of the approaches mentioned in the section on symptom presentation which may have relevance in all patient consultations. In order to give a flavour rather than an exhaustive overview of these treatments two common symptoms, incontinence and pain, and two common conditions essential hypertension and asthma are chosen as illustrations.

Incontinence

Incontinence is one of the most distressing symptoms, both to patients and to relatives, and can be associated with various forms of brain damage or neurological disorder or may result from surgical interventions.

Engel (1977) has successfully treated a considerable number of adult patients with faecal incontinence due to organic disorders using biofeedback. Biofeedback techniques are based on the assumption that amplification of feedback from biological processes, that are normally undetectable, will allow the person to control these processes. There is ample evidence that normal healthy subjects can control palmar sweating, muscular contractions, EEG activity, peripheral blood flow, etc. if given appropriate feedback from electronic monitoring devices. The techniques have been applied clinically, e.g. to tension and migraine headaches, cardiac arthythmias, and neuromuscular impairments, with some success.

Engel postulates that the patients fail to control their faecal flow due to failure to co-ordinate the action of the internal and external anal sphincters. Using rectal balloons, he gave patients feedback on the activity of both sphincters by monitoring balloon distension. He then trained patients to close the external sphincter when the internal sphincter was distended by inflating the internal balloon. During training the patients could see the graphical records of their sphincter activity and were praised for successful control. Gradually the records were withdrawn until they could control the shpincter without any visually aided feedback. The treatment took between one and three sessions of about two hours each. Twenty-eight out of 40 patients achieved at least a 90 per cent decrease in frequency of incontinence which continued during an extended follow up period. Given that the patients' problems were usually of many years duration, this was a considerable success rate for a brief treatment.

A variety of techniques have been used in the treatment of enuresis based on the variety of causes. For example a patient whose primary difficulty is restricted movement may be incontinent because it takes too long to get to the toilet and may simply benefit by being seated nearer to the toilet or having a commode nearer the seat. On the other hand, a demented patient may be incontinent because he or she forgets to go to the toilet and may benefit by regular prompting or carrying a small alarm which signals at regular intervals. Similar approaches may be used where organic impairment interferes with normal afferent signals or where the interval between initial urge and bladder evacuation is brief. The treatment aims to train habits of toileting dependent on time rather than bladder signals.

A further form of habit training that has been applied with adults with chronic brain syndrome as well as its original application with children is the bell-and-pad method of treating nocturnal enuresis. Urine completes a circuit causing a bell to ring, thus wakening the sleeping bed-wetter. Over many nights, the sleeper learns to wake earlier and earlier until he wakes in time to go to the lavatory.

Thus where incontinence arises as a symptom there may be psychological methods available to overcome it.

Pain

Many of the conditions discussed throughout this book will have pain as an important symptom. As mentioned previously, the context and especially the social context will influence the expression of pain and thus may be important in the patient's presentation to their doctor. Are there psychological methods of reducing pain as a continuing symptom?

Most techniques of pain relief involve a psychological component. The doctor's suggestion and the patient's expectation that pain will be relieved are fundamental to the placebo response which probably facilitates even the most potent analgesics. For example, it has been estimated that half the pain relief achieved by morphine is due to placebo effects.

Experimental investigations have shown how important the suggestion of pain relief can be. For example, the use of audio-analgesia in dental treatment is only effective when the patient is told that the music will reduce the pain; the same music without the analgesic suggestion is not so effective.

When we consider treatments that are exclusively psychological, three approaches are currently being used. First, there are treatments designed to reduce muscle tension as the source of pain. This is illustrated by the use of bio-feedback of frontalis muscle EMG as a means of reducing tension headache or using analagous feedback for back or shoulder pain. Secondly, pain relief may be achieved by anxiety reduction approaches; if the severity of pain experienced is directly related to the threat or distress associated with the pain, then techniques which reduce this threat should reduce the pain. The suggestion of pain relief may work in this way and the effectiveness of techniques such as hypnotic analgesia and relaxation training may be due to anxiety reduction. Alternatively cognitive techniques, where the patient may be trained to interpret the pain in a different, less threatening, way may allow pain reduction. These techniques are at a more experimental stage in development and have been studied in acute, especially surgical, rather than chronic pain. The assumption is that what the patient thinks about the pain leads to the distressing severity. For example, if a pain in the chest is interpreted as the onset of a heart attack the pain will be worrying and unnecessarily severe whereas if it is interpreted as a temporary pain associated with exercise which will disappear quite quickly then the pain itself may be less severe. Obviously such cognitive techniques would have to be appropriately tailored to the patient's condition.

In addition to muscle tension reduction and anxiety reduction techniques, there are operant conditioning techniques and these are used particularly with chronic pain that seems unduly severe for the organic pathology. Inappropriate pain behaviour may be maintained by the responses of other people in the patient's environment. If patients get all the attention of their families, doctors, nurses, etc. when they express pain or ask for help then these behaviours will become more frequent whereas if healthy coping responses are reinforced, these will predominate. For example, complaining of pain may bring medication, attention, etc. If medication is given contingent on pain complaint it may reinforce these complaints, whereas if it is administered on a time basis these behaviours are not reinforced. An important treatment programme based on this operant hypothesis was first introduced by Fordyce *et al.* (1968) who removed the positive rewards for pain behaviour and instead rewarded healthy behaviour. Pain medication was given on a time basis, the timing corresponding closely to the patient's spontaneous demands. Activity levels in specific tasks, such as walking, were monitored and targets set for the individual. Success was graphed and verbally rewarded and goals gradually increased. Staff and family were discouraged from attending to the patient when expressing pain and encouraged to reinforce healthy activity including success in reaching targets. One of the first patients treated in this way had an 18-year history of back pain, was taking narcotic medication and was active for only two hours per day on average before treatment. After seven weeks of treatment she was taking no narcotic medication, was walking two miles per day and was working for about two hours in occupational therapy. With continuing outpatient treatment she became independent and active at home. Other programmes in the United States report similar success, showing reductions in reported pain, reductions in analgesic medication and increases in activity levels.

Thus in addition to the psychological component of many forms of pain relief there are specific psychological techniques, the choice of technique depending on whether the pain is thought to be maintained or exacerbated by muscle tension, by anxiety or by reinforcement. (Further discussion of pain treatment can be found in Katz and Zlutnick (1975), Williams and Gentry (1977), or Prokop and Bradley (1981).)

Essential hypertension

The possibility of psychological treatments for essential hypertension is important because hypotensive medication may have unpleasant side-effects, treatment is being recommended at lower levels of blood pressure, resulting in more patients being treated for longer periods, and compliance with pharmacological treatments under these circumstances for a condition that is often symptomless is poor.

Psychological approaches to the treatment of essential hypertension have adopted two main strategies. First, the biofeedback approach gives subjects direct information about their blood pressure (or a physiological index that varies with blood pressure) with a view to bringing it under voluntary control. This has not been very successful and it has proved technically difficult to provide continuous feedback of blood pressure using non-invasive techniques. Fortunately successful reductions in blood pressure appear to be associated with general relaxation and stress reduction and these techniques have been more fully developed with patients.

Thus the second approach involves a general programme of stress management. Studies of hypertensives show that they are likely to have exaggerated blood pressure reactions of longer duration than those of normotensives in response to a wide variety of stress, e.g. stressful interviews, mental tests, saline injections, cold pressor tests. Based on the hypothesis that their response to stress is of aetiological significance, a programme which teaches patients to modulate their responses to stress should reduce blood pressure. Various attempts to teach relaxation or to control physiological parameters of stress using biofeedback have shown some success, but amongst the most successful is Patel's work, with patients in general practice.

Patel and North's (1975) treatment involved educating patients about stress reactions, including film information about 'fight or flight', followed by training in relaxation using direct instructions and the use of biofeedback, usually skin conductance. When the patients were achieving some skill in relaxation, they were directed to incorporate relaxation into their daily lives, especially at points where they might be stressed or hurried, e.g. while driving they would relax while stopped at red traffic lights or when the telephone rang they would relax momentarily before lifting the receiver. Treatment taking 12 sessions of approximately ½ hour duration produced reductions in blood pressure from an average of 168/100 to 142/85 which were maintained at follow-up. A control group of similar patients showed no change over a similar number of sessions with no stress management training.

Further research on Patel's and similar treatments have led to optimism that it may be possible to offer such a treatment as an alternative to long-term medication.

Asthma

As with essential hypertension, the medical treatment of asthma may involve long-term treatment with drugs with unpleasant side-effects or even the dangerous side-effects of steroid therapy. Therefore the search for psychological treatments is worthwhile. A further similarity is the presence of psychosomatic theories about the symptomatology, and evidence that psychological factors can trigger symptoms. A treatment approach which reverses or interrupts this causal pathway seems attractive.

Asthma has been shown to be precipitated by emotional arousal, by suggestion (e.g. if the patient believes an inhalation contains an irritant broncho-constriction results) and the presence of the patient's family. The role of psychological factors, in precipitating asthma was investigated by Purcell *et al.*

(1969) who studied the role of the parent–child relationship in a group of 13 children for whom psychological factors were thought to be the main precipitants of their asthma. The children were studied in three phases. In the first and third they lived at home normally with their parents. In the second phase, they lived at home, but with substitute parents, i.e. maintaining the same physical environment, but removing any precipitating factors of the relationship between the child and his parents. The separation phase showed considerable improvements; they had fewer asthmatic attacks, wheezed less, required less medication, and had improved lung function compared with the phases when they lived with their parents. This evidence illustrated the role that psychological factors can play in eliciting such symptoms. Another group of children whose asthma was considered to be precipitated by infective or allergic factors did not benefit from the separation phase.

One of more interesting approaches to treatment was the use of systematic desensitization by Moore (1965). Sytematic desensitization is one of the behavioural techniques used successfully in the treatment of phobic patients, training a relaxation response, incompatible with the previous response of fear. In asthmatics relaxation was seen as incompatible with bronchial constriction. The procedure uses a graded hierarchy of images associated with asthma graded from mild breathing difficulties up to a full asthmatic attack. The patient is trained to relax and then is instructed to imagine each step in the hierarchy, starting with the mildest difficulties, while maintaining relaxation. Further hierarchies deal with specific irritants for that subject, e.g. a hierarchy going from 'you are invited to a party' to 'you are in a very smoky crowded room'. The treatment produced improvements in lung function when compared with a control group who received relaxation alone.

More recently there have been further attempts to treat asthmatics with systematic desensitisation, relaxation, biofeedback, and operant conditioning. The results to date have been rather mixed, but research continues. While pharmacological treatments continue to be ineffective for some asthmatics, the possibility of a psychological alternative must be explored.

Other conditions

Incontinence, pain, essential hypertension, and asthma illustrates some of the diversity of techniques and conditions treated. Similar examples of treatment of neuromuscular impairment, epilepsy, cardiac arrhythmias, spasmodic torticollis, migraine, Reynaud's disease, and so on could also illustrate this very attractive, exciting, but as yet rather undeveloped aspect of treatment. As things stand there may be patients or conditions, such as borderline hypertension in a young person or obesity, where a psychological treatment may be the treatment of choice, or the first line of treatment before another more dangerous or irreversible treatment is attempted.

CONCLUSION

Psychological factors play a complex role in chronic disease. This has been known for centuries, but the research describing the precise relationships between psychological factors and disease processes which might allow prevention and treatment is at an early stage. Whereas behavioural factors have long been recognized as important in heart disease, the evidence that specific individuals, those displaying Type A behaviours, are particularly susceptible has set the stage for preventive action by indicating the population at risk and hinting at the specific behaviours which make them vulnerable. Similarly, the knowledge that patients do not always obey doctors' advice is not new, but the fact that this is not due to some unchangeable aspect of the patient's personality and that it can be improved by some simple changes in doctors' consulting styles is a relatively recent finding.

The long-term span of chronic disease means that the interaction between psychological factors and the disease can be even more complex than in acute conditions. What are the implications for those caring for patients? First, it may be possible to predict from a healthy patient's behaviour that they are at risk and thereby to consider some preventive action. Secondly, changes in cognitive abilities, emotional states, styles of behaviour, etc. may be symptomatic of chronic disease. Thirdly, presentation of physical or psychological symptoms may be influenced by emotional or interpersonal factors including the doctor's response, and may therefore be misunderstood. Fourthly, over the months or years of the disease, consultations frequently deal not with the disease itself, but with the patient's response to the disease including emotional adjustment, coping mechanisms such as active information seeking or denial and changes in the patient's behaviour such as loss of independence or sexual dysfunction. Fifthly, the patient's family or friends may seek similar consultations to alleviate their anxieties, to get information about the patient's condition, and to ask for advice about the patient's behaviour and how to behave toward the patient; their behaviour may affect the course of the patient's behaviour and disease. Sixthly, a recurrent problem is that of ascertaining whether advice and recommendations are being followed and if not, what the

Table 2.2. *Summary of the relationship between psychological factors and chronic disease*

1. Risk behaviours
2. Psychological changes as symptoms
3. Emotional and interpersonal influences on symptom presentation
4. Emotional responses, coping mechanisms, and behaviour change in response to chronic disease
5. Responses of important others
6. Compliance with advice
7. Psychological treatments

barriers to compliance are. Finally, the doctor might wish to be aware of psychological interventions, especially where physical treatments may be of long duration and have unpleasant or even dangerous side-effects. These implications are listed in Table 2.2. This is a relatively new and active area of research and, while some of the treatments have been described above in a tentative way, it seems likely that the major investment of effort and money, particularly into cardiovascular disease, should produce clinically useful treatments in the near future.

REFERENCES

Becker, M. H. and Maiman, L. A. (1975). Sociobehavioural determinants of compliance with health and medical care recommendations. *Medical care* **13**, 10–24.

Boyle, C. M. (1970). Differences between doctor's and patient's interpretations of some common medical terms. *Br. med. J.* **ii**, 286–9.

Byrne, P. S. and Long, B. E. (1976). *Doctors talking to patients.* HMSO, London.

Engel, B. T. (1977). Fecal incontinence. In *Behavioural approaches to medical treatment* (ed. R. B. Whilliams and W. D. Gentry). Ballinger, Cambridge, Mass.

Fordyce, W. *et al.* (1968). Some implications of learning in problems of chronic pain. In *Behaviour therapy and health care* (ed. R. C. Katz and S. Zlutnick). Pergamon, Oxford.

Friedman, M. and Rosenman, R. H. (1974). *Type A behaviour and your heart.* Knopy, New York.

Hallauer, D. S. (1972). Illness behaviour – an experimental investigation. *J. chron. Dis.* **25**, 599–610.

Hawton, K. (1982). Sexual problems in the general hospital. In *Medicine and psychiatry: a practical approach* (ed. F. Creed and J. Pfeffer). Pitman medical, London.

Henry, J. P. and Stephens, P. M. (1977). *Stress, health and the social environment: a sociobiological approach to medicine.* Springer, New York.

Holmes, T. H. and Rahe, R. H. (1967). The social readjustment rating scale. *J. psychosomat. Res.* **11**, 213–18.

Katz, R. C. and Zlutnick, S. (eds.) (1975). *Behaviour therapy and health care.* Pergamon, Oxford.

Ley, P. (1977). Psychological studies of doctor–patient communication. In *Contributions to medical psychology,* Vol. 1 (ed. S. Rachman). Pergamon, Oxford.

McDaniel, J. W. (1976). *Physical disability and human behaviour* (2nd edn). Pergamon, Oxford.

Melsack, R. and Wall, P. (1982). *The challenge of pain.* Penguin, Harmondsworth, Middlesex.

Moore, N. (1965). Behaviour therapy in bronchial asthma: a controlled study. *J. psychosomat. Res.* **9**, 257–76.

Parkes, C. M. (1975). *Bereavement: studies in grief in adult life.* Penguin, Harmondsworth, Middlesex.

Patel, C. and North, W. R. (1975). Randomised controlled trial of yoga and biofeedback in the management of hypertension. *Lancet* **ii**, 93–5.

Pattie, A. H. and Gilleard, C. J. (1979). *Manual of the Clifton Assessment Procedures for the Elderly (CAPE).* Hodder & Stoughton, London.

Prokop, C. K. and Bradley, L. A. (eds.) (1981). *Medical psychology: contributions to behavioural medicine.* Academic Press, New York.

Purcell, K., Brady, D. *et al.* (1969). Effect on asthma in children of experimental separation from the family. *Psychosomat. Med.* **31**, 144–64.

Ray, C., Lindop, J., and Gibson, S. (1982). The concept of coping. *Psychol. Med.* **12**, 385–96.

Robinson, J. O. (1969). Cited in Goldstein, I. B. (1981). Assessment of hypertension. In *Medical psychology: contributory to behavioural medicine* (ed. C. K. Prokop and L. A. Bradby). Academic Press, New York.

Rutter, B. M. (1979). The prognostic significance of psychological factors in the management of chronic bronchitis. *Psychol. Med.* **9**, 63–70.

Sackett, D. C. and Haynes, R. B. (1976). *Compliance with therapeutic regimens.* Johns Hopkins University Press, Baltimore.

Williams, R. B. and Gentry, W. D. (eds.) (1977). *Behavioural approaches to medical treatment.* Ballinger, Cambridge, Mass.

World Health Organization (1980). *International classification of impairment, disability and handicap.* Geneva.

3 Social aspects of chronic disability

The biological phenomena of a disabling condition – for example, the fact that a person born with trisomy 21 will have the clinical features of Down's syndrome – have about them an invariability. But the social aspects of chronic disability depend to a very real degree on human volition. Whether something is a social problem is significantly determined by people choosing that it should be so defined, and the extent and manner in which it is a problem is thus relative to a particular culture. There are basically three components of the social aspects of chronic disability: the social problems of the disabled, the social policies designed to meet such problems and the implementation of these policies in the practical delivery of services. While there do exist certain matters of social definition which are comparatively timeless and universal they tend to be fairly self-evident and, once mentioned, perhaps rather uninteresting – the fact that the disabled being biologically deviant are also very generally regarded as socially deviant, and are therefore frequently stigmatized, is an example. More interesting are the local and time-bound realities; we shall describe here the social aspects of chronic disability in Britain in the 1980s.

The culturally relative nature of social reality may be illustrated at once. We discuss below the important relationship between chronic disability and poverty; but both the government which held office between 1976 and 1979 and that which took office in 1979 are known to have worked intermittently at a Green Paper on a comprehensive disability income which, when published, may substantially alter what is described in that section of this chapter.

It is not only the more obviously variable matters such as the administrative decisions of government that are subject to a fluctuating definition of social reality, but also more fundamental concepts such as the nature of poverty and its significance in the life of society at large. Indeed, there are disabled people who would argue that the very disability itself does not constitute a problem for them but rather for society at large, insofar as that society has failed to make appropriate provision for their characteristics. Clearly this is one area of medical concern where an approach which takes seriously the 'whole-person-in-context' is surely mandatory.

DEFINING THE FIELD

A minor irritation in the growing literature on disability has been the inconsistency with which have been used terms such as defect, impairment, disablement, and handicap and adjectives like primary and secondary, intrinsic, and extrinsic. The point is that there are some important conceptual distinctions to be made, but the words used for them differ among authorities. The most substantial epidemiological work in the field has been that of Harris and her colleagues (1971); the definitions of these workers are to be recommended for general use and are adopted here. They may be illustrated from the example of a child with congenital heart disease: this may lead to inadequacy of oxygenation ('impairment') and shortness of breath which in time leads to restricted mobility ('disability') which may further result in loss of schooling ('handicap'). The definitions of these workers are:

Impairment: lacking all or part of a limb or having a defective limb; having a defective organ or mechanism of the body which stops or limits getting about, working or self-care.
Disability: loss or reduction of functional ability.
Handicap: the disadvantage or restriction of activity caused by disability.*

The broad principles are, however, clear. Impairment is a physical attribute of the individual – though not every example of that kind of defect is to be included. For example, most members of the population have lost at least one tooth and a substantial proportion have some deficiency of visual accommodation – but these ordinarily constitute little disability and less handicap. However, some attribute of the individual is required as a necessary, but not sufficient, element in each of the concepts impairment, disability, and handicap. The other elements belong not to the individual but to the context within that individual finds himself and to the interaction between individual and context. This three-part scheme:
  1. The properties of the individual;
  2. The properties of the social context;
  3. The properties of the interaction between the two;
is a convenient way of organizing a good deal of general material on the social aspects of disability.

Factors belonging to the individual

An important contribution by Agerholm (1975) offers a scheme of classification of the individual attributes – she calls them intrinsic – which comprehensively define the field (Table 3.1). Unfortunately she refers to these attributes as handicaps, whereas in the Harris scheme they would be called disabilities, or sometimes impairments.

*The word handicap originates from a seventeenth century game of chance 'hand'i'cap' in which a closed hand, full or empty, was withdrawn from inside a cap. Later it came to be used to describe measured disadvantages imposed on the better competitors in a game or race to reduce their chances of winning. In this century it has been used increasingly to describe the long-term disadvantages which reduce an individual's chance in competition with his peers in ordinary life situations (Agerholm 1975).

Table 3.1. *Classification of intrinsic handicaps: key handicaps and components. (After Agerholm (1975))*

Key handicaps	Handicap components
1. Locomotor handicap (the locomotor handicapped)	A Impaired mobility in environment B Impaired postural mobility (relation of parts of body to one another) C Impaired manual dexterity D Reduced exercise tolerance
2. Visual handicap (the visually handicapped)	A Total loss of sight B Impaired (uncorrectable) visual acuity C Impaired visual field D Perceptual defect
3. Communication handicap (the communication handicapped)	A Impaired hearing B Impaired talking C Impaired reading D Impaired writing
4. Visceral handicap (the viscerally handicapped)	A Disorders of ingestion B Disorders of excretion C Artificial openings D Dependence of life-saving machines
5. Intellectual handicap (the intellectually handicapped)	A Mental retardation (congenital) B Mental retardation (acquired) C Loss of learned skills D Impaired learning ability E Impaired memory F Impaired orientation is space or time G Impaired consciousness
6. Emotional handicap (the emotionally handicapped)	A Psychoses B Neuroses C Behaviour disorders D Drug disorders (including alcoholism) E Antisocial disorders F Emotional immaturity
7. Invisible handicap (the invisibly handicapped)	A Metabolic disorders requiring permanent therapy (e.g. diabetes, cystic fibrosis) B Epilepsy, and other unpredictable losses of consciousness C Special susceptibility to trauma (e.g. haemorrahic disorders, bone fragility, susceptibility to pressure sores) D Intermittent prostrating disorders (e.g. migraine, asthma, vertigo) E Causalgia and other severe pain disorders
8. Aversive handicap (the aversively handicapped)	A Unsightly distortion of defect of part of body B Unsightly skin disorders and scars C Abnormal movements of body (athetosis, tics, grimacing, etc.) D Abnormalities causing socially unacceptable smell, sight, or sound
9. Senescence handicap (the senescence handicapped)	A Reduced plasticity of senescence B Slowing of physical or mental function of senescence C Reduced recuperative powers of senescence

One further point may be made here in relation to the Harris definitions. This is that they put an excessive emphasis on locomotor disability. The public stereotype of the disabled person is a young, male adult in a wheelchair; yet the largest group of the disabled are women, and over pensionable age. Those classified in the Agerholm terminology, as having intellectual, emotional, or invisible disabilities are also much more numerous than the Harris survey suggested or is generally believed (Weir 1981). In terms of social policy and social provision this has tended in recent years to lead to an emphasis on access where valuable gains have certainly been made:

. . . as if when people with disabilities can get inside buildings, they will automatically be integrated. With this image of disability dominant, integration becomes a spatial rather than a social and economic problem . . . (Walker 1981*a*).

This quotation comes from a book by members of the Disability Alliance, a federation of some 60 organizations concerned with handicap which was formed in 1974 in part specifically to press for a broader view of the social problems experienced by people with handicaps.

The social world of people with disabilities

Agerholm proposes a concept of *extrinsic* handicap – a disadvantage arising from an individual's environment or circumstances. The points to be stressed here are: *first* (as already indicated) these matters are subject to social definition – they are as they are because of human choice, and in principle could be otherwise; *second,* there exist social conditions which would constitute a disadvantage to anyone whether healthy or disabled; and *third* such conditions tend in fact to press particularly hard on those with intrinsic disability.

The remainder of this chapter is chiefly to do with a number of the most important areas of social disadvantage as they affect people with disabilities. These are:

Poverty and financial provision.

Educational requirements and provision that is age appropriate (including further education).

Employment problems and opportunities.

Accommodation, including households (whether in ordinary or special housing) and group living in residential care.

Personal mobility ranging from international travel to turning a gas tap or the page of a book.

Leisure activities including sports, etc. and holidays.

It will be apparent, however, that although these are discussed separately below there exist in practice strong links between them. For example, the lack of employment opportunities has important implications for financial status, which in turn, may clearly affect housing, the arrangements for assisted mobility, and many other matters.

We must note one other topic ommitted from the list – the question of social *attitudes*. This matter belongs partly to sociology and partly to psychology. Social context is not only material but also personal: the family, neighbours, employers, shop-keepers, professional helpers and others who surround us. Society displays rather regularly a tendency to hold a particular set of attitudes towards those of its members who are sick or disabled. The essential psychological mechanism underlying this phenomena is that of stereotyping – the tendency once a person is identified as having one characteristic to attribute to him or her a constellation of other characteristics which, rightly or wrongly, are believed always accompany it (thus, all wheelchair users may be treated as though stupid – 'Does he take sugar?'). And the essential social outcome of stereotyping is obviously towards enhancing the deprivation, both actual and experienced, of the person with disability. Such deprivation all too easily flows over into attitudes that are socially dismissive and rejecting.

The author's view is that it is unhelpful to consider these social problems in terms of 'the special needs of the handicapped'. In a very important sense people with handicaps have no special needs; rather, they share our common needs – for life-support, recognition by others, education and work, happiness and self-fulfillment, and the like. It is simply that meeting such needs is in some ways more difficult. A wider adoption of this emphasis 'same needs; different provision' might help to avoid some of the social stigmatizing mechanisms. However similar the words may look, to be in the medical sense an invalid ought not to entail becoming socially invalidated.

Interactional matters

Professional practice with and on behalf of the individual disabled person and his family is (as in many other fields) partly the delivery of a general policy which naturally is concerned with collective provision. In this chapter we must deal with social problems and social policies at a collective level. Indeed, there are some advantages in doing this; such an approach draws attention to common aspects which cut across medical categorizations. If restricted mobility makes it impossible for a single person to reach the local shops, the consequences for self-care may be much the same whether the restriction is produced by pulmonary insufficency, severe arthritis, blindness, or brain failure. In addition, some of the problems of the handicapped will be solved only by collective action – the changing of social policy through political processes.

However, although there may be intrinsic disabilities which are handicapping despite any variation in the social context and extrinsic disabilities which are handicapping despite any variation in the persons who experience them, in practice and for the individual it is the matching (or, more often, the mis-match) between a set of personal characteristics and a set of social conditions which is the vital concern. In an important sense *handicap is essentially an interactional concept*. This emphasis differs from that adopted by Harris *et al.* (1979) in defining handicap as the disadvantage '. . . caused by disability'; in equal measure, we may consider it caused by society.

Good professional practice in this area is therefore – not surprisingly – a question of close attention to the particularities of the individual's relations with his environment. Such attention should be:

(i) **Broad**: People with handicaps frequently complain that others tend to treat them as though their handicap were their most important, if not indeed their only, significant characteristic.

They therefore ask all concerned not to underestimate the handicapped as a person and to appreciate that those with handicaps reflect the spread of intelligence, interests, motivations, application and activities of the general population (Evidence to a Working Party of the Central Council for Education and Training in Social Work 1974, p. 16).

This is reminiscent of the characterization by Mathers (1970) of a health-enhancing, as opposed to a disease-attacking, orientation to medical practice.

(ii) **Detailed**:

They indicated that they expected their helpers to be knowledgeable about the nature, process and characteristics of handicapping conditions and their effects on them and their families. . . . They were highly critical also of the information given them by professionals and helpers about services, rights, etc. (Evidence to a Working Party of the Central Council for Education and Training in Social Work 1974).

(iii) **Assertive**:

The families of those with handicaps stressed their need for workers to be able and willing to give actual practical assistance and not just verbal advice particularly in stressful circumstances. . . . They welcome particularly those workers who were willing to fight for them. They appeared to value workers who were assertive and demanding on their behalf. They usually interpreted this as an expression of 'caring' on the part of workers (Evidence to a Working Party of the Central Council for Education and Training in Social Work 1974).

(iv) **Collaborative**: this important matter requires more extended discussion.

For some years the world of the disabled has become increasingly articulate and organized; much instructive collaboration is with disabled people themselves. Traced in terms of formal societies and organizations, the historical progession has been from the foundation of bodies *for the disabled* (for example, the National Association for Mental Health) to bodies of *groups of disabled people* and their families (Disabled Income Group, Spastics Society, Possum Users Association – and many others) and to bodies specifically concerned with breaking down barriers *between people with and without disability*. Part of society's responses to the increasing pressure on behalf of, and by, people with disabilities is that their world has become increasingly complex – and the demands on the expertise of professional advisers correspondingly great. Fortunately, directories and other useful tools have been developed. One example of such a resource is: *Directory for the disabled: a handbook of*

information and opportunities for disabled and handicapped people, edited by
Ann Darnbrough and Derek Kinrade. No practice library should be without a
copy of the current edition of this publication. A number of similar reference
books are also available.

Good professional practice in this area also necessitates a good deal of trans-
professional collaboration which may involve the entire multi-disciplinary
clinical team. The contribution of nurses is not further discussed in this
chapter, and that of physiotherapists and occupational therapists will be
considered later. What of social workers? The general practitioner's liaison is
likely to be chiefly with social workers from the local authority area team,
although hospital-based social workers may be involved in work with some
chronically disabled patients. The social caseworkers' expertise is generally a
combination of social care planning with a function of advice giving, emotional
support, counselling, or psychotherapy. Essentially, their role is to do with the
patient's psycho-social adjustment which may of course be improved from
either side – that is, by manipulation of the social environment or by enabling
relevant change in the individual's attitudes or behaviour. Social workers thus
often have a key role in co-ordinating services, both those to which they have
direct access because (like home helps or family aids) they are provided through
the Social Services Department and those (like most financial benefits, and
housing, educational, or occupational provisions) for which the social worker
will negotiate on the patient's behalf. These responsibilities derive in part from
the obligations laid upon local authority social services departments by the
National Assistance Act, 1948 and the Chronically Sick and Disabled Persons
Act, 1970. Before the Seebohm reorganization social work practice in this area
was the responsibility of Welfare Department, and it is widely recognized that
throughout most of the decade from 1970 other preoccupations of the social
services departments led to relative under-provision for work with the disabled.
In the 1980s there is some evidence of a redressing of balance in these matters.

Despite these other areas of activity, however, it remains true that a
considerable amount of power and responsibility for many aspects of the life of
the disabled other than the strictly medical rests upon doctors. Indeed, the
Disability Alliance, which is not uncritical of this role, assert that it 'dominates
much of the administration of benefits and services' – for example, in controlling
access to attendance and mobility allowances, housewives' non-contributory
pension and industrial disablement pension, and to such services outside the
NHS as certain residential and day care resources, special education, and the
like (Walker 1982).

FINANCIAL CONSIDERATIONS

If there were one point in this chapter to be singled out for special emphasis it
would be the strong association in Britain in the 1980s between chronic disability

and poverty. The strength and importance of this association can scarcely be over-stressed. Although provision for the disabled – as, indeed, for everyone – in our society is partly in cash and partly in the form of other kinds of material aid and in personal services, money is in an important sense plainly the key to most of life's opportunities.

This association is not new. Following the dissolution of the monasteries, through which the churches' care for the disabled had for centuries been made available, provision was made under the Elizabethan Poor Law, 1601 and these arrangements persisted unchanged until the Poor Law Amendment Act, 1834. The principle throughout this time, based upon the association of disability with poverty, was the necessity for some relief for the poor, but also upon the need to minimize public expenditure. During most of the nineteenth century there was no statutory provision for the disabled except that for which they were eligible under the poor laws. They were less harshly treated than able-bodied paupers, although as Topliss (1979) indicates this also was true of widows, orphans, and the elderly so that disability itself was not officially recognized. When specific recognition came (in the Report of the Royal Commission on the Blind, the Deaf and Dumb, etc. of the United Kingdom, 1889) the economic principle still applied in that educational provision for blind and deaf children, introduced in 1893, was advocated on the grounds that the number of paupers would thereby be reduced.

The provision of workshops for the disabled following the Boer War and retraining centres after the First World War – for servicemen, although the civilian blind were shortly afterwards included among those eligible – were also based largely in the economic principle. The same is true of the more extensive provision introduced for service personnel and civilians following the Second World War. It is suggested by many that the Chronically Sick and Disabled Persons Act 1970 represents the first legislative departure from the operation of this principle, although others argue that its very uneven implementation is evidence of the covert persistence of such a principle in the public administration.

The continuing association of disability and poverty is well documented. The OPCS survey (Harris *et al.* 1971), despite its deficiencies, was significant in showing that some 30 per cent of people with disabilities were living on supplementary benefit, and that a further 7 per cent – about 250 000 people – were entitled to benefits but not drawing them. This survey also established a further point of critical importance, namely that, in general, the greater the degree of disability the greater the poverty. The independent survey of household resources and standards of living carried out by Professor Peter Townsend in 1968–69 (Townsend 1979) confirmed these findings. Expressed in a slightly different way, this study demonstrated that of those living below the supplementary benefit level, those with even minor disability (11 per cent) appeared twice as frequently as the non-disabled. And those with appreciable or severe disability aged 15 and over who were living at or below that state's poverty line were about three times the number of the non-disabled. Furthermore, comparing those having no incapacity with those severely incapacitated, Townsend showed that the proportion living in a near poverty rose from 24 per cent to 58 per cent as the severity of incapacity increased. Finally, an analysis of the General Household Survey carried out by Hayward on behalf of the Royal Commission on Income Distribution and Wealth (1978) also disclosed the same relationship – about half the families in which the head was permanently disabled were living on incomes close to the state definition of poverty.

It should be noted that all these researchers take as the standard of comparison the state's definition of entitlement to supplementary benefit. This is of course based on no more than the sum prevailing at any time for mere subsistence; it takes little account of the fact that, for the disabled, their's may be a permanent and unimprovable state of affairs, or that disability almost always entails expenditure above the normal. Moreover, these studies take no note of the disabled living in residential institutions.

Mechanisms of poverty

In the explanation of this matter there are three broad areas for consideration:

1. The social norm is that income is received in exchange for work done, but the disabled have restricted access to the employment market.

2. State social security benefits are generally inadequate, inequitably distributed and too difficult to obtain.

3. The expenditure of people with disabilities are necessarily higher than those of comparable members of the population.

The following account draws on that of Walker (1982).

Low income and wealth

Even when in work, there is evidence that the disabled are more likely than the non-disabled to be in low-paid occupations. In a survey in 1964, it was shown that disabled incomes were some 25 per cent below the national average (Sainsbury 1970). Buckle (1971) reporting on part of the OPCS investigation of 1969, showed that half of those with impairments who were in work had incomes below 42 per cent of the national average. A Department of Employment Survey (1973) of wage rates in sheltered factories and workshops and in training centres reported that 19 out of 25 local authority workshops and 24 out of 32 run by voluntary bodies paid rates at about half of the average earnings for male manual workers. And similar conclusions were reached by the Royal Commission on Income Distribution and Wealth (1978) and by Townsend (1979).

Townsend also reports on measures of wealth:

More of the incapacitated than of the non-incapacitated for each major age group were in debt or had no assets or had less than £100 . . . Fewer were owner-occupiers, held a personal bank account, owned a car or had personal possessions other than furniture or clothing (such as jewellery, silver and antiques) worth £25 or more.

Clearly, part of the explanation of these figures lies in the diminished capacity for work of many disabled people. And this factor is likely to be the more significant when impairments are multiple; a single impairment may be coped with or compensated for by the person concerned and his family but two impairments seem more than twice as daunting to all concerned. Part of it may be due to the attitudes of employers and other workers or the public at large – which may or may not be justified. And a further part of the explanation may be the paucity of suitably adapted work places, or of the relevant training provision. The result is to make a high proportion of people with disability dependent on state benefits.

Social security benefit

The benefits to which disabled persons may be entitled fall into four broad categories: contributory benefits, non-contributory benefits, industrial injury benefits (and war pensions), and supplementary benefits. The following description is very selective, for fuller details see Lynes (1981).

(a) *Contributory benefits* derive from the National Insurance Scheme, and recipients must therefore qualify in various ways to be 'in benefit'. They include: *Invalidity pension* (£31.45 in 1982–3) which replaces sickness benefit after 28 weeks and is payable as long as an incapacity for work continues: *Invalidity allowance* (three rates £2.20–6.50 in 1982–3) payable in addition; varies with the age at which incapacity began. Medical certification is required.

(b) *Non-contributory benefits* are of frequent relevance to disabled people and their families. They include: *Non-contributory invalidity pension* (£19.79 in 1982–3) for those incapable of working (including married women unable to do normal housework) for at least 28 weeks. *Attendance allowance* (£26.25 or £17.50 in 1982–3). The higher rate is for those requiring attendance both day *and* night; the lower for those requiring attendance only by day or night. Decisions are made on the basis of medical recommendation after examination arranged by the DHSS and the disability must be so severe as to require frequent or prolonged attention in connection with the disabled person's bodily functions or *continual* supervision in order to avoid substantial danger to himself or others. Darnbrough and Kinrade (1979) comment '. . . it is all too easy to be refused the allowance not because the facts do not justify payment but because they are inadequately presented'. *Invalid care allowances* (£19.70 in 1982–3) payable for a person of working age other than a married woman who does not work but cares for a disabled person who must, however, be in receipt of attendance allowance or constant attendance allowance. *Mobility allowance* (£18.30 in 1982–3) for physically disabled persons between the age of 5 and 65 (or those over 65 who are already receiving it) who are unable or virtually unable to walk (see below)

(c) *Industrial injuries* benefits are payable in respect of conditions which arise from accidents at work or industrial disease, and they are, on the whole, more generous than the above. Benefits include: *Disablement benefit* (£53.60 in

1982–3 for 100 per cent assessment). *Unemployability supplement* (31.45 in 1982–3). *Special hardship allowance* (£21.44 maximum in 1982–3). *Constant attendance allowance* (£21.50 in 1982–3). *Exceptionally severe disablement allowance* (£21.50 in 1982–3). Quite substantial numbers of disabled people benefit from payments under this category. There is also a substantial, though declining, group who derive a similar range of benefits from war pensions.

(d) *Supplementary benefits* exist partly to top up benefits of the kind noted above, which are in fact often quite inadequate, and partly to meet needs which are not covered by such benefits. The Social Security Act 1980 (which includes an amended version of the fundamental legislation, the Suuplementary Benefits Act 1976) provides that every person in Great Britain of or over the age of 16 whose resources are insufficient to meet his requirements 'shall be entitled to benefit'. Entitlement is decided (subject to appeal) by officials known as benefit officers and is governed by an extensive range of detailed regulations which (since November 1980) have substantially reduced the scope for the exercise of discretion. Nevertheless, some regulations still include clauses such as 'when it is reasonable in the circumstances' or 'is the opinion of the benefit officer' and there is then a chief supplementary benfits officer and a system of local tribunals with an appeal to the Social Security Commissioners to ensure a reasonable degree of consistency.

A number of general points will be apparent. First, the rates are by no means particularly generous. Second, the system is enormously complex. Each of the above resources is hedged about with its own set of criteria as to entitlement. The change in 1980 to a system of legally enforceable and publically available regulations from one depending on the discretion of individuals whose judgements were always prone to vary and which sometimes seemed arbitrary to the point of injustice has, however, been generally welcomed.

Third, many disabled persons and their families are compelled to be dependent upon some combination of benefits – and, indeed, some combinations may extend beyond those listed above to include also benefits such as rent and rate rebates. Nor do such combinations always act in a simple additive fashion; for example, benefiting from rent and rate rebates renders a person ineligible for any supplementary benefits; invalidity benefit cannot be paid if certain other national insurance benefits or training allowances are being received, and so forth. Fourthly, some benefits are contributory, others not; some are means tested, others not; and some are taxable as income while others are not. Fifthly, as well as a recognition of need, the pattern of benefits available may reflect with little rationality the place or circumstances in which the disablement occurred, the type of disability and the age of onset of the disability or the current age of the person concerned.

Public policy has paralleled the wishes of many disabled people in pointing to the desirability of their living at home. Socially, households are very clearly economic units and the law (for the purposes of Supplementary Benefit calculations) recognizes an 'assessment unit' whose requirements and resources must be aggregated. Thus the relative deprivation experienced by many disabled persons in Britain tody must also affect other family members. Some recognition of this fact appears in the shape of Income Tax allowances – the Blind Person's Allowance, the Dependent Relative Allowance and the House-keeper Allowance – and also in the form of additions where there are dependent adults or children in a number of the social security benefits listed above. In addition, there are a number of specific benefits for care-givers – the Attendance Allowance, the Invalid Care Allowance, and, relevant in some circumstances, Family Income Supplement.

Many people with disability are known not to be receiving the full extent of their entitlement, partly because of the shame felt to be attached to what people of sensitivity consider to be 'handouts', but sometimes because of mistaken or perverse decisions by officials. It is not, in the present author's view, the place of the doctor to be expert in this field, but it is important for medical persons to understand the general nature of their patients' problems in this area and to be able to refer them to competent Welfare Rights advice. This may be obtainable through specialist Welfare Rights agencies or through organizations such as The Disability Alliance or the Child Poverty Action Group (for details see Darnbrough and Kinrade 1979).

Finally, we must again note that entitlement to many of these benefits depends at some point on medical certification and frequently upon the patient, or their responsible relative, having full, accurate, and early medical information. Medical certification may be simply a matter of providing in a relatively informal fashion supporting evidence upon which a benefits officer may reach a decision; others are a statutory formality. It is worth taking the trouble to discover the precise form of the official requirement and, so far as clinical judgement allows, to match this in drafting the recommendations. Further, where it appears that the resulting decision is unjust to the patient the possibility of an appeal is worth consideration. It should also be borne in mind that responsibility for the initial application for many benefits rests with the potential beneficiary and that since some benefits are not payable until a qualifying period has elapsed, there are good reasons for sharing with the patient or responsible relative the full extent of the likely disability and the prognosis as early as possible.

Some of these medical certificates attract a fee which is negotiated on behalf of the profession through the Civil Service Department – for more complete details and information concerning the current rates readers should consult a resource such as the British Medical Association's Members' Handbook.

Additional expenditure

This is clearly a matter which depends on the particulars of the individual case – several autibiographical accounts exist in the literature (e.g. Sanders 1981) as well as more systematic surveys (Baldwin and Glendinning 1981). It is necessary, however, for doctors to be aware of the influence of this factor in accounting for the relative financial hardship of many handicapped persons.

Several sources of additional expenditure can be distinguished: *Ordinary items:* extra food to meet special diets, allergies, difficulties in swallowing, weight problems – or simply to make life pleasanter for people in chronic discomfort. Extra clothing and bedding because of incontinence, destructiveness, discharge or dribbling, wear from calipers or other appliances. Extra fuel bills almost always accompany immobility. Extra transport costs – taxi fares may, for example, be unavoidable for people not able to make use of other forms of public transport. Higher telephone bills. *Less regular expenditure:* one illustration: a survey in 1975 showed that one third of a sample of families had moved house on account of a disabled child. Housing adaptations are not always wholly paid for out of public funds – in another study, the average amount paid by families for this purpose in 1976–78 was £363 (Bradshaw 1980). *Other necessary articles:* cars, washing machines, freezers, telephone, and the like, which might ordinarily be regarded as luxuries, are for many disabled persons and their families necessities – especially if a policy of home-based rather than institutional care is being properly pursued. While the initial cost of such items may be met by Supplementary Benefit payments, maintenance costs and the replacement of items which wear out rapidly because of heavy usage may attract less financial support. *'Crisis' costs:* admission of a disabled person to a limited period of hospital or other residential care, or a period of deterioration, may be associated with loss of earnings among the family members, additional fares, costs of child minding, and the like, as well as lapses in control over budgeting.

Although beyond the scope of this chapter, it may be remarked in conclusion that the Disability Alliance holds that the solution to these multiple financial problems lies in the establishment of a single, simple, and comprehensive disability income guaranteed as of right, universal rather than selective in operation, and based upon need rather than on such accidental features as the place and type of disability, the person's earnings record, or the age of the individual concerned. Provisional costing for such a scheme has been produced (Wilson 1981). It is perhaps a combination of the dismissive attitude of the able-bodied society with a fear that public expenditure might somehow pass out of control that has so far prevented the implementation of this policy.

EDUCATIONAL PROVISION

This topic must be considered in terms of pre-schooling, provision for disabled people of normal school age, and further education. The following section draws heavily upon the relevant chapters in Darnbrough and Kinrade which should be consulted for further details.

The basic rights are enacted in the Education Act, 1944 and the Education (Scotland) Act 1945 together with subsequent legislation which, in 1970 in

England and Wales and 1974 in Scotland, abolished the concept of 'ineducability' for children with mental handicap and brought the responsibility for meeting their needs in an appropriate fashion into line with that of every other child, whether disabled or not, as a duty of local education authorities. The present position is that, although the report on Special Education Needs (Warnock 1978) recommends that statutory categorization of children with handicaps should be abandoned, it still remains.

The essential point is of course that where need exists for special educational provision, this should be recognized as early as possible; education authorities have a duty in law to 'ascertain' children who require such provision. Medical practitioners – both in primary care and community medicine as well as in hospital practice – may obviously have an important role in this process, along with parents and other care-givers, teachers, psychologists, social workers, and members of a large range of other disciplines. Ascertainment in England and Wales applies to children of two years of age and over, in Scotland to children of any age, and it may indeed be of crucial importance to children whose disability involves some learning difficulty to arrange for pre-school provision from the earliest feasible age.

Parents have a right to ask that their child be ascertained and the education authority is bound to comply unless it believes the request to be unreasonable. Once placed in a special school, however, the child cannot be withdrawn by the parents without the agreement of the LEA though they have a right to appeal to the Secretary of State. There is an important debate in the educational world between those who believe special schooling to be the most effective form of provision and those who advocate integration of disabled children into ordinary schools – either in special classes or into the general classrooms. Darnbrough and Kinrade (1979) take the view that all these alternatives should be available in order to provide the maximum flexilbility in placing the individual child, but in practice this is unlikely to be possible within a single LEA. On the other hand, LEAs have the power to arrange for a child to attend a school in another area or a non-maintained special school, many of which are run by voluntary organizations and are excellent because they have been able to confine themselves to their limited chosen task without too much influence by political pressures. In such cases, the LEA is empowered to pay fees and board and lodging if necessary and to meet the costs of reasonable travelling.

A comprehensive list of references to literature useful to parents, and of societies and organizations appropriate to a wide range of disabilities, is given in Darnbrough and Kinrade (1979).

Concerning further education for the disabled these same authors write:

Acquired skills and knowledge can also mean the difference between a life-sapping, mundane round of drudgery known as earning a crust, and a fulfilling involvement as a happily employed person. For a person who becomes disabled, further education of one sort or another may be essential in order to alter course to accommodate specific handicaps.

Disabled persons share the ordinary eligibility for mandatory and other LEA awards, and authorities are empowered to make an additional allowance (at present up to a maximum of £180 per annum) to award-holding disabled students who incur as a result of their disability extra costs 'related to study'. Most colleges and universities will go to considerable trouble to accommodate disabled students, and many have special equipment (page-turners, aids to reading, writing and so on) to facilitate this. Darnbrough and Kinrade (1979) give particulars of useful organizations such as the National Bureau for Handicapped Students, the Association of Disabled Professionals, the Open University Adviser to Disabled Persons and the particularly wide range of resources for the blind and partially sighted. For those whose disabilities are such that some form of residential vocational training is appropriate, four colleges exist: Finchdale College, Durham; Portland College, Mansfield; Queen Elizabeth's Foundation, Leatherhead; and St. Loye's College, Exeter. The facilities offered by each are summarized by these authors, who also give details of other residential provisions for disabled students. A survey carried out in 1981 showed that only 18 per cent of a sample of nearly 190 persons leaving St. Loye's over a four-year period had not at some time been in employment (Jowett 1982).

EMPLOYMENT

We have already noted the relative deprivation experienced by people with disabilities in relation to work; for instance, at a time when the general level of unemployment was 10.1 per cent (Manpower Services Commission, March 1981) the figure for the disabled was 15.3 per cent. General practitioners will be well aware of the psychological importance of work:

. . . it gives people a sense of purpose and competence, it makes tham feel needed; it provides a change of environment so that they may appreciate their home better when they return to it in the evening, it brings them into contact with a different range of people from their friends at home and may lead to further interests and social activities . . . (Warnock 1978).

There are some specific provisions, deriving in the main from the Disabled Persons (Employment) Acts of 1944 and 1958. The intention of these is 'to secure for the disabled their full share within their capacity of such employment as is ordinarily available' (Tomlinson 1943). The 1944 Act established a voluntary register of those:

substantially handicapped on account of injury, disease (including a physical or mental condition arising from imperfect development of any organ, or congenital deformity, in obtaining or keeping employment or work on his own account otherwise suited to his age, qualification and experience; the disablement being likely to last for 12 months or more.

It also set up the quota system – an employer with more than 20 employees is legally required to employ persons registered as disabled to the extent of 3 per cent of his workers. In addition, certain occupations were reserved for the registered disabled, powers were provided to establish sheltered work (Remploy) and to subsidize local authority and voluntary agency sheltered workshops, and a staff of Disablement Resettlement Officers was provided within what is now the Manpower Services Commission's Employment Service Division.

These services still exist, although it should be noted that Manpower Services Commission recommended in 1981 that the quota system should be abandoned in favour of statutory general duty on employers to take 'reasonable steps' to promote equality of opportunity in employment for disabled people, together with a code of practice and educational measures aimed at persuading employers to find work for disabled persons. As a group, the disabled are of course very vulnerable to the general pressures produced by unemployment. Topliss (1979), quotes the illustration of the figures for people registered blind in 1972. In the Northern Region (which had a high level of unemployment) the number of blind persons returned as being incapable of work considerably exceeded those in work – and of the latter nearly one half were considered fit only for sheltered employment, whereas at the same time in London those incapable of work were less than half those in employment – 76 per cent of whom were in open employment. Nevertheless, medical practitioners may still find themselves called upon to certify disabled people for registration.

Also within the scope of the Employment Services Division are the 27 Employment Rehabilitation Centres, through which some 14000 persons annually pass on courses of 6–8 week's duration. Tax-free allowances plus free meals, assistance with fares and a lodgings allowance are payable. These Centres provide not only guided rehabilitation to ordinary working conditions for those previously in work but also assessment and vocational guidance for handicapped school leavers. An ERC course is obtainable on medical recommendation through the Disablement Resettlement Offices.

A further provision through the Employment Service Division is sheltered work for that minority of disabled persons unable to cope with open work conditions but nevertheless able to be in employment outside their homes. Examples include: *'Enclaves':* the arrangement whereby an independent body or a local authority employs the workers, is paid for the work done and receives a government subsidy. A number of local authorities have parks and gardens enclave schemes which provide particularly for those disabled through residual mental illness or through mental handicap. *Remploy:* this is a government supported company which has 87 factories and provides about 8000 jobs, chiefly in furniture, leather goods, or textiles production and the associated management and administration. Remploy is also responsible for the Blind Advisory Service which exists to support over 50 workshops for the blind run by local authorities, the Royal National Institute for the Blind and other voluntary bodies. *Financial assistance:* special assistance in travel costs for getting to work may be available to some disabled persons. Grants can be made to employers for adaptations to premises and equipment (ramps, special toilet facilities, etc.) on behalf of a specific disabled employee. Special aids such as jigs or other modifications to tools, electric typewriters, telephone attachments, braille rulers, and micrometers can be had on permanent free loan. Currently there is an experimental job induction scheme which offers a grant to employees who take on a disabled person for a trial period in order to assess his or her suitability for a job.

In addition, there exist a wide range of provisions by the National Health Service, local authorities, and voluntary bodies which provide employment through rehabilitation schemes, day centres and the like.

Finally, an unknown number of disabled persons, make a substantial contribution towards being self-supporting by self-employment in their own homes – a group which include some of the most severely disabled such as the members of the Mouth and Foot Painting Artists Association.

ACCOMMODATION

Most people with disabilities live in private households but there is no direct relationship between the severity of type of disability and the kind of accommodation in which such persons find themselves. Topliss (1979) gives the figures shown in Table 3.2.

Table 3.2. *Accommodation of disabled persons (1977 figures)*

	No. in private households	No. in institutional care
Under 65 years	1 453 000	76 000 (5 per cent of the total)
Over 65 years	1 783 000	267 000 (13 per cent of the total)

Housing for the disabled

The OPCS Survey (Buckle 1971) suggested that 25 per cent of the disabled persons interviewed lived in accommodation that required 'substantial improvement' or even that the person should be re-housed. This was not in general because the property itself was substandard but because the everyday needs of people with disability require special provision if they are not to be subject to additional, extrinsic, handicap. Less than 5 per cent were in specially built accommodation, though where it exists this is usually very satisfactory. Some 40 per cent were in owner-occupied housing, and these tend to be in the worst-quality places; just over 20 per cent are in privately rented accommodation, and the remaining one-third are local authority tenants whose housing is generally the best. It is officially recognized, however, that 'there is an urgent need for housing authorities to do much more for people who are physically handicapped and to help housing associations to do much more' (Department of the Environment 1974).

The Chronically Sick and Disabled Persons Act 1970 requires local authorities to consider the housing needs of those registered (by the authority itself – not the Department of Employment), to provide assistance with adaptations and 'extra facilities to secure their greater safety, comfort or convenience' and to notify to the Minister plans for including special housing for the disabled in their housing developments. On the latter point, it may be noted that between 1970 and 1973 there were notified 1281 such dwellings – 0.5 per cent of all housing applications, the disabled being about 6 per cent of the population.

The implementation of this part of the Act has been rather uneven principally for two reasons: local authorities vary in the comprehensiveness of their registration and there was, especially in the early days, uncertainty about precisely what costs should be met from the budget of the local authority's housing department and what from the social services department. The distinction is that between 'adaptations' and 'aids'. Housing authorities are responsible for extensions and structural alterations: wider doors, ramps, alterations to provide a suitable bathroom or WC and the like. 'Aids' may include a very wide range of equipment and gadgets to help disabled people to make use of the bathroom, lavatory, kitchen, or bedroom and living room accommodation. Assessment of the kind of need may be made by social workers, or – better, and more frequently – by occupational therapists based either in local authority social services departments or in hospital, and the equipment itself is available through the departments where the authority is satisfied that such provision is necessary. The special expertise of occupational therapists extends to the recommendation of suitable aids (and often the development of new ones) but – at least as importantly also help and encourage-ment to the beneficiaries in learning to make the best use of what is available. The aim is to achieve an optimal matching between the particular skills and disabilities of the individual concerned and the environment within which he lives.

Voluntary organizations have an important role also in these matters, notably the Disabled Living Foundation which provides a constantly up-to-date advisory service concerning aids and equipment. This is very necessary in a field where engineering and other technologies have made great advances in recent years. There are corresponding bodies in Northern Ireland, Scotland, and in Wales – more detailed information is given by Darnbrough and Kinrade (1979).

Living at home is not, however, only a matter of the physical environment, but also of the personal environment. Indeed, there is an important sense in which a disability is a family problem (Baldwin and Glendinning 1981). It is beyond the scope of this chapter to discuss the psychological aspects of this matter, a good introduction to which may be found in Topliss (1979) who remarks that they are 'likely to be of far greater significance than the material disadvantages'. Note should be made, however, of the importance of help and support for care-givers; the real costs of community care are largely borne by the relatives of those who receive it. Medical care of the disabled is clearly a matter of 'family practice' and relief for the care-givers through the use of day centres, intermittent or holiday admissions, and of such domiciliary support and Home Helps and laundry service must be considered. Associations or Societies concerned with specific impairments often offer relatives a useful measure of support and advice, and there is now an Association of Carers.

Finally, a difficult problem concerning the accommodation of disabled people and their families in private facilities may come to the notice of the general practitioner. This is the question of what becomes of the surviving family members when a disabled person dies or moves into life-long residential care, and the house has been extensively and expensively modified. Plainly, such situations can give rise to serious conflicts of interest and require careful advice and considerable counselling.

Residential care

Although a small minority of the disabled, those in residential care tend to be a particularly disadvantaged group. The essence of the solution to the state of affairs is embodied in the comment 'Residential care should become the preferred form of treatment for those for whom it is provided' made by a Working Party of the Central Council for Education and Training in Social Work (CCETSW 1974). The emphasis here – the preferred form of treatment – contrasts with ideas of residential care as being residual (the 'last resort') and to do with what some authors have called 'warehousing' (Miller and Gwynne 1972), that is, the maintenance of people in status quo rather than the pro- motion of change. It may be objected that many people with disabilities, though by no means all, are on a deteriorating course and that 'treatment' or 'change' are unrealistic aims, but this argument may be countered by pointing to the avoidance of institutionalization, the maintenance of a high level of functioning for as long as possible, symptom relief and assisting people to make a constructive and 'good' death as being perfectly proper therapeutic objectives.

How this approach to residential care is to come about is beyond the scope of this chapter to discuss in detail, but in the author's view two principles are of the greatest importance. These are: a much more flexible use of domiciliary, day care, and residential resources (partly a matter of policy and planning, and partly of professional practice) and a much higher level of professional expertise throughout the staffs of residential institutions (partly a matter of personnel management and partly of education and training). Considerable progress has been made on these matters in recent years, though more needs to be done.

Some of this residential provision is in the National Health Service – in psychiatric or mental subnormality hospitals, units for the younger chronic sick, certain orthopaedic and trauma units, geriatric hospitals, and so forth – over the policies of which medical practitioners have a good deal of influence. Other provision is in the local authorities which are required under the National Assistance Act, 1948 to provide residential accommodation for the elderly and infirm as well as having a range of statutory obligations concerning child care which are not infrequently invoked on behalf of disabled children, and per- missive powers under the Mental Health Act, 1959 to provide hostels for the mentally subnormal and the mentally ill. Still other provision is in the hands of voluntary organizations, some of which, such as the Leonard Cheshire Foundation (the largest provider of accommodation for the severely physically disabled and chronically sick adults) and the Richmond Fellowship (30 hostels and group homes for people with psychiatric problems), operate on an extensive scale. In relation to local authority and voluntary provision it is unusual for medical practitioners to have a controlling decision over their residential work, but they may often influence such matters to the benefit of patients with chronic disability.

For further discussion see King *et al.* (1971), Walton and Elliot (1980), Jansen (1980), Clough (1981).

MOBILITY

This area of functioning attracts particular state provisions which are considered below, but three general comments must be made on it. First, as already indicated, the social handicaps of people with disabilities are much broader than this although the public sterotype, and to some extent government policy, has elevated mobility problems to a position of prominence in thinking about disablement. Second, the concept of mobility is itself wider than may first appear. Clearly it has to do with disorders affecting motor function, but it also is influenced by sensory impairments. Blindness is an obvious cause of restricted mobility: deafness less so. It also has to do with impairment of motivation as in chronic mental illness, or an incapacity to find one's way as in subnormality or dementia.

Third, mobility problems effect the whole range of kinds of movement from fine finger movements up to international travel and at every level examples may easily be found of the marginal nature of the adjustment of many disabled people – a small increase or decrease of capacity for movement may have dis- proportionately large effects on the individual's total adjustment to the environment. There is an obvious contribution of physiotherapists and speech therapists (taking speech defects to be a form of mobility problem, as they clearly are in some instances) to the amelioration of spasticity and pain and to the recovery of function and re-training following paralysis. It depends upon a careful functional assessment of the problems and the consistent application of a treatment programme directed partly at the individual concerned, but where necessary devising environmental modifications to achieve an optimal matching between person and situation and thus a maximum degree of self-management.

It is neither necessary nor possible to detail in full the extraordinary range of aids to mobility now available. At the level of fine movement they include such items as: large-handled cutlery, toothbrushes, and safety razors; free-hand trays; drinking aids and specially designed plates; long-handled shoe horns; lazy tongs; spring-loaded scissors; stockings and dressing sticks; specially designed footwear; walking sticks; frames and crutches. Also relevant to this level of movement are such matters as special forms of gas and water taps, and household adaptations such as raised toilet seats, higher or lower working surfaces, and high-level electricity points. At a grosser level of movement 'geriatric' or other especially designed chairs, mechanically or electrically adjustable beds, commodes, and a variety of lifters and hoists, hand or electrically operated wheelchairs, and so on have obvious relevance.

Outside the living accommodation, mobility is also partly a function of the individual and his various resources and partly of the environment. The environmental aspects range from broad considerations of planning (the siting of residential homes and sheltered housing in relation to hills, to shops and recreation facilities, bus and other transport routes and to other housing) to smaller-scale features of the built environment like the lowering of kerbs at road junctions, and the duty to make access possible for the disabled to public buildings and toilets. Disabled car-parking spaces and the 'orange badge' scheme are related provisions.

Also relevant, are provisions in the non-built environment. 'Trying to board a pay-as-you-enter bus – up the steep steps, through the narrow entrance, while fumbling for change and clutching parcels, children, walking-stick, crutches – requires the agility of a mountain goat!' (Darnborough and Kinrade 1979) – and these authors go on to point to examples such as the San Francisco underground and the Los Angeles bus system where entrances are accessible to wheelchair users. The limited attention paid to such matters as the design of public transport arrangements in Britain reflects, no doubt, the relative lack of political and economic leverage of the disabled and elderly. The most imaginative provision is made by airlines and, to some extent, by British Rail.

There are also some financial provisions related to mobility.

Mobility allowance

A taxable benefit payable in addition to other social security benefits to those with 'inability or virtual inability' to walk – which means that the ability to move on foot is so impaired that the person cannot make real progress, or that the exertion would constitute a danger to life or lead to serious deterioration in health. The disablement must be likely to persist for at least one year and the applicant must be able to be moved (with help) without endangering life, and must be capable of appreciating his surroundings. New applications may be made in respect of people from 5 to 65 years of age, but extensions of an existing allowance may be allowed up to age 75. A clearly formulated medical recommendation is required.

Motability

This is a name of a voluntary organization which was set up in 1978 when the mobility allowance (which is payable to disabled passengers as well as to

disabled drivers) replaced the preceding arrangements for the issue of government cars, including the single-person three-wheeler car (the notorious 'trike').
The whole of the mobility allowance has to be paid to the organization in
addition to any other costs of the arrangement, which may be considerable and
have to be paid in a lump sum at the outset. In return a car from a limited list of
choices is made available on what is, in effect, a three- or four-year lease.
Insurance, accident costs (but not maintenance) and excessive mileage are
additional costs.

War pensioners

Separate arrangements exist which are in general more generous than the
above. A car, adapted where necessary, a three-wheeler (so long as these are
still available) or a private car allowance may be provided. For further details,
see Darnbrough and Kinrade (1979).

Other provisions

Many people with restricted mobility including all those in receipt of a mobility
allowance, are exempt from Vehicle Excise Duty; there are concessions on
tyres, some car purchase and car-hire charges and on tolls and ferries; there are
specialist insurance brokers for the disabled; car conversion is an important
area of consideration, embracing not only controls but such matters as swivel
seats and roof-mounted hoists; there are special arrangments for disabled
driver training. Here also, Darnbrough and Kinrade (1979) give full particulars.

Finally, we must note the arrangements which it may be possible for disabled
people to make concerning holidays in Britain or abroad. Travel and tour
operators are increasingly making provisions for people with a wide range of
disabilities on an integrated basis; it is plainly necessary to give advance notice
and important to describe fully the help which is needed. The disabled person is
normally expected to provide for himself any special equipment and personal
assistance required, but there are few opportunities for group holidays for
unaccompanied disabled persons where volunteer staff are available. Under the
Chronically Sick and Disabled Persons Act, 1970 local authority social service
departments may give financial assistance to enable persons registered as
disabled to have aholiday, and they may also be able to offer some help in
making the arrangements.

HOLIDAYS AND LEISURE ACTIVITIES

Darnbrough and Kinrade (1979) provide a comprehensive list of specialist
interest holidays, of a house-exchange scheme for those living in adapted
housing, and of a considerable range of voluntary and other holiday organizations which cater for the disabled. The Automobile Association, the Royal
Association for Disability and Rehabilitation, and MIND all publish holiday
guides. The same authors also give country-by-country information relevant to

overseas holidays, noting travel agents, sources of information concerning access and the arrangements for medical treatment while on holiday.

In respect of leisure activities in general, it is perhaps important to note the danger of too readily thinking of the disabled in terms of their filling time only with such activities rather than undertaking a 'proper' job. It is, of course, true that for many people with disabilities the everyday 'personal maintenance' activities take up more time and energy than they do for the non-disabled. Also, as we have seen, the disabled are likely to be particulary at risk of unemployment. In addition, leisure activities for disabled and non-disabled alike are an obvious source of zest for living. Nevertheless, there is plainly a risk that an excessive emphasis on leisure activities for the disabled may be subtly stigmatizing or degrading.

That said, the available facilities in this area are quite extensive. There is a permissive power under the Chronically Sick and Disabled Persons Act, 1970 for local authorities to provide radio, television, library, and similar facilities, as well as 'lectures, games, or outings'. In practice, the availability of such provision varies greatly from one locality to another and they are exceedingly vulnerable everywhere to financial stringencies. On the voluntary side, such well-known bodies exist as the British Sports Association for the Disabled as well as a host of organizations catering for special interests. Darnbrough and Kinrade (1979) provide a list including details of organizations, facilities, and relevant publications or activities from amateur radio, angling, and archery through the alphabet to wheelchair dancing, wine making, writing, and yoga. Those with responsibility for counselling the disabled – especially, perhaps, the newly disabled and their families – may find this a useful stimulus to the imagination.

A FINAL WORD

This chapter has surveyed the major components of the social aspects of disability. Considerable emphasis has been given to the social policies designed to assist such people in meeting their common human needs; and indications have been given of ways in which general practitioners and their colleagues of other disciplines may translate these policies into the delivery of services for individual patients. Is there a single concept within which all this might be summed up?

We suggest that the key word is normalization. Originating during the 1970s in Scandinavia, and largely in respect of institutionalized and mentally handicapped children (Nirje 1970), this concept is of wider application. Of course, it is not intended to deny the reality of the physical or mental impairment or to promote unrealistic expectations of a person who is disabled. But it is to say that 'normal' behaviour cannot be encouraged in abnormal conditions such as hospital or segregated education (Gunzburg 1970) or other circumstances of deprivation. Taking a robustly interactional stance, the argument of this chapter is that the ideal of normalization is one to which all should aspire for the whole world of handicap. Partly this will mean continued efforts to make such provision for the disabled that their state could be as like as possible that of 'normal' peopl; and partly it will be a matter of redefining the world of the normal until there is ordinarily within it a respected and recognized place for people with disabilities. Not until these processes have been accomplished will there exist a state of integration which we could regard as socially healthy.

REFERENCES

Agerholm, M. (1975). Handicaps and the handicapped. *Jl R. Soc. Hlth* 1, 3–8.

Baldwin, S. and Glendinning, C. (1981). Children with disabilities and their families. In *Disability in Britain: a manifesto of rights* (ed. A. Walker and P. Townsend). Robertson, Oxford.

Bennett, A. F., Garrad, J. M., and Hall, T. (1970). Chronic disease and disability in the community: a prevalence study. *Br. med. J.* iii, 762.

Boswell, D. M. and Wingrove, J. M. (1974). *The handicapped person in the community.* Tavistock, London.

Bradshaw, J. (1980). *The family fund: an initiative in social policy.* Routledge and Kegan Paul, London.

Buckle, J. R. (1971). *Work and housing of impaired persons in Great Britain.* HMSO, London.

Central Council for Education and Training in Social Work (1974). *People with handicaps need better trained workers.* Paper No. 5. CCETSW, London.

Clough, R. (1981). *Old age homes.* Allen and Unwin, London.

Darnborough, A. and Kinrade, D. (1979). *Directory for the disabled: a handbook of information and opportunities for disabled and handicapped people.* 2nd edn. Woodhead-Faulkner for the Royal Society for Disability and Rehabilitation.

—— (1973). *Sheltered employment for disabled people.* London.

Department of the Environment (1974). Circular 1974/75.

Gunzburg, H. C. (1970). The hospital as a normalizing training environment. *J. ment. Subnorm.* 16, 71–83.

Harris, A. I., Cox, E., and Smith, C. R. W. (1971). *Handicapped and impaired in Great Britain.* HMSO, London.

Jansen, E. (ed.) (1980). *The therapeutic community.* Croom Helm, London.

Jowett, S. (1982). *Young disabled people: their further education, training and employment.* NFER-Nelson.

King, R. D., Raynes, N. V., and Tizard, T. (1971). *Patterns of residential care.* Routledge and Kegan Paul, London.

Lynes, T. (1981). *Penguin guide to supplementary benefits,* 4th edn. Penguin, Harmondsworth.

Mathers, J. R. (1970). Psychiatry and religion. In *Religion and medicine: a discussion* (ed. M. A. H. Melinsky). SCM Press, London.

Miller, E. J. and Gwynne, G. V. (1972). *A life apart.* Tavistock, London.

Nirje, B. (1970). The normalization principle – implication and comments. *J. ment. Subnorm.* 16, 62–70.

Royal Commission on the Blind, Deaf and Dumb, etc. of the United Kingdom (1889). Report 5781. HMSO, London.

Royal Commission on the Distribution of Income and Wealth (1978). Report No. 6. Lower incomes. Cmnd. 7175. HMSO, London.

Sainsbury, J. (1970). *Registered as disabled.* Bell, London.

Sanders, D. (1981). The meaning of disability. In *Disability in Britain: a manifesto of rights* (ed. A. Walker and P. Townsend). Robertson, Oxford.

Tomlinson Report (1943). Report of the Interdepartmental Committee on the Rehabilitation and Resettlement of Disabled Persons. Cmnd. 6415. HMSO, London.

Topliss, E. (1979). *Provision for the disabled,* 2nd edn. Blackwell, Oxford.

Townsend, P. (1979). *Poverty in the United Kingdom.* Allen Lane, London.

Walker, A. (1981*a*). Disability rights and progress of the IYDP. In *Disability in Britain: a manifesto of rights* (ed. A. Walker and P. Townsend). Robertson, Oxford.

—— (1981*b*). Disability and income. In *Disability in Britain: a manifesto of rights* (ed. A. Walker and P. Townsend). Robertson, Oxford.

—— (1981*c*). Beyond the International Year of Disabled People. In *Disability in Britain: a manifesto of rights.* Robertson, Oxford.

—— and Townsend, P. (eds.) (1981). *Disability in Britain: a manifesto of rights.* Robertson, Oxford.

Walton, R. G and Elliott, D. (1980). *Residential care: a reader in current theory and practice.* Pergamon, Oxford.

Warnock, M. (1978). *Special education needs.* Cmnd. 7212. HMSO, London.

Weir, S. (1981). Our image of the disabled and how ready we are to help. *New Society* 7–10.

Wilson, J. (1981). The cost of a comprehensive income scheme. In *Disability in Britain: a manifesto of rights* (ed. A. Walker and P. Townsend). Robertson. Oxford.

4 Implications for practice

Theo Schofield

INTRODUCTION

In Chapter 1 Hasler described the size and nature of the problem of providing care for patients with chronic illness. He discussed the advantages of providing this care in general practice, and argued that providing care of a high standard will require changes in attitude, developments in practice organization, and more appropriate medical education both undergraduate and postgraduate. In this chapter we will discuss these necessary changes in more detail.

ATTITUDES

Cartwright and Anderson (1981) found that 50 per cent of doctors did not enjoy their job very much and thought that 50 per cent of their consultations were trivial. They did not explore the nature of these consultations but Pendleton (1981). in an interview study of the factors that could predict both patient and doctor satisfaction after a consultation, found that doctor satisfaction was greatest when the doctor was dealing with new acute physical problems, and that doctors felt less sympathetic and less satisfied the more often they had seen the patient before with the same problem. Patients were also less satisfied by these consultations, and the study demonstrated that the major component of patient satisfaction seemed to be relief and that patients with chronic problems were unlikely to feel relieved, since the problem would not be cured.

These findings are disturbing though not perhaps surprising. Medical students and many junior hospital doctors spend most of their time in departments providing care for acute episodes of illness. They rarely stay in one department long enough to experience the long-term nature of many patients' problems, and discharge can be too easily equated with cure. Such education may not only equip the doctor with inappropriate knowledge and skills, but may also provide him with inappropriate standards and ideas of his role as a doctor.

Pendleton and Schofield (1982) have argued that to maintain motivation, general practitioners need to have clearly defined sense of purpose and standards to which they aspire, and also be receiving feedback on their own performance. In the context of chronic disease this means, for example, aiming for the prevention of the complications of the disease rather than its cure;

aiming to encourage patients to take responsibility for their own illnesses; aiming to minimize the degree of handicap the patients' disabilities cause them, and aiming to help families adjust and adapt to one of their members having a chronic illness. This is not a comprehensive list of aims, and one of our difficulties is to define them in such a way that we can either measure or make judgements about our degrees of success in achieving them. There is ample evidence, however, that if we do not receive appropriate encouragement then our motivation, our performance and the quality of care that we provide, will inevitably decline.

ACCESSIBILITY

In a survey conducted by the Oxford Region Course Organizers and Regional Advisers (1983) 25 patient organizations and 86 community health councils were asked what they considered to be the important features of general practice, and what were the main causes for concern. Fifty per cent were concerned about access to the doctor, either in his surgery or on home visits. Other comments, that are relevant to discussion later in this chapter, were the doctors' ability to communicate effectively, good working relationships between the doctor and other professionals, and the knowledge of services, benefits, and self-help groups available to patients.

Patients with chronic diseases have particular problems with access to their doctor. Many of course will still be in full-time employment, but their illness may make their hold on their job more tenuous, and this may be exacerbated by frequent visits to the doctor during working hours. Getting time off work is also frequently more difficult for hourly paid rather than salaried workers.

Logan *et al.* (1978) showed that provision of specially trained nurses at work to care for exployees with asymptomatic and uncomplicated hypertension significantly improved their blood pressure control. This solution runs the risk of fragmenting patient care. It suggests the probable value of appointment systems that allow patients at work to be seen in the early morning or evening, or at weekends.

Millard, in Chapter 3, points out that patients with chronic diseases are more likely to have problems with mobility and are less likely to be able to afford private or public transport. These difficulties may be alleviated by seeing patients at times when relatives or friends with cars are available to bring them to the surgery; by encouraging and supporting a volunteer driver service or by willingness to visit patients in their own homes. Pereira Gray (1977) reviewed the evidence that there was a steady and progressive downward trend in the number of home visits to patients by their doctors, and argued the case for their value, because of the different quality of the doctor–patient relationship on the patient's home territory, and because of the much wider range of information about patient available in their homes:

The full impact of chronic handicap on patients is best evaluated at home. . . . If we go to see for ourselves what difficulties our patients face, we are often led away from our traditional over-emphasis on drug treatment and find other ways of helping.

CONTINUITY OF CARE

Balint, in his book *The doctor, his patient and the illness* (1957) first described the doctor–patient relationship as a mutual investment company with the general practitioner gradually acquiring valuable capital invested in his patient and vice versa, the patient acquiring a very valuable capital bestowed in his general practitioner. The Second European Conference on the Teaching of General Practice (1974) in their description of the work of the general practitioner, included the *'use of prolonged contact to provide repeated opportunities to gather information at a pace appropriate to each patient, and to build up a relationship of trust which could be used professionally.'* However, despite these declarations of good intent, there is considerable evidence (Aylett 1976; Pereira Gray 1979) that with the changes and developments in group practice organization, patients are less likely to see the same doctor at each consultation in general practice. This not only affects the quality of the doctor–patient relationship, but also the outcome of the consultation. For example, Ettlinger and Freeman (1981) found that personal contact and identification with their doctor predicted the degree to which patients would comply with the treatment that he had prescribed.

RECORDS

Continuity of care does not just mean seeing the same doctor on each occasion. It involves the transfer and accumulation of information from one consultation to the next. This is the essential function of the patient's medical record. Good records will also allow the management of the patient's problems to be reviewed and also assist in communication between partners and other members of the health-care team.

In the past decade, reform of general practitioner records has generated enormous activity both in the literature and in practice. Many new systems have been developed, some based on the existing 7½ × 4 inch medical record envelope, for example the Aldeburgh system (Tait 1977) and others using A4 records, for example, Hawkey *et al.* (1971), Zander *et al.* (1978).

One major stimulus to these changes has been the work of Dr Lawrence Weed who in 1969 described the Problem-Orientated Medical Record system. It was initially designed for use in teaching hospitals but has since been adapted for use in general practice. There are three elements to this system, the data base, problem list, and the continuation record, each of which are relevant to the care of patients with chronic diseases. The data base contains fixed and slowly changing information, including the patient's marital status and occupation. The problem list at its simplest can be a list at the front of the notes or can be subdivided into personal or family history and active and inactive problems. The essential point is, however, that it should contain not only records of precise physical diagnoses, for example, myocardial infarct, but also contain problems such as unexplained chest pain and relevant social and psychological problems, described at the level of their understanding.

The continuation record is structured into:

1. Subjective information obtained from the patient.

2. Objective information obtained by observation, examination, or investigation.

3. An assessment of the patient's problem, which is expressed not as a differential diagnosis, but at the level of understanding of the problem at that time, and includes psychological and social factors.

4. A plan which includes not only the treatment given but also other management; records any investigations planned and most importantly, the information given to the patient in the consultation.

At first sight, this system may appear cumbersome and the adaptability and effort required in practice to sort a patient's records in chronological order, construct problem lists, and alter habits of recording, cannot be under-estimated. On the other hand, it is hard to see how we can provide continuous and comprehensive care for patients, particularly with chronic disease, unless all this information is readily available at each consultation.

Two other features of the medical records of patients with chronic disease deserve discussion.

Flow sheets

For many chronic diseases flow sheets can assist both recording and management and one such card for diabetics is described by Stewart in Chapter 7. These cards have two major advantages. The first is that they can prompt action by the doctor, for example, collecting information, performing examinations or giving explanations at each consultation. Every action does not necessarily take place, however, at every consultation and this can be reflected in the design of the flow chart, which can be divided into (i) the initial phase of diagnosis and intitiation of treatment; (ii) routine regular review; (iii) major review at intervals when some of the base-line procedures may be repeated.

The second advantage of flow charts is that they can set targets, for example, blood pressure or diabetic control, and the pattern of care and the degree of achievement of these targets can be seen more readily, if the information is presented in chart form.

Repeat prescription records

Many patients with chronic diseases are receiving regular prescriptions and the extent of repeat prescribing in practice has recently been reviewed by Drury

(1982). Bolden (1980) identified seven factors that were considered important in the design of a repeat prescription system.

1. It should enable any patient requiring repeat medication to obtain a prescription within 24 hours of requesting it.
2. Prescriptions should be prepared with meticulous accuracy without errors.
3. There should be a built-in recall system which is clear to patients and staff.
4. It should be apparent to any doctor using the medical records what drugs the patient is currently taking and when they obtained the last supply.
5. The system should be designed to be as simple and cheap as possible.
6. The system should enable a doctor to audit his or her repeat prescribing in the practice.
7. It should be possible to check a patient's request for repeat medication against their supplies and their compliance.

Three methods of organizing repeat prescriptions have been advocated. The commonest is the repeat prescription card held by the patient. The major defect of this system is that the card may not be available when changes in medication are made at a consultation and this discrepancy would not become apparent unless the repeat prescription is checked against the patient's record on every occasion. They are also not available to the practice for audit. They can, however, be used to give the information to the patient, but to do this they need to include space for such information as intended action and possible side-effects of each drug, the time of day they should be taken, and what to do if doses are accidently omitted.

Some practices use a repeat prescription register which is checked each time a patient requests a repeat prescription. This has the advantage that it can be used as a method of patient review and repeat prescribing audit, but again, the information may not be available or be updated at each consultation.

The third system which may be used in combination with the other two is a regular prescription record in the patient's notes. It usually lists the drug given, the dose, quantity to be prescribed, the recall interval and a record of each repeat prescription. It can also be designed to include drug hypersensitivities and adverse reactions. As long as it is updated when changes are made or repeat prescriptions given, this system comes closest to meeting Bolden's objectives, particularly if there is also some system for the purpose of audit of identifying those patients who are receiving repeat prescriptions.

DISEASE REGISTERS

Repeat prescribing is only one facet of the management of patients with chronic illnesses that we may wish to review, and this is one of the reasons for keeping a register of these patients in the practice. Other advantages are to provide information for planning services. (For example, if we wished to have a diabetic clinic, how many patients would be involved?) and also to be able to offer groups of patients specific services (for example, influenza vaccine for patients with chronic heart and chest disease and diabetes.)

The first essential step for any practice contemplating setting up a disease register is to decide which diseases they wish to include in the register and the purposes for which they intend to use the information. Having decided which patients must be included, the next step is to identify them. This can be done from memory, which is unreliable, from repeat prescriptions which excludes patients who are no longer receiving treatment, or from consultations which excludes those patients who are no longer being seen. A more laborious, but more reliable method is to review all the patients' records, perhaps at the time when they are being summarized.

We have found that the number of patients with certain chronic diseases that were identified by reviewing all 8000 patient records in the practice (Harris and Schofield, unpublished data; Table 4.1) significantly exceeded the number of patients that were expected to be found using the rates in the Second National Morbidity Survey (1974) which collected its data at the time of each consultation. These results were not due to differences in the age, sex, or social class make-up of the practice and suggested that a proportion of patients with chronic disease were not receiving continuing care in general practice. Examination of our records confirmed this hypothesis.

The register may be kept in a variety of formats, the choice of which depends particularly on the uses to which the information is likely to be put. The simplest format is a list of patients' names under each disease kept either in a loose-leaf folder or on cards. This list can then be used to identify the patients' records from which further information can be obtained. Additional information can be included on the card. If, for example, the practice intends inviting patients with diabetes to a diabetic clinic, or to have influenza vaccine, including the patient's address means that the register can be used without the records; while if the practice intends to use the register for audit, entering the patient's date of birth or date of diagnosis may be helpful. If the practice already has an age/sex register, one format that overcomes some of these difficulties is to attach coloured tags to the tops of the cards of patients with particular diseases.

A disease register not only needs to be created, it also needs to be maintained. The practice needs to ensure that new diagnoses made either by the general practitioner or in hospital are entered on to the register, and that when the patient leaves the practice or changes adress, the details of the register are altered. It therefore needs to be clear in the patient's records that their name is also contained in the disease register. Using the age/sex register as the basis for the disease register eliminates this difficulty.

Maintaining the practice registers and some items of information from the patient's records on a microcomputer has substantial advantages in the field of chronic disease. There can be automatic linkage between the practice register

Table 4.1. *Comparison of record-based and consultation-based morbidity data in selected diagnostic groups*

	Review of 8000 practice records*		Second National Morbidity Study 1970–71†
	No. of recorded patients	Recorded patients/ 1000 patients on list	Recorded patients/ 1000 patients on list
Myxoedema	32	3.9	1.0
Diabetes mellitus	107	13.0	4.5
Gout	68	8.3	1.6
Pernicious anaemia	13	1.6	1.4
Schizophrenia	28	3.4	1.4
Epilepsy	104	12.7	2.9
Glaucoma	24	2.9	0.9
Hypertension	302	36.8	19.1
Chronic bronchitis	146	17.8	11.5
Asthma	144	17.6	10.2
Rheumatoid arthritis	62	7.6	5.0
Osteoarthritis	130	15.9	18.2

*Harris, G. and Schofield, T. P. C. Unpublished data.
†Office of Population Censuses and Surveys (1974).

and the disease register; much more information can be readily stored and analysed, for example, the date and reading of the most recent blood pressure; and a wide variety of outputs can be produced, for example lists of patients due or overdue for recall; word-processed letters addressed to the patients with adhesive labels to address the envelopes; and analyses of follow-up and control for audit.

RECALL SYSTEMS

One response to the problem, variously described as non-compliance, non-adherence, or default, is to set up a recall system whereby patients who do not attend when expected can be identified and sent reminders or requests to attend. This is particularly relevant in conditions which are asymptomatic, for example, hypertension, or those that may be insidious in onset, for example pernicious anaemia following gastrectomy; or those that by their very nature make patients less able to attend, for example, chronic schizophrenia or myxoedema. Some doctors may reject this approach as being too paternalistic, a view with which Ivan Illich (1982) would concur, but on the other hand it can be seen as consistent with our responsibility to provide all necessary medical services for a defined list of patients.

PATIENT EDUCATION

The same dilemma also applies to our approach to patient education. The terms 'communication' and 'education' are frequently used interchangeably and indiscriminately and much health education, which is properly the promotion of understanding and the facilitation of choice, is in fact health persuasion which, has as its goal, not informed choice, but a particular behaviour or set of behaviours which are considered to be in some way desirable by the persuader. The slogan 'Look after yourself' may in fact mean 'Doctor yourself', which as Illich (1982) remarked is the ultimate slogan in a medicalized world.

There is, on the other hand, considerable evidence (Cartwright and Anderson 1981; Oxford Region Course Organizers and Regional Advisers 1983) that patients are critical about the amount of information they are given by their doctor, not only about the disease and its management, but also about other services, benefits, and self-help groups available to them.

How then should general practice respond? Pendleton *et al.* (1983) have argued that each consultation is part of a cycle of care and that the patients' understanding of their problem is not only a major determinant of whether and how they present their problem, but is also a major factor in the consultation's outcomes. They have included exploring the patients' own ideas and concerns about their problem, sharing the doctor's understanding with the patient, and involving the patient in the management and essential tasks for each consultation. Tones (1982) went beyond the consultation and described the way the doctor and the health care team can develop a co-ordinated approach to health education. This would involve the identification of groups of patients either with chronic diseases or at special risk, choosing relevant educational objectives and then selecting appropriate members of the team and educational methods to achieve them. For example, patients with diabetes might receive information about their disease from their doctor; help with self-monitoring from the practice nurse; dietary advice from the dietician, and explore their own and their families' attitudes to the disease in a group discussion resourced by the health visitor. These activities could also be co-ordinated with the facilities of the British Diabetic Association which is one example of the many self-help groups available for patients with chronic diseases. The objectives of this educational method would be not only to help patients understand their disease more fully and be more involved in their own management, but also to make more appropriate and perhaps fuller use of all the facilities available, including even their own doctor.

One form of patient education which is particularly relevant to a number of the chronic diseases discussed later in this book is the ability to persuade patients to give up smoking. This is discussed more fully by Fowler (1982). Effective persuasion depends on working with the patient's own health beliefs. The health belief model described by Becker *et al.* (1974) describes five elements of these beliefs:

1. People vary in their overall interest in health and their motivation to look after it. This element has been called 'health motivation'.

2. With reference to any specific problem patients vary in how likely they

think they are to contract it. This element has been called 'perceived vulner-ability'.

3. Patients vary in how dire they believe the consequences of contracting a particular illness would be, or of leaving it untreated. The term 'perceived seriousness' describes this belief.

4. Patients weigh up the advantages and disadvantages of taking any particular course of action: the element of 'perceived costs and benefits'.

5. These beliefs do not exist ready formed for all possible problems. They are prompted or aroused by a variety of so-called 'cues for action', such as a new symptom, a television programme, or a visit to the doctor.

In the case of smoking therefore it is necessary for the doctor to explore the patient's motivation to stop: their ideas about the possible consequences, and whether it might ever happen to them; the difficulties that the patient might have in stopping, but also its possible benefits; and whether there is any particular reason, for example, a recent chest infection, for the patient to decide now to give up smoking. The effectiveness of this advice has been shown to be reinforced by giving the patient the 'give up smoking' leaflet published by the Health Education Council which is also based on the same health belief and behavioural principles (Russell *et al.* 1979).

THE HEALTH CARE TEAM

Health education is only one example of the contribution that all the members of the health care team can make to the care of patients with chronic disease. The value and organization of the health care team in primary care has been fully reviewed by Marsh and Kaim-Caudle (1976) and Pritchard (1978). Pritchard has more recently (1979) argued that the health care team functions in two distinct ways. The first is the patient-centred microteam which includes any professional helpers involved in caring for a particular patient; it also includes the patients themselves and the patients' own supporters such as their spouse or their daughter. The second is a management-orientated macroteam concerned with developing policies and services within the practice. The patients' input into this team may be provided by a patient participation group. Both types of team also have the important function of providing support for individual members of the team.

Apart from a willingness to provide this support when required, we as general practitioners should have a knowledge of, and a respect for, the skills and pro-fessionalism of the other members of the team. We should be able to refer patients appropriately, but continue to maintain our own relationship with our patients and be able to continue to collaborate in the best interests of our patients. There may be occasions when we are not involved in the microteam, but we are frequently required to at least co-ordinate the management team, which requires us to develop skills in communication, teamwork, and management.

SPECIAL CLINICS

Stewart in Chapter 7 has described the setting up and organization of a special clinic for patients with diabetes in general practice. One disadvantage of asking all patients to attend at a set time is that it may make the problem of access that have already been discussed more difficult. However, the advantages in the improved patient care and a more efficient use of the practice team are impressive. This has been confirmed by a recent published report from Glyncorrwg Health Centre by Wojciechowski (1982).

PERFORMANCE REVIEW

To be able to maintain both motivation and performance, it is essential that general practitioners, and indeed all professionals, are able to obtain feedback on their work. The commonest source of this feedback is from their own patients, but patients have a need to believe in their doctors. They get used to their doctor's usual ways of working and see only a limited range of alternative style, and fear that criticism will decrease their doctor's motivation to help. They believe (like many doctors) that patients should not question doctors' decisions. Paradoxically, some patient satisfaction may be brought about by factors which may be harmful to the patient's health, for example, repeat prescribing and the creation of doctor dependence.

Where then is our feedback to come from, and by whose standards should we be judged? Three aspects of medical audit have been described (Donabedian 1966); the structure which refers to the setting in which care is provided and the resources available; the process which describes the methods by which decisions are made and actions taken; and outcome which refers to the achievements of care. It is beyond the scope of this chapter to describe the development of audit or performance review in general practice and it has been reviewed fully by Mourin (1976) and Stevens (1977). A further method of performance review looking at a doctor's actual work in practice has recently been proposed (Royal College of General Practitioners 1981) but it is fair to say that none of these methods has been widely accepted and practised. Freeling and Burton (1982) for example, had an average of attendance at an audit group of 14 general practitioners out of the original 350 who were invited.

The answer to these questions must be that the setting of standards and the review of performance should be undertaken by general practitioners themselves and the development of acceptable and effective methods remains one of the most urgent tasks facing general practice.

CONCLUSIONS

In Chapter 3, Millard quoted the Working Party of the Central Council for Education and Training in Social Work, in saying that good professional practice for handicapped persons should be broad, detailed, assertive, and collaborative. The same criteria must apply to the care that we as general practitioners provide for all our patients with chronic illnesses, and in this Chapter I have described some of the major changes in attitudes, education, and organization that will be required if we wish to achieve these aims in practice.

REFERENCES

Aylett, M. J. (1976). Seeing the same doctor. *Jl R. Coll. gen. Practrs* 26, 47–52.

Balint, M. (1957). *The doctor, his patient and the illness.* Tavistock, London.

Becker, M. H. (1974). The health belief model and personal health behaviour. *Hlth Educat. Monogr.* 2, 236.

Bolden, K. J. (1980). Repeat prescription system. *Jl R. Coll. gen. Practrs* 30, 378.

Cartwright, A. and Anderson, R. (1981). *General practice re-visited.* Tavistock, London.

Donabedian, A. (1966). Evaluating the quality of medical car. *Hillbank Mem. Fund Q.* 44, 166–206.

Drury, V. W. M. (1982). Repeat prescribing. A review. *Jl R. Coll. gen. Practrs* 32, 42–5.

Ettlinger, P. R. A. and Freeman, G. K. (1981). General practice compliance study: is it worth being a personal doctor? *Br. med. J.* 282, 1192–4.

Freeling, P. and Burton, R. H. (1982). General practitioners and learning by audit. *Jl R. Coll. gen. Practrs* 32, 231–8.

Fowler, G. (1982). Smoking in *Preventive medicine in general practice* (ed. M. Gray and G. H. Fowler) pp. 133–48. Oxford University Press.

Hawkey, J. K., Louden, I. S. L., Greenhalgh, G. P., and Bungay, G. T. (1971). New record folder for use in general practice. *Br. med. J.* 4, 667–70.

Illich, I. (1982). Medicalization and primary care. *Jl R. Coll. gen. Practrs* 32, 463–70.

Leewenhorst Working Party (1977). Statement by a Working Party Appointed by the Second European Conference on the Teaching of General Practice 1974. *Jl R. Coll. gen. Practrs* 27, 117.

Logan, A. G., Campbell, N. P., Milne, R. J., Achber, C. and Haynes, R. B. (1978). Usefulness and feasability of treating hypertension at the worksite using specially trained nurses. In *Abstracts of the 5th Scientific Meeting of the International Society of Hypertension,* Paris 12–14 June. Congrès-Services, Paris.

Marsh, G. and Kairn-Caudle, P. (1976). *Team care in general practice.* Croom Helm, London.

Mourin, K. (1976). Auditing and evaluation in general practice. *Jl R. Coll gen. Practrs* 26, 726–33.

Office of Population Censuses and Surveys (1974). *Morbidity statistics from general practice. Second National Study 1970–71.* HMSO, London.

Oxford Region Course Organizers and Regional Advisers Group (1984). *Priority objectives for vocational training.* In preparation.

Pendleton, D. A. (1982). Doctor/patient communication. D.Phil. thesis, University of Oxford.

—— (1983). Doctor/patient communication: A review. In *Doctor patient communication* (ed. D. A. Pendleton and J. C. Hasler). Academic Press, London.

—— and Schofield, T. P. C. (1983). Motivation and performance in general practice: *The Medical Annual*. Wright, Bristol.

Pereira Gray, P. J. (1978). Feeling at home. *Jl R. Coll. gen Practrs* **28**, 6–17.

—— (1979). The key to personal care. *Jl R. Coll. gen. Practrs* **29**, 666–78.

Pritchard, P. (1978). *Manual of primary health care*. Oxford University Press.

—— (1979). The development of team working in primary health care.

Royal College of General Practitioners (1981). *What sort of doctor?* RCGP, London.

Russell, M. A. H., Wilson, C., Taylor, C., and Baker, C. P. (1979). Effect of general practitioners advice against smoking. *Br. med. J.* **ii**, 231.

Stevens, J. L. (1977). Quality of care in general practice. *Jl. R. Coll. gen. Practrs* **27**, 455–66.

Tait, I. (1977). The clinical record on British general practice. *Br. med. J.* **ii**, 683–8.

Tones, K. (1982). *Beyond the consultation: the health education role of the primary health care team*. MSD Foundation, London.

Wojciewchowski, M. T. (1982). Systematic care of diabetic patients in a general practice. *Jl R. Coll. gen. Practrs* **32**, 531–4.

Zander, L. I., Beresford, S. A. A., and Thomas, P. (1978). *Medical records in general practice*. Occasional Paper 5. RCGP, London.

Part II

A number of important chronic diseases are considered in this part. At the end of each chapter is included a Performance Review Check list, to suggest to general practitioners criteria they might like to use in carrying out audits in their own practices. There is also a list, where appropriate, of important Patient Organizations and literature for patients.

5 Asthma

Ian Lister Cheese

INTRODUCTION

This account of the care of patients with asthma is biased towards those practical aspects which are important if effective care is to be achieved in general practice. It is a personal account reflecting the style, beliefs, and experience of one family doctor. But it owes much to discussion with colleagues in the Oxford Region, in hospital and in general practice, and to authoritative writings which have been freely tapped to draw the current paradigm. Most influential among the latter are those from the Cardiothoracic Institute and Brompton Hospital, London. The experience owes most to patients and often to their parents. They have done their part not just willingly but with enthusiasm and responsibility. Without these the approach described could not work. Except where they aid clinical understanding details of physiology, pathology, and immunology have been given scanty attention and biochemistry and neurology have not been considered at all. Although of fundamental importance and great interest they are actually of little practical concern to the family doctor. Not considered either are the fascinating but poorly understood influences of the non-physical environment. Rarely is it possible to assess or manipulate such factors although the opportunity may be given to observe them.

Long-term care of the asthmatic by a family doctor may derive initially from knowledge of the family constitution and dispositions, knowledge which allows a unique advantage, that of predictive awareness. Then follows diagnosis of asthma, its assessment and individual treatment all made more sure by the use of dependable physiological measurements. Lastly, by thoughtful tutorship, day-to-day and long-term management is devolved securely to the patient himself, aided in a child by his parents.

The foundations of this method, the means of its application and the requirements of a doctor and his practice to achieve it are the central matter of this chapter.

In asthma there are effective and safe treatments and ways to discover who might benefit from them. There are well-tried methods for appraising the clinical state and its fluctuations and there is fairly common agreement on the proper responses to make when asthma worsens.

THE IMPACT OF ASTHMA

At one time the impact of asthma on a patient and his family discouraged use of the term unless it was unavoidable, hence the gentler evasive terms 'wheezy bronchitis' or just 'wheeziness'. These terms are still used, both as the legacy of an obsolete reticence and also because wheeziness in very young children is commonly believed not to hold the same significance as asthma. This belief is justified only in the first years of life. After three years it is very often wrong and proper treatment thereby denied. 'Not all that wheezes in childhood is asthma' is true but in practice much of it is or will be.

Until about 15 years ago the severely asthmatic child was different from his peers. He was smaller, he did not play games, he was 'delicate'. Even before modern treatments this unhappy caricature of the childhood asthmatic must have been uncommon because the severely asthmatic child requiring intensive treatment is rare today. But that image is still recalled by parents and reinforced by some doctors.

Despite great advances asthma remains troublesome and is a cause of much disruption of life. At best there is the unmeasurable burden of intermittent treatment. At worst, fortunately in only a few, there is imperfect control of symptoms, repeated threats of severe asthma, and the drawbacks of systemic steroid therapy.

Childhood asthma inhibits participation in games and is the commonest cause of absence from school, accounting for nearly 30 per cent. The effect on educational, social, and physical attainment can be surmised.

The parents of an asthmatic child often suffer repeated interruptions of sleep besides the anxieties provoked by chronic illness. The effects of the disease on family and personal lives are a private burden only occasionally admitted as the counterpart of the child's illness.

Patients and their parents are, or ask to be, or should be, well-informed. They know that asthma runs in families and often are aware of collusion with sensitive skin. Their beliefs are readily shared with the doctor. It seems to the writer that they attribute too much significance to allergy and emotion as 'causes' of asthma but they recognize the association with infection (or upper respiratory symptoms which may simulate infection and which may have the same essential origin as asthma). It is obvious to all that asthma is a condition which may last for years and a plan of management leading to self-care requires an extended dialogue. This should clarify patient's beliefs, rectify faulty ones, and by description and explanation appropriate to the patient and a commitment to responsive support, permit confidence, and an independent near normal life for the patient and his family.

Consultations might naturally assume a tutorial form in which the allotment of time is substantial (in a moderately severe asthmatic 1–1 ½ hours spread over 6–12 weeks) but as acceptable management is achieved the frequency of consultations falls. In succeeding years this initial investment is amply repaid. It is an investment too for other partners in the practice because its successful outcome greatly diminishes out-of-hours and emergency calls.

DEFINITION OF ASTHMA

The historical recognition of asthma is of episodic wheezy breathlessness, a description now superseded by clinical definitions which require evidence of wide variability of expiratory air-flow, either spontaneously or in response to external influences among which are included particular treatments.

A recent definition by Scadding expressed in functional terms is succint: 'asthma is a disease characterized by wide variations over short periods of time in resistance to flow in intrapulmonary airways'.

A definition should not exclude a small but important group of patients whose air-flow is diminished and apparently fixed, changing in some, but not all, only when corticosteroids are administered. This may represent a stage in the disease earlier manifested in more typical ways.

Lately has grown the concept of an inherent disposition to variable bronchial hyper-activity to numerous and external stimuli. From this concept new definitions may eventually be derived.

PHYSIOLOGY OF ASTHMA AND MEASUREMENT OF RESPIRATORY FUNCTION

In asthma the airways narrow and on expiration tend increasingly to close. This may be countered to a degree by expiration from an increased lung volume which increases the distending pressure of airways and opposes their closure. Among changes observed in lung function tests are, therefore, those of expiratory obstruction, reduced peak expiratory flow (PEF), and forced expiratory volume in the first second (FEV_1) and increased residual volume (RV). Vital capacity (VC) is reduced proportionally less than FEV_1 so FEV_1/VC is diminished. An increase in total lung capacity (TLC) is not always seen because it reflects the net change in VC and RV.

With worsening asthma tidal volumes fall. To maintain ventilation the respiratory rate increases and with it the work of breathing and of the heart.

When less than 70 per cent of VC remains to be expired expiratory flow does not increase continuously with increasing alveolar pressure, that is the pressure generated in expiration; it levels out. This defines the maximum expiratory flow at a given residue of vital capacity, and above a certain level of effort it becomes independent of effort. When more than 70 per cent of VC remains, expiratory flow is effort dependent, but tests of maximum flow still yield consistent results, arguing that subjects do in fact exert maximum force.

Tests of forced expiratory flow are conveniently represented using the maximum expiratory flow/volume relationship. Air-flow and lung volume changes are measured continuously during forced expiration (Fig. 5.1).

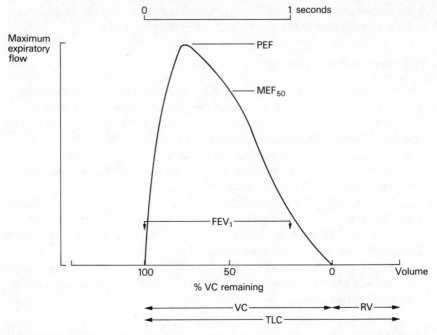

Fig. 5.1. Respiratory function tests and the maximum expiratory flow–volume curve.

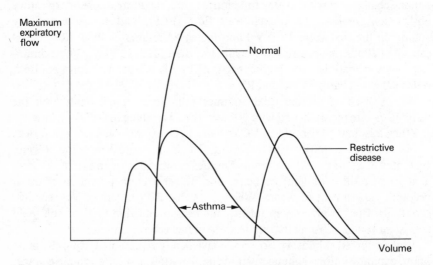

Fig. 5.2. Respiratory disease and the maximum expiratory flow–volume curve.

Expiratory flow is reduced in other conditions (Fig. 5.2) but not with the variability peculiar to asthma.

The determination by spirometry of FEV_1 and VC and their ratio allows a fuller assessment but in practice one wishes to discover the possibilities of effective treatment and only rarely is this helped by more subtle tests.

The common tests of respiratory function are summarized in Table 5.1. It is clear that measurement of peak flow is uniquely suited to the day-to-day management of reversible airways obstruction. Other techniques, whatever their usefulness and importance, really do not meet this practical requirement.

PEF is thought to represent flow in proximal airways (of more than 2 mm diameter) where even large changes may be asymptomatic. Conversely changes in smaller airways, even if producing symptoms, may not be detected by measurements of PEF.

It is likely that hyperinflation with increased RV is more closely related to obstruction of smaller airways, its symptoms being inspiratory dyspnoea and a sense of tightness. Thus it may be found that both topical steroids and bronchodilators in those with airways obstruction may produce marked symptomatic benefit without improvement in PEF but with increased VC and reduced RV.

Despite these limitations to the usefulness of PEF measurements, fluctuating or progressively worsening levels do confirm the presence of pathological changes throughout the bronchial tree.

Frequently during the early stages of worsening asthma, marked symptoms are absent until PEF is reduced to 50–60 per cent normal. Thus useful premonitory changes in PEF are often seen before symptomatic changes and measurement is extremely helpful down to unrecordable levels.

PATHOLOGY OF ASTHMA

The most obvious pathological features are recurrent excessive contraction of bronchial smooth muscle, oedema of bronchial mucosa, and secretion of viscid mucus.

The first usually resolves spontaneously or with treatment but it is likely that in many patients mucosal and exudative changes persistently obstruct small airways (of less than 2mm diameter) although their effects are detectable only by elaborate tests.

Less obvious but important in severe asthma and detectable even after symptomatic recovery are changes in the distribution of ventilation which without compensatory redistribution of perfusion results in hypoxaemia. Hyperventilation cannot fully redress the imbalance although it does initially produce a fall in arterial P_{CO_2}.

AETIOLOGY OF ASTHMA

It is common knowledge that asthma runs in families. In 50–75 per cent of children with asthma there is a family history of the disease or other manifes-

Table 5.1. *Some tests of pulmonary function*

Measurement		Method	Notes

Peak expiratory flow	(PEF)	Mini-Wright peak flow gauge
		Wright peak flow meter
			Instrument simple, cheap, portable, robust
			Useful throughout clinically important range
			Except
			    (i) in severe asthma (PEF <1 l/s)
			    (ii) in young children
			    (iii) in frail subjects
			Detects presymptomatic change
			Easily used by patients aged 5–85 +
			Frequent measurements possible
			Manoeuvre may worsen bronchoconstriction
			    (but heighten test sensitivity)

Forced expiratory volume in first second	(FEV$_1$)	Spirometer	As above Instrument expensive, not portable* Useful until PEF< 0.5 l/s May be related to vital capacity
Vital capacity	(VC)	Spirometer	A fundamental measure of lung function Influences maximum expiratory flow
Total lung capacity and Residual volume	(TLC) (RV)	Plethysmograph Gas dilution Gas wash-out	Specialized time-consuming laboratory techniques
Maximum expiratory flow – lung volume		Pneumotachograph and spirometer or plethysmograph, etc.	Specialized laboratory technique Gives much information on lung dynamics

*There are now miniature devices, although costly.

tation of hyper-irritability such as eczema, episodic rhinitis, or hay fever. This state of hyper-irritability is often called, perhaps with too narrow a view, hypersensitivity.

The association occurs also in patients. Thus 50 per cent of atopic infants have asthma or rhinitis, 5 per cent of those with hay fever have asthma, and 40 per cent of children with asthma have eczema.

In one study comparing first-degree relatives of asthmatic patients with those of controls the likelihood of the former developing asthma before the age of 50 was 18 per cent, of the latter only 1.3 per cent.

In homozygous twins concordance for asthma, although not complete, is much higher than in dizygotic twins where it is similar to that between other siblings. This suggests that an hereditary element disposes to a particular kind of response to external influences.

In recent years has evolved the concept of an inherited disposition to variable bronchial hyper-reactivity in response to certain factors. The expression of the asthmatic disposition is contingent on events in the physical and social environment and modified by events which seem intrinsic (Table 5.2). Some at least of these are related to the passing of time, body-time, in which the most obvious variation is diurnal. It has been demonstrated that this depends on the individual's daily rhythm rather than solar time, and is related to sleep. The rhythmical change is normally present but in may asthmatic subjects is much exaggerated. Subclinical worsening of asthma has been shown in some to occur in REM sleep. Asthma may also worsen, usually subclinically, in the premenstrual phase.

Certain factors are well known and often demonstrable, others are less easy

Table 5.2. *Factors which may provoke asthma*

(i) Infection: most commonly viral respiratory infections
(ii) Exercise: of particular kinds, intensity, and duration
(iii) Allergens
    Domestic
        Natural: ubiquitous, especially house-dust mite, pollens,
            moulds, feathers, furs, dander. Some foods
        Artificial: several drugs and chemicals (e.g. tartrazine)
    Occupational
        Possibly causal in 2% of asthmatics but very important in
        certain industries
(iv) Irritants: dust, mechanical stimuli, cigarette smoke, cold air,
            humidity change, chemicals (e.g. sulphur dioxide in
            drinks: by inhalation)
(v) Specific drugs: β-antagonists, non-steroidal anti-inflammatory drugs,
            especially aspirin
(vi) Hyperventilation: including sustained laughter but uncommon
(vii) Intrinsic
        (a) Central neurological: often, but not always, regular
            and predictable
        (b) 'Psychological': usually unpredictable

---

to identify. Fortunately effective treatment does not always depend upon this identification but in some instances, for example in the recognition of occupational asthma or of asthma due to particular kinds of exercises but not others it may be of great importance.

The nature of the asthmatic disposition is not known, neither is the mode of its inheritance, but some mechanisms of its expression have been revealed. At the investigative level there is knowledge of the biochemical events within bronchial smooth muscle and epithelial cells and of the humoral, cellular, and neurological influences upon them, although of central neurological processes virtually nothing is known.

THE ONSET OF ASTHMA

Asthma may begin at any age. The onset is most commonly in childhood and early adult life but there is no age at which it may not appear for the first time.

PREVALENCE OF ASTHMA

Numerous epidemiological studies testify to the difficulty in making a diagnosis without vigorous, albeit simple, measurements. Surveys of prevalence in diverse communities produce widely different results. Nevertheless with notable exceptions a consistent tendency emerges. The prevalence of asthma in Britain in 1.5–5.1 per cent in children and 2–5.4 per cent in older subjects.

Because small airways are more readily obstructed by secretions, wheeziness is common in infants and does not necessarily indicate bronchial hyper-reactivity. But it still has prognostic value (Table 5.3).

Table 5.3. *Wheeziness in infancy: prognostic significance*

Age (years)	Wheeziness (%)	Subsequent asthma (%)
0–1	50	3–7
1–3	30	18
3+	10	42

From Clark and Godfrey (1977).

Of course the likely prognosis is influenced by dispositions which may already have been recognized. In one study involving the follow-up of eleven-year-old children 3.5 per cent were thought to be asthmatic and 8.8 per cent in addition had wheezy bronchitis. Such figures describe a cumulative prevalence. In the previous twelve months 2 per cent of these children had experienced asthma and 2.9 per cent wheezy bronchitis. This is a period prevalence. These statements beg the question, of course, of how one distinguishes between the two conditions, if indeed they are different. In adults the epidemiological problems are compounded by the additional respiratory diseases of later life, chronic bronchitis and emphysema.

Asthma is the commonest major chronic disorder of childhood but its prevalence is much the same at all ages, about 5 per cent. It need be acknowledged only that the disorder is very common. There will be about 100 asthmatic patients in a practice of 2000. If its recognition is uncertain in epidemiological studies, asthma is without doubt missed in some patients and although a less likely error it may be wrongly diagnosed in others. The writer's experience is that it is commonly undiagnosed at all ages and least likely to be recognized in the elderly when wheeziness is less often a symptom than breathlessness and other plausible but inadequate diagnoses are made.

PROGNOSIS IN ASTHMA

Most asthmatic children, 70–80 per cent, have mild asthma with infrequent attacks and long remissions. A minority whose asthma is more frequent and of longer duration tend to be boys with more severe infantile eczema an earlier onset of asthma and a close family history of asthma.

Numerous studies from which the following conclusions are taken show that most children improve:

1. Bronchial reactivity diminishes in most through the ages of 7 to 14 to 21 years.

2. 65 per cent have less severe attacks at the age of 14 years than at 10.

3. 70–90 per cent have stopped attacks by 10 years of age.

4. 80 per cent have stopped by puberty.

5. 68–89 per cent of mild asthmatics have not wheezed after the age of 10 years but of more severe asthmatics all wheezed after 10.

6. In hospital clinics the numbers requiring continuous therapy or follow-up fall.

7. Of children with an onset of asthma before aged 13 years, 71 per cent are free of asthma by 20.

On the other hand long-term studies deny the optimism implied. Of asthmatic children reviewed after 20 years only half were quite well. Half of the remainder had recurrent or established asthma and the rest had symptoms including those of hay fever.

Death is rare in asthma although in England and Wales 45 children and a total of 1500 patients die each year. Many authorities believe that with better care fewer would die.

Much commoner is acute severe asthma which is usually the state in which worsening asthma fails to respond to normally adequate doses of bronchodilators properly delivered. Even children with mild asthma are not spared acute severe asthma, but it is much more likely to occur in the minority of children whose asthma is unremitting or in whom episodes are frequent.

In adults there is less likelihood of spontaneous cure. Fewer are helped by sodium cromoglycate and most of the elderly are found to require topical corticosteroids.

Although chronic bronchitis and emphysema (chronic 'irreversible' obstructive airways disease) occur with asthma it is not known if the disorders are causally related, nor is it known whether modern treatments of asthma have had any influence upon these other disorders.

There have been great advances in the treatment of asthma but perversely they have had no influence overall on mortality. Admissions to hospital for asthma have increased and this is due partly to self-referral systems which are actually used by patients with less severe asthma on admission.

Undoubtedly some patients present with devastatingly severe asthma of sudden onset. Most do not. Given the effective treatments now available there have been numerous inquiries into the management of patients admitted with acute severe asthma. These inquiries repeatedly conclude that many episodes of acute severe asthma occur in patients who are wrongly diagnosed, inadequately treated, imperfectly tutored, or in whom the severity of the clinical state is not recognized. It is difficult to refute such conclusions.

If these life-threatening, alarming and wasteful episodes are to be prevented the task is clearly that of the family doctor. There are now available knowledge and methods to make it possible but there are also common difficulties such as the inability of many patients to perceive worsening asthma, failure of compliance, and the occasional fulminant nature of some attacks.

CLINICAL FEATURES

Episodic wheeziness accompanied or not by shortness of breath or cough should always alert the doctor to the possibility of asthma. Wheeze may be absent and this is true at any age. In children recurrent cough, especially at night, is a common presentation frequently misdiagnosed as 'bronchitis'. Not every child with recurrent cough has asthma, however. Cough, dyspnoea, and wheeze after exercise are often not mentioned. Very young children simply do not exercise in spells long enough to produce symptoms and in schoolchildren where they do occur they often pass before being noticed by an adult as significant.

The episodic nature of the disorder with symptoms occurring particularly at night may be elicited only on persistent enquiry. Unless nocturnal symptoms are sought a crucial feature may be overlooked. This is especially likely in a subject who seems perfectly well in the daytime even to the extent of having normal simple lung function tests. The episodic pattern may be seasonal and besides asthma earlier bouts of hay fever or rhinitis may be recalled.

Dyspnoea alone or paroxysmal nocturnal dyspnoea are insufficiently well known as features of asthma and incidental findings of hypertension or cardiac disease may lead to a wrong or incomplete diagnosis and occasionally to disastrous treatment.

The family history, or in ideal general practice an intimate knowledge of the family, may give essential pointers. This is true also of the elderly where even more information is to be gained from the succeeding generations. There are instances when adults will deny the possibility of asthma especially if it has never occurred previously and there is no earlier family history.

EXERCISE-INDUCED ASTHMA (EIA)

A notable characteristic of asthma is marked increase in airways obstruction after exercise, although sometimes evident before exercise ceases. Initially, as in normal subjects, a small unsustained decrease in obstructon due to sympathotonic effeçts is seen.

The phenomenon is important because (i) it is a cause of impaired exercise tolerance; (ii) it provides a diagnostic test; (iii) it allows standardized measurements of bronchial reactivity in research studies; (iv) it supplies an approximate guide to treatment.

Among healthy children 92 per cent show a post-exercise fall in PEF of less than 10 per cent and 98 per cent of less than 15 per cent, but 33 per cent show none. If a child has a fall in PEF of more than 10 per cent he probably has asthma, of more than 15 per cent then almost certainly; but a fall of less than 10 per cent does not exclude asthma. 80 per cent of asthmatics have a fall of more than 10 per cent. On further testing the figure rises to 91 per cent.

EIA has been valuable in research. For example it has been used to demonstrate variable bronchial reactivity in the asymptomatic relations of asthmatics, identical twins, wheezy babies, and relations of wheezy babies. It reveals that the disposition is quantitative not qualitative.

In one standard test the patient runs for 6–8 minutes to breathlessness and a pulse rate of up to 180/min in children and 150/min in adults (which is not always possible in the unfit). PEF is measured before and at intervals during and after exercise for 10–20 minutes.

EIA is an approximate guide to treatment in that the fall in PEF tends to be greater in more severely affected patients. EIA is prevented by prior administration of sodium cromoglycate or bronchodilator but reversed only by the latter.

There is good evidence that the major stimulus for EIA is heat loss from bronchial mucosa precipitated by the hyperpnoea of exercise and increased by reduction of temperature and water content of inspired air.

DIAGNOSIS AND ASSESSMENT OF ASTHMA

The history and clinical features will often place the diagnosis of asthma beyond doubt. In other instances it may be no more than a strong suspicion and in a few there may be persistent uncertainty. A measured assessment of airways function is then required. The range of variation in airways flow is continuous, little being demonstrable in normal subjects, more in those related

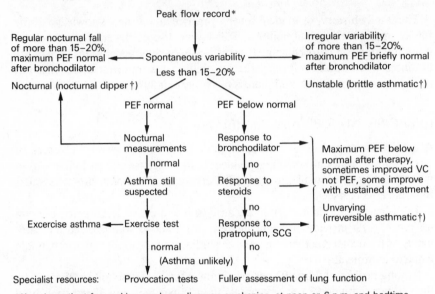

Fig. 5.3. Diagnosis of asthma. Determination of the pattern of variability.

* Kept by patient for working week: readings on awakening, at noon or 6 p.m, and bedtime.
† Turner-Warwick (1977).

to asthmatic patients, and most in the frankly asthmatic. Further, the degree of variability changes in given subjects with time and circumstances. Between subjects in whom airways flow shows only slight variability and those whom we designate asthmatic the distinction is arbitrary, but from a clinical point of view it is usually quite clear who has significant asthma and who does not.

It is widely accepted that variability in PEF of 15–20 per cent or more between readings which are consistent at any one time is diagnostic of asthma. This degree of variability has been chosen from studies on patients and other subjects in exercise tests and less formally on numerous individual occasions.

In practice it is usually found that when asthma is present the variability is well outside normal, although there are patients who seem to have unvarying airways obstruction.

Initially measurements of PEF or FEV_1 measured at different times of day for a week may give unequivocal information. Repeated measurements of PEF which are most easily made by patients at home may demonstrate spontaneous and predictable changes or changes in relationship to accidental external stimuli.

If no change is found but PEF is below normal then two questions arise. Are there other causes such as reduced lung volume or vital capacity, or extra-pulmonary airways obstruction, and is there reversibility with specific treatment?

The commonest specific test of reversibility is the response to bronchodilators. The writer administers salbutamol as a powder (200–400 µg) from a 'Rotahaler' or with even greater certaintly as a nebulized aerosol (5–10 mg), with measurement of PEF before and 10 minutes afterwards. These forms of administration require little or no patient skill whereas that from a metered aerosol is rather unsure even with practice.

If the PEF lies within normal limits then provocation tests might be applied. Of these the response to exercise under standardized conditions is valuable, safe, and easily reversible if necessary. Other provocation tests are not appropriate outside the specialized laboratory for they must be administered with practised skill.

At ages when measurements cannot be made the symptoms of episodic cough or wheeze and their prevention by treatment may be enough to make a confident diagnosis, to be confirmed later when measurement is possible. PEF and FEV_1 can usually be measured satisfactorily from the age of five and sometimes earlier.

Lastly in those patients in whom the reduction in airways function seems resistant to bronchodilators yet the discovery of asthma might yield a treatable handicap a trial of systemic corticosteroids is nearly always justified. An important reservation is that chronic bronchitis may also benefit and more subtle studies of lung function may be needed to determine the contribution of asthma.

The objective information so acquired, together with the patient's account is usually sufficient to decide whether or not intrusive treatment is needed. Almost invariably treatment is pharmacological.

Forms of treatment may be prophylactic or responsive. If prophylactic then they may be selective. For example, a small number of patients, particularly children, have asthma after exercise and at no other time, and others only seasonally. The former may be treated with sodium cromoglycate taken before exercise, or bronchodilator taken before or afterwards. The writer prefers a bronchodilator because it seems always effective whereas SCG will occasionally fail and in any case is ineffective if given after exercise. In some subjects the frequency of attacks or their persistence when untreated leads to the establishment of continuous preventive treatment. The choice of continuous treatment is a matter of judgement and any of the main groups of drugs, bronchodilators, SCG, topical or systemic corticosteroids may be appropriate.

In other patients it will be decided that treatment be given only when asthma becomes symptomatic and it is useful to distinguish between relapses which are mild and those which are or may become severe.

It is possible that prophylactic treatment is advised too often and for too long in many patients, although from the best of motives. The writer is inclined to think that a more responsive form of supervision combined with regular review might still achieve the same aims and yet spare needless rather intrusive therapy for some patients, especially children. Withdrawal of prophylaxis could be attempted at shorter intervals than those adopted for example following the original trials of SCG which were dominated by patients with more severe perennial asthma in whom the alternative treatment was with systemic corticosteroids.

Against this view it has been shown that in asymptomatic patients with normal VC, FEV_1, PEF, more searching measurements of function, e.g. RV, specific airways conductance, P_{aO_2}, often reveal persistent abnormalities. Whether the likelihood is then increased of further episodes or worsening chronic disease is not known. Neither is it known of continuous treatment in the asymptomatic patient yields long-term benefits.

CLASSIFICATION OF ASTHMA

The limits of present knowledge have encouraged numerous classifications of varying usefulness (Table 5.4). None describes or predicts all features of asthma. The author favours a scheme which stresses the very inconsistency of the disorder whilst recognising the different characteristics of airflow obstruction remarked by Turner-Warwick (Fig. 5.4).

Table 5.4. *Some classifications of asthma*

Extrinsic atopic	IgE mediated
Extrinsic non-atopic	Specified hypersensitivity to external allergens. Not IgE mediated
Intrinsic	Unspecified hypersensitivity: association with autoimmune disease and aspirin sensitivity
Exercise	
Associated with chronic bronchopulmonary disease	
From Clark and Godfrey (1977)	
Brittle	Irregular variability, achieving normal PEF with bronchodilator
Nocturnal	Regular fall in PEF
Irreversible	
Group 1 Never achieve normal PEF but show reversible component	
Group 2 Irreversible PEF but reversible VC	
Group 3 Improved PEF with sustained treatment (e.g. steroids)	
From Turner-Warwick M (1977)	

Children (described at age 14).

A Intermittent mild	Not more than 5 episodes
B Intermittent moderate	More than 5 episodes but none within 12 months
C Intermittent severe	Continuing episodic asthma
Intermittent very severe	Very frequent asthma, remissions
D	less than one per month, or
Chronic unremitting	chronically unremitting
From McNicol and Williams (1973)	

Children	**Treatment**
A Mild intermittent	Intermittent brochodilator
B Severe intermittent	Intermittent courses of steroids
C Moderate perennial	Sodium cromoglycate
D Severe perennial	Topical steroids
E Very severe	Systemic (oral) steroids
From Clark and Godfrey (1977)	

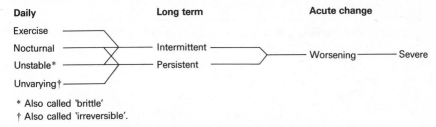

Fig. 5.4. Classification of asthma reflecting temporal characteristics.

CERTAIN FEATURES OF ASTHMA AND THEIR CONSEQUENCES

Asthma seems a wayward disorder. It can change quickly, sometimes with devastating suddenness. None the less there are good reasons for believing that it worsens commonly over several days. Unfortunately many patients are not aware of deterioration until it is marked, with PEF reduced to perhaps 50 per cent of normal. Without sensitive forms of continuous assessment matched by the organization of a willing effective response for all patients their confidence and that of the family doctor are insecure.

There is yet no means of predicting accurately: (i) which treatments will be effective; (ii) whose established treatment might fail; (iii) which patients, for obscure reasons, do not take treatment appropriately or seek advice; (iv) who might suffer acute severe asthma.

The occurrence of acute severe asthma may be thought a failure of care, not just a failure of attention or treatment although each may contribute, but rather a failure of the whole programme of care in which patient education towards self-care is a major part. Not all patients, of course, are teachable and not all who are behave predictably; and there are people who regardless of advice, guidance, and support frustrate the most diligent concern. But these are few.

MANAGEMENT OF ASTHMA

Assessment of lung function

It is now almost self-evident that without continued measurements of lung function the management of a disorder as capricious as asthma is haphazard and uncertain. The measurements most often made derive from forced expiration. Tests of maximum flow although subject to limitations considered earlier have the overwhelming advantage of simplicity.

The ready availability of the Mini-Wright Peak Flow Meter, the reproducibility of measurements made by it and the simplicity of interpretation should have transformed the management of this disease.

Table 5.5. *Uses of peak flow measurements*

(i) To confirm a diagnosis of asthma
(ii) To assess its pattern and severity
(iii) To evaluate treatment
(iv) To monitor its natural history
(v) To establish patient self-care
(vi) To exclude asthma

In the continuing care of patients with possible, likely or proven asthma in general practice measurements of PEF have many uses (Table 5.5).

Diary cards are kept as a form of assessment complementing physiological measurements and in children under five years of age and those unable to perform forced expiratory manoeuvres they are an alternative. But their use is time-consuming and most patients are unwilling to keep them for long periods.

Radiology

The chest X-ray may be helpful and occasionally is vital.

1. Uncomplicated asthma. Over-inflation is found in over 25 per cent of children and 20 per cent of adults.

2. Complications of asthma: pneumothorax (rare in children), pulmonary collapse; infiltrations, especially aspergillosis, tuberculosis.

3. Differential diagnosis: emphysema, cystic fibrosis; obstructive airways lesions (neoplasm, foreign body); cardiac causes (left heart failure, mitral valve disease).

4. Latent tuberculosis, especially if systemic corticosteroids are to be used.

Allergy studies

Their part is limited. The identification of many ubiquitous allergens is of no practical value but recognition of a few particular ones may be helpful. This information permits avoidance and sometimes an opportunity for hyposensitization.

1. Horses, pets: most patients choose to keep their animals and bear the consequences.

2. House-dust mite: attempts well short of obsessional to reduce the population are worth a simple trial.

3. Pollen, especially grass pollen: hyposensitization may be helpful.

4. Foods: possibly milk, eggs, fish, nuts, chocolate in children but not very important; preservatives and additives – sulphur dioxide (inhalation rather than ingestion?), sodium benzoate, tartrazine, especially aspirin-sensitive asthmatics; occupational exposure to grain, flour, coffee, castor beans.

5. Occupational allergens: these are being identified more frequently (although responsible in only about 2 per cent of asthmatics). As a preventive measure it is prudent to counsel atopic children respecting future employment.

6. Drugs (sensitivity to aspirin and related drugs is not immunological): occupational asthma with pharmaceutical agents is well described but uncommon.

Drugs, their uses and their administration

Three main groups are bronchodilators (β_2-agonists and xanthine derivatives), sodium cromoglycate (SCG), and corticosteroids topically or sytemically. In addition there are anticholinergic drugs (ipratropium) and calcium antagonists but their place is not yet clear.

Bronchodilators are short-acting, from 3–8 hours depending on the individual the status of his asthma and the formulation of the drug. They are given as sole therapy in intermittent asthma, as supplementary therapy in persistent and worsening asthma, and as specific therapy in EIA. Used intensively they are the keystone of treatment in acute severe asthma.

SCG was a notable advance when first introduced in the treatment of moderate and severe perennial asthma. It is safe, prevents unacceptable asthma in about two-thirds of children (but fewer adults) given it regularly, and although it does not seem to restore normal function in most asthmatics its original success in sparing many children from systemic corticosteroids gave it great importance. The main disadvantage is the need for six-hourly administration. It fails in about a fifth during the first year and afterwards in about a third. Unfortunately its beneficial effect may not be known for several weeks although it may be obvious in the first fortnight. Not infrequently it causes irritative bronchoconstriction but this may be prevented by a bronchodilator.

Preparations of safe very active topical corticosteroids have not, curiously, displaced the high position of SCG, especially in hospital paediatric practice. Undoubtedly there is disquiet, so far unjustified, about the use of topical corticosteroids in children.

Topical corticosteroids (beclomethasone, betamethasone) are an important advance. They have outstanding properties: (i) they are often the only alternative to systemic steroids; (ii) they need to be taken only twice or even once daily; (iii) they seem to reduce nocturnal variability; (iv) they give sustained improvement to many 'irreversible' asthmatics; (v) the dose can be titrated readily against PEF and the ideal dose thereby determined.

A disadvantage is their propensity to cause oropharyngeal thrush but this is a minor problem.

Systemic corticosteroids (prednisolone, prednisone by mouth, hydrocortisone parenterally) are used to supplement other treatments, normally topical corticosteroids when they alone are inadequate. The combination often permits a lower dose of systemic corticosteroids. They are used in deteriorating asthma to prevent acute severe asthma, and in acute severe asthma where their use is widely thought to be essential although this belief has been questioned.

None of these agents (with the possible exception of ipratropium) is effective in wheezy infants below 12 months. Fortunately at this age the disorder is

(a)

Drug	Administration				
	Oral solution	Oral slow release	Aerosol	Powder	Nebula
Ipratropium			●		●
Sodium cromoglycate SCG			●	●	●
Systemic steroid	●				
Topical steroid			●	●	
Xanthine	●	●			
β_2-agonist	●	●	●	●	●

(b)

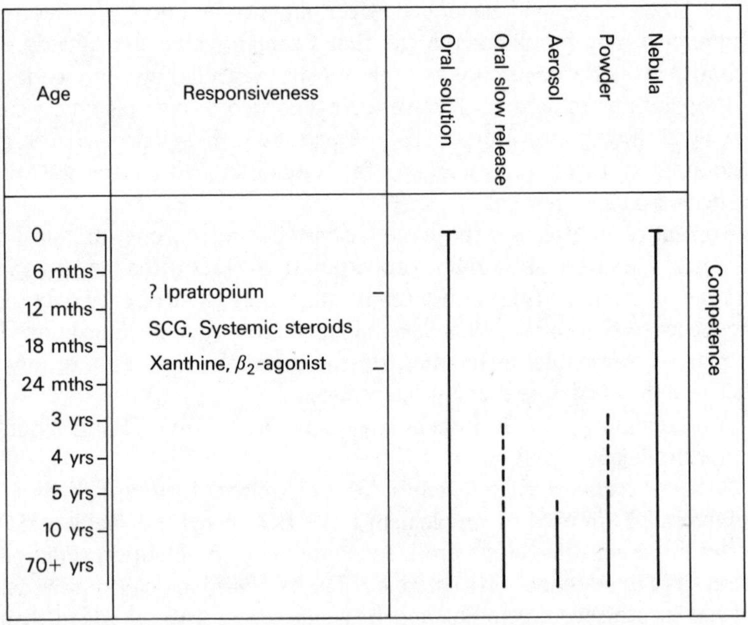

Fig. 5.5. (a) Administration of drugs in asthma. (b) Ages of responsiveness and competence.

usually not severe or prolonged but it does cause anxiety and occasionally hospital admission is needed for supportive treatment. Thereafter SCG and steroids become effective and after about 18 months bronchodilators.

In older children the problem is one of administration of drugs and the methods available then and later are illustrated in Fig. 5.5.

Nebulized aqueous aerosols

A notable change in many practices, following current hospital practice, is the increased use of nebulizers to deliver bronchodilator (and SCG and ipratropium) in worsening asthma. The method has been employed for many years in Australasia both in hospital and domiciliary care.

It often allows effective delivery to peripheral airways when because of airflow obstruction, tiredness, impaired co-ordination, want of skill or infancy there is inadequate penetration by metered aerosol or dry powder.

In very severe asthma it may fail because of mucus plugging and this is an indication for parenteral aminophylline or β_2-agonist.

There is concern that unsupervised use of nebulizers might lead to experiences similar to that of the 1960s when increased reliance by patients upon aerosol sympathomimetics delayed the administration of steroids in worsening asthma which probably accounted for the increased mortality in asthmatic patients at that time.

Order of treatment (Table 5.6)

The writer's preference is for swift control rather than prolonged assessment of a drug with a high prospect of failure. Thereafter the potency and intensity of treatment can be reduced under supervision. If a patient presents with worsening asthma corticosteroids are introduced forthwith.

A bronchodilator is used for mild intermittent asthma. In persistent asthma which limits moderate activity, where there is adequate bronchodilator responsiveness and maximum PEF more than about 70 per cent of normal then a choice is made between SCG and inhaled corticosteroids added to the bronchodilator.

Acute severe asthma

This describes worsening asthma which is usually found to be progressively less responsive to bronchodilators. Diminished responsiveness is not always apparent, for example when asthma has not been diagnosed previously or when it results from stopping treatment especially with steroids, or when an attack has been neglected or so fulminant that there has been no opportunity for treatment.

Symptoms may not appear until PEF has fallen to 50 per cent of normal and worsening restriction of a patient's normal physical activity indicates asthma of a degree requiring prompt action.

Table 5.6. *Guide to pharmacological treatment of asthma*

Severity	Features	Treatment	Notes
Intermittent asthma	Cough, wheeze occasionally certain exercises may be limited maximum PEF near normal	Infrequent bronchodilator	commonly nocturnal – use slow-release bronchodilator exercise induced – β_2-agonist, SCG are preventive wide choice of preparations
Persistent asthma	Frequent cough, wheeze, dyspnoea sleep often disturbed moderate activity restricted bronchodilator of limited effect maximum PEF< 70% normal	Regular bronchodilator add SCG 80–160 mg daily or beclomethasone 200–1600 µg daily	4–6 hourly (oftener in some patients) 6 hourly (sometimes 4 hourly) 12 hourly: after 2 weeks reduce weekly to maintenance dose
Worsening asthma	Cough, † wheeze, ‡ dyspnoea continually sleep increasingly disturbed quiet activity limited bronchodilator progressively less effective	Bronchodilator 2–4 hourly add prednisolone 10–50 mg daily and subsequently beclomethasone 200–1600 µg daily	nebulizer may be an advantage 6–12 hourly, withdrawing over 4–18 days 12 hourly: after 2 weeks reduce weekly to maintenance dose
*1A	maximum PEF< 60–70% normal pulse increased 90/min adult		
1B	110/min child		
Severe asthma 2A	Dyspnoea severe, continuous much increased respiratory effort difficulty speaking wheeze may be absent	Oxygen (28%) and hydrocortisone 50–250 mg i.v. and aminophylline 100–500 mg i.v. and/or salbutamol 5–20 mg by nebulizer and commence prednisolone 10–50 mg daily	bronchodilators worsen hypoxaemia no risk of respiratory depression 3 mg/kg
2B	sleep much disturbed difficulty getting up		6 mg/kg Slowly
3	bronchodilator ineffective as normally administered		amount delivered uncertain. If tremor or palpitations pause.
4	PEF becomes unrecordable pulse 100–150/min adult 120–160/min child pulsus paradoxus > 10 mm Hg	Admit to hospital if Grade 2A (Sherwood Jones)persists	**VITAL** Give hydrocortisone, bronchodilator before journey Oxygen in ambulance

*Sherwood Jones Grade. ‡Wheeze may be slight. † Cough may be absent. See also Fig. 5.4.

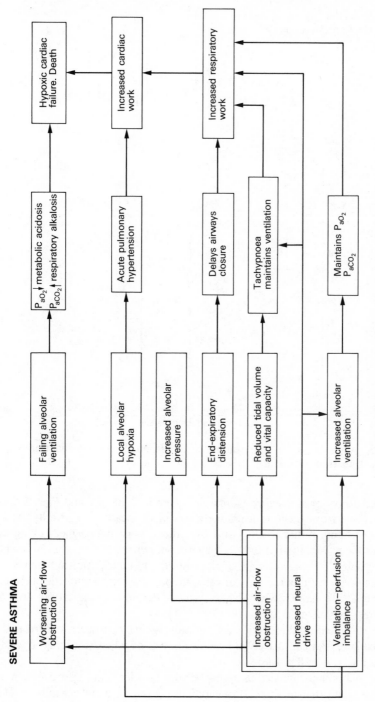

Fig. 5.6. Asthma: adaptive changes and consequences.

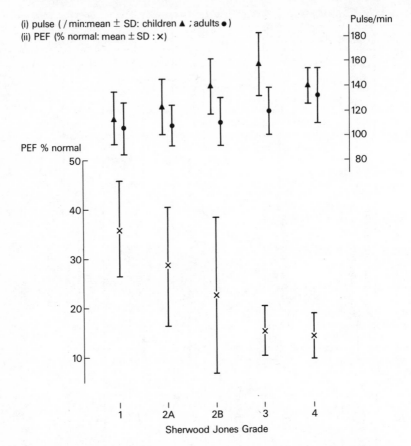

(i) pulse (/ min:mean ± SD: children ▲ ; adults ●)
(ii) PEF (% normal: mean ± SD : ×)

Pulse/min

PEF % normal

Sherwood Jones Grade

Fig. 5.7. Acute severe asthma: features at admission. Sherwood Jones grading of severity. Data from Arnold *et al.* (1982).

The features of worsening asthma are given in Table 5.6 and Figs. 5.6 and 5.7. No one feature allows a uniquely confident measure of severity. Many, each correlating rather weakly with the others, must be weighed taking into account the possibility that asthma may worsen swiftly, often within 24 hours.

Fortunately the clinical decision is less subtle. The anticipation and prevention of more severe asthma is a duty of care and because one therapeutic decision is simple and safe, namely when to give systemic steroids, the indications need not be distressingly obvious.

The early self-administration of steroids is one approach to care and is adopted here. Patients are given Prednisolone to be taken according to written instructions (Fig. 5.8 p. 106).

If bronchodilator inhaled as aerosol or dry powder is not effective then it is pointless using that method. Bronchodilator given by nebulizer might still be

Table 5.7a. *Clinical grading of severity of asthma. (After Sherwood Jounes)*

Grade	Severity of asthma
1A	Patient able to carry out housework or job with moderate difficulty. Sleep occasionally disturbed
1B	Patient only able to carry out housework or job with great difficulty. Sleep frequently disturbed
2A	Patient confined to chair or bed but able to get up with moderate difficulty. Sleep is disturbed with little or no relief from inhaler
2B	Patient confined to chair or bed and only able to get up with great difficulty. Unable to sleep. Pulse rate over 120/min
3	Patient totally confined to chair or bed. No sleep. No relief from inhaler. Pulse rate over 120/min
4	Patient immobilized and completely exhausted

Note: Sherwood Jones recommends admission to hospital once patient reaches Grade 2A. From Clark and Godfrey (1977).

Table 5.7b. *Simplified Sherwood Jones grading of asthma*

Grade	
1	Able to work with difficulty
2	Almost confined to chair, moving with difficulty
3	Confined to bed
4	Moribund

After Hetzel *et al.* (1977).

effective by reaching otherwise inaccessible peripheral airways in adequate dose and often the response is dramatic. It may, however, be small or not sustained and then bronchodilator must be given parenterally. In the earlier stages of worsening asthma the power of steroids to restore bronchodilator responsiveness is almost beyond doubt. Indeed no other agent can achieve this (except the passing of time). Steroids may halt and reverse the detioration and it is their timely administration for which the general practitioner should be responsible, preventing established severe asthma in which mucus plugging of small airways is a crucial factor and the benefits of steroids are rather less sure.

Unfortunately a number of patients are unable to perceive the severity of asthma and others misjudge the failing response to bronchodilator. Some have had inadequate guidance in anticipation of worsening asthma. Such patients eventually present in a more advanced state and a willing reaction from the doctor and his practice assumes even greater importance.

Information which should be recorded both for immediate care and for hospital colleagues who might need it is summarized (Tables 5.6 and 5.8). Table 5.6 describes treatment schedules currently used by the author.

Admission to hospital is wise when: (i) there is a wish for alternative care by the doctor, patient, or parent; (ii) domiciliary treatment fails to improve on Sherwood Jones Grade 2A (Tables 5.7a and 5.7b).

VENTOLIN relieves asthma for 4 – 6 hours. Taken before exercise it will prevent asthma afterwards.

If VENTOLIN is needed more often than usual (every 2 – 4 hours) asthma is getting worse. It needs a different treatment *that day.*

See Card 2

PHYLLOCONTIN SA taken before sleep helps night-time asthma.

BECOTIDE taken twice a day prevents asthma but *must be taken regularly*.

VENTOLIN is less important. It gives additional help for 4 – 6 hours but usually is not needed.

If VENTOLIN is needed more often than usual (every 2 – 4 hours) asthma is getting worse. It needs a different treatment *that day.*

See Card 2

INTAL prevents asthma but *must be taken regularly* 3 – 4 times a day even when you are well. It usually prevents asthma which follows exercise.

VENTOLIN will give additional help for 4 – 6 hours and prevent exercise asthma but usually it is not needed.

If VENTOLIN is needed more often than usual (every 2 – 4 hours) asthma is getting worse. It needs a different treatment *that day*.

See Card 2

CARD 2

WORSENING ASTHMA Use of PREDNESOL to prevent severe asthma

Even before wheeze, tightness, shortness of breath, and the need to take VENTOLIN more often there may be cough or symptoms of a cold. Any of these may warn of worsening asthma.

Then (i)　Measure peak flow
　　　(ii)　if it is below 50 – 60 % of normal for patient take twice the usual dose of VENTOLIN

This guide is not too sensitive to acceptable variations nor too insensitive to significant deterioration. The response to bronchodilator provides a critical test.

(iii)　measure peak flow after 10 minutes and 2 hours
(iv)　if either is no better take PREDNESOL Adult 20 mg (30 – 50 mg/day) Child 5 – 10 mg (10 – 30 mg/day) It is not realistic to be more precise. The dose for individuals is found empirically.
(v)　phone doctor for further advice.

These examples describe the author's practice. There are numerous other drugs with similar pharmacological actions (see British National Formulary, current edition).

Fig. 5.8. Information and instructions for patients. Examples.

Table 5.8. *Acute severe asthma: useful information*

History	see performance review check list
(i) Asthma diagnosed?	
(ii) Duration, pattern, severity	
(iii) Treatment	Table 5.6
(iv) Acute severe asthma	
(v) Hospital admission	} Tables 5.10 and 5.11
(vi) Compliance	
Current episode	
(i) Symptomatic change	
(ii) Duration, pattern, severity	Tables 5.10 and 5.11
(iii) Treatment by patient	
— response	} Table 5.6 and Fig. 5.8
(iv) Treatment by doctor	
— response	
Objective features	
(i) Sherwood Jones grading	Table 5.7
(ii) Capacity to speak	
(iii) Respiratory work	
rate	
accessory muscles	
hyperinflation	
(iv) Wheeze	
(v) Breath sounds	
(vi) Pulse	Fig. 5.7
(vii) PEF, (FEV$_1$)	Fig. 5.7
(viii) Arterial paradox	Table 5.9
(ix) Dehydration	

Table 5.9. *Arterial paradox (systolic fluctuation, pulsus pradoxus). When asthma is more severe than Grade 1A or PEF less than 20 per cent normal paradox is usually more than 10 mm Hg. If paradox is more than 20 mm PEF is usually less than 35 per cent normal*

(a) Probability of PEF value for given degree of paradox

Paradox (mm Hg)	PEF (% normal)		
	35	40	45
15	80	88	88
20	95	95	100

(b) Probability of paradox exceeding 10 mm Hg for given PEF value

PEF (% normal	Paradox> 10 mm Hg (%)
25	62
20	78

Data taken from Knowles and Clark (1973) and Shim and Williams (1978).

Table 5.10. *Admission with acute severe asthma*

(a) Previous factors

Factor	% of patients (i)	(ii)	(iii)
Chronic asthma	62	–	–
Admission previously	50	–	78
Admission preceding year	35	–	46
Acute episode preceding year	–	51	–

(b) Duration of onset

Onset less than	% of patients (i)	(ii)
1 h	–	13
24 h	66	46

Data from: (i) Cooke *et al.* (1979); (ii) Arnold *et al.* (1982); and (iii) McKenzie *et al.* (1979).

Table 5.11. *Death in asthma*

(a) Previous factors

Factor	% of patients (i)	(ii)
Duration of asthma 10 years	80	
Chronic asthma	67	
Admission previously	64	62
Admission in preceding year	21	34
Reluctance to seek help or unreliable	67	
Currently off work with asthma	67	

(b) Duration of onset of final episode of asthma

Final episode less than	% of patients (i)	(ii)
30 min	–	23
1 h	26	–
2 h	26	34
8 h	–	61
12 h	63	–
24 h	79	78

Data from: (i) British Thoracic Association (1982); and (ii) Macdonald *et al.* (1976).
46 per cent had known history of rapidly progressive attacks.
Other surveys have shown 24 h duration in 70.6, 66, but also in 18.5 per cent.

Specialist hospital care offers: (i) for the doctor shared burden of responsibility, and relief of anxiety for all; (ii) assessment of P_{aO_2}, P_{aCO_2}, and their attempted correction; (iii) administration of optimal doses of oxygen, bronchodilator, steroids; (iv) recognition and correction of pneumothorax; (v) fuller assessment of lung function; (vi) controlled ventilation if necessary.

Information and instructions for patients

Lucid, concise, and unambiguous written information and instructions are an indispensable part of care. If written on a card in the surgery and addressed personally they seem to be more valued and more compelling than a printed document.

Such information needs to describe two circumstances: (i) routine treatment and its purpose; (ii) recognition of worsening asthma and its treatment.

These requirements are met in the printed examples (Fig. 5.8).

Smoking

Inhaled cigarette smoke rather unexpectedly does not greatly irritate the airways of either asthmatic or normal subjects. Most show some bronchoconstriction one minute after inhalation but not after 3–10 minutes. However, asthmatic smokers do have lower lung function than asthmatic non-smokers.

Surprisingly, too, at least among hospital outpatients one-quarter are smokers and one-quarter ex-smokers.

The long-term effects of smoking on asthma are not known, but it seems likely that some individuals are more susceptible and suffer chronic airways obstruction.

Common indications for specialist referral

Non-urgent
  (i) Disquiet
       (a) Of patients, parents
       (b) Of doctor, who wishes to share care, and perhaps make arrangements for self-admission
  (ii) For diagnosis and assessment
       (a) Uncertainty of diagnosis
           other respiratory disease: emphysema, chronic bronchitis, cystic fibrosis.
           cardiac disease: left ventricular failure, ischaemic heart disease, hypertensive heart disease, mitral valve disease.
       (b) Atypical features present
           constitutional illness, weight loss, abnormal chest X-ray, abnormal blood picture, raised ESR, possibility of malignant disease, connective tissue disorder, tuberculosis, aspergillosis
       (c) Assessment of allergic factors: often at patient's wish
       (d) Assessment of possible occupational factors

(iii) For treatment
    (a) Unfamiliarity with treatment regimes
    (b)When complicated by or complicating associated disorders needing treatment,
      e.g. ischaemic heart disease, hypertension, diabetes, degenerative and inflammatory musculoskeletal disease, tuberculosis, aspergillosis, affective disorder, peptic ulceration
(iv) Escalation of treatment
    (a) Systemic corticosteroids in childhood
    (b)Potentially harmful doses of systemic corticosteroids in adults
(v) Failure of treatment
    (a) Wrong treatment
    (b)Imperfect techniques of self-administration
    (c) Non-compliance
    (d)Unstable (brittle) asthma (uncommon, but difficult to control)
    (e) Steroid unresponsiveness (uncommon)
    (f) Unrecognized precipitants, e.g. allergens, drugs, e.g. aspirin, β-blocker
    (g) Unrecognized features, e.g. as in (ii)
    (h)Consideration of changed environment in children (rare)

Urgent
(i) Acute severe asthma
    (a) Failure of domiciliary treatment
    (b)Wish for alternative care by patient, parent, or doctor.
(ii) Wheeziness in infants (including broncholitis, bronchitis)
    (a) When accompanied by exhaustion, dehydration
    (b)When anxiety of parent or doctor requires it

Uses of peak expiratory flow (PEF) measurements

PEF measurements in diagnosis and assessment

It is widely accepted that variability in PEF of 15–20 per cent warrants a diagnosis of asthma. Readings of PEF recorded by a patient at intervals during 12–16 hours of day are often all that is required to make a diagnosis and with it the initial assessment of severity. A regular diurnal variation is found in most patients although in unstable (brittle) asthma the variation is quite erratic and in unvarying (irreversible) asthma not spontaneously demonstrable.

In other patients, in over 90 per cent of children, and probably most adults when they can perform the test, a fall in PEF may be demonstrated after appropriate exercise. Often diminished airways flow may be reversed by inhalation of a bronchodilator. But there are some adults in whom this manoeuvre fails and a course of systemic cortocosteroids is necessary in order to demonstrate reversibility. There may then be doubt whether one is dealing with asthma or chronic bronchitis, but by practical criteria valuing relief of symptoms the distinction is actually of little importance.

The ranges of PEF (and FEV$_1$, VC) in normal subjects with respect to age, sex, and height are well documented and provide a valuable guide.

PEF measurements in the determination of treatment

A judgement on treatment having been made the response should be measured. The measurement is most easily done by the patient who keeps a record of PEF whilst treatment is given and then withdrawn. Various treatments given separately and if necessary in combination, may be compared and it soon becomes clear which are effective and acceptable. This method also allows the rejection of superfluous treatments because in many instances the addition of further therapy to a main one makes an insignificant clinical difference. Demonstration of a measureable change in lung function may be of not the slightest practical importance. Lastly, this method will allow the rejection of harmful treatments or otherwise unacceptable ones.

PEF measurements to monitor natural history

Asthma is a capricious disorder. It may appear without warning, or established treatment may fail, and mild asthma may swiftly worsen and become acutely severe.

Measurements of peak flow taken regularly or at times when the soundness of lung function is in doubt will reveal these changes and allow a patient to modify treatment and seek advice. Conversely, natural remission is common especially in the young. The tendency for asthma to remit is, of course, discovered by most subjects themselves but a deliberate withdrawal of treatment whilst lung function is observed may allow natural resolution to be detected earlier. Even after prolonged remission asthma may recur. It has been found that in 36 per cent of patients who have been symptom free for a year or longer asthma will recur ten years or more later.

PEF measurement and self-care

Asthma is a disorder particularly well suited to self-management by patients. Its pattern and severity and the effectiveness of treatment may all be assessed at home with precision using a peak flow meter. Moreover, this actively leads to a much clearer understanding and acceptance of the disorder. It encourages independence and a closer approach to normal life. The measurement of peak flow can be made by almost all patients including children from about five years. The records made early in assessment demonstrate to patient and doctor which particular readings are of value. For the great majority of patients only two readings a day are necessary. It is scarcely reasonable to expect most children or indeed most adults to take readings more often and it is fortunate that those made first thing in the morning and last thing at night are usually adequate when there is evidence of relapse. Patients soon learn when readings are necessary as a routine or with symptomatic change and within a short time the wise occasional use of measurements is all that is required.

It is possible to show which measurements confirm or refute failing benefit from treatment and above all which may predict the onset of acute severe asthma, the major indication for change of treatment and prompt advice.

PEF measurements in the exclusion of asthma

It is not at all unusual for patients to claim that asthma is worsening when in fact symptoms are associated with an inappropriate increase in lung volume, sometimes with increased ventilation, but with no evidence of airways obstruction. This may be a response to or expression of anxiety. It is possible also that the perception of dyspnoea or of the urge to inspire is exaggerated in these patients.

Occasionally an asthmatic patient will present with symptoms which are those of chest infection rather than of asthma. Measurement to exclude significant airways obstruction is valuable, reassuring both patient and doctor and ensuring proper treatment.

PROFESSIONAL AND EDUCATIONAL REQUIREMENTS OF THOSE CARING FOR ASTHMATIC PATIENTS

Medical training almost exclusively in the hospital setting gives little practical guidance into and no experience of long-term care in asthma. (There is, of course, experience in the management of acute severe asthma.) This part of care, the largest by far in extent and in total cost, is experienced only in the formative years of vocational training and early appointment in general practice. Such is true of most disorders in medicine requiring continued care.

This unpreparedness has led in a variety of common disorders to critical enquiry by many general practitioners anxious to establish ways of doing things better.

Through informed group discussion, ideally with a specialist resource available, measurable standards of care may be agreed and their acceptance and effectiveness determined by subsequent audit.

Requirements of the practice

Because asthma can worsen in hours it is vital that any patient with asthma should know when to seek advice from his doctor and to know that he will not be impeded. A patient should be able to describe his condition and the reception staff understand and respond confident that the doctor will do likewise. Early consultation over the telephone may allow new treatment to be initiated before the patient is seen. Even better is assurance of ready access to a responsive doctor. It is found that well-guided patients do not abuse this facility, and it is never a burden on the practice: indeed late requests for advice become less frequent and management correspondingly less taxing.

Reception staff are quick to learn which conditions in medicine demand swift recognition but to teach these things is the responsibility of doctors.

The equipment needed for the management of asthma throughout a practice is not elaborate. Ideally most patients should have their own peak flow gauge and many will buy one (costing today about £12). Others may be given by charitable organizations and yet others purchased by a practice for loan. The cost is small for the gain in confidence, peace of mind, and clinical satisfaction.

A spirometer is occasionally very useful because it does permit measurement of FEV_1 and VC and if PEF is reduced intractably these other values may reveal the nature of other causes.

Of great value in treatment and sometimes convenient in diagnosis is the portable electric air pump and nebulizer. Indeed it has transformed the management of lesser grades of acute severe asthma especially in children. Suitable instruments cost about £80–120 (although a recently introduced foot-pump is much cheaper) and are much used in practices which have them.

PERFORMANCE REVIEW CHECK LIST

General

1. Can the practice identify all its asthmatic patients?
2. Does the practice have a policy for the detection of asthma and its general management?

Patients on treatment

1. How many of the following were recorded during the initial assessment? Allergies, smoking habits (of parents, if a child), triggering factors, daily variability, family history, and social consequences.
2. How many of the following measurements are recorded at initial and subsequent assessment? Weight, height, chest shape, and peak flow rate?
3. Is there any record of the patient's (or parents') ideas or the information given to the patient?
4. Are the current drugs and dosage clearly recorded?
5. Are the effects of those drugs on peak flow rates recorded?
6. What proportion of patients on treatment have recorded peak flow rates more than 30 per cent below that expected for their sex and height?

Emergencies

1. Is there a practice policy for the management of acute asthma?
2. Is there a record of patient instructions for action when the breathing deteriorates?

PATIENT ASSOCIATIONS AND SELF-HELP GROUPS

The Asthma Society and Friends of the Asthma Research Council (12 Pembridge Square, London W2 4 EH; tel. 01-229-1149) co-operates with the medical profession in patient education through meetings, pamphlets, and its journal. It provides aid for those with asthma and their families, spreads knowledge about asthma, and raises funds for research sponsored by the Asthma Research Council. In Britain there are now about 70 branches.

Local charities and individuals will often give generously and enable instruments to be bought to allow improved care. In asthma appropriate and desirable aids are peak flow gauges, portable nebulizers, and portable oxygen equipment.

PATIENTS' BOOKS AND LEAFLETS

The Asthma Research Council and its affiliated charity publish many pamphlets, are associated with a series of little books, especially for children, and publish *Asthma News*. Useful booklets have been prepared by pharmaceutical companies. For those who wish to learn more the volume by Lane and Storr *Asthma: the facts* is enticingly written and very comprehensive.

The following list is representative

The Asthma Research Council, 12 Pembridge Square, London W2 4EH
Ten facts about asthma
Do you or your family suffer from asthma?
Coming to terms with asthma Paul Buisseret (1975)
Understanding your asthma Sean Hilton (1981)
Asthma at school (for teachers with asthmatic pupils)
Asthma and pregnancy
Will my child grow out of asthma?
I have asthma Althea (1982) (a booklet for children)

The Chest, Heart and Stroke Association, Tavistock House North, Tavistock Square, London WC1
Asthma: twenty questions and the answers
Our child has asthma: some parent questions answered

Pharmaceutical companies
Childhood asthma: a guide for parents and children Schering Chemicals Ltd.
A patients guide to the treatment of asthma by inhalation Fisons Ltd.
Asthma and exercise Fisons Ltd.
House dust mite Fisons Ltd.

Other publications
Asthma: the facts D. J. Lane and C. A. Storr (1979). Oxford University Press
Your child with asthma S. Godfrey (1975). Heinemann Health Books

FURTHER READING

Aretaeus. On asthma. Willis, T. Of an asthma. In *Classic descriptions of disease,* 3 edn (ed. R. H. Major). Thomas Springfield, Ill. (1945).
British national formulary, No. 4. British Medical Association and Pharmaceutical Society of Great Britain (1982).
Clark, T. J. H., and Godfrey, S. (eds.) (1977) *Asthma.* Chapman and Hall, London.

Forgaca, P. (1978) *Lung sounds.* Baillière Tindall, London.
—— (1981). *Problems in respiratory medicine.* MTP, Lancaster.
Lane, D. J. and Storr, A. (1979). *Asthma: the facts.* Oxford University Press.
Osler, W. (1892). *The principles and practice of medicine.* Pentland, Edinburgh.

USEFUL REFERENCES

Anderson, S. D., McEvoy, J. D. S., and Bianco, S. (1972). Changes in lung volumes and airways resistance after exercise in asthmatic subjects. *Am. Rev. resp. Dis.* **106**, 30–7.

Arnold, A. G. and Lane, D. J. (1982). Letter. *Br. med. J.* **285**, 1570.

—— —— and Zapata, E. (1982). The speed of onset and severity of acute severe asthma. *Br. J. Dis. Chest* **76**, 157–63.

Bacon, C. J. (1978). Nebulised salbutamol in treatment of acute asthma in children. *Lancet* i, 158.

Bellamy, D. and Collins, J. V. (1979). 'Acute' asthma in adults. *Thorax* **34**, 36–9.

British Medical Journal (1977). Another look at asthma. *Br. med. J.* **ii**, 414.

—— (1978*a*). Diet and asthma. *Br. med. J.* **i**, 669.

—— (1978*b*). Allergy to house dust mite in childhood asthma. *Br. med. J.* **ii**, 589.

—— (1978*c*). Asthma in children. *Br. med. J.* **ii**, 716–7.

—— (1980*a*). Hyposensitisation to house dust mites. *Br. med. J.* **i**, 589–90.

—— (1980*b*). Aspirin sensitivity in asthmatics. *Br. med. J.* **281**, 958–9.

British Thoracic Association (1982). Deaths from asthma in two regions of England. *Br. med. J.* **285**, 1251–5.

Clark, T. J. H. and Hetzel, M. R. (1977). Diurnal variation of asthma. *Br. J. Dis. Chest* **71**, 87–92.

Cochrane, G. M. and Clark, T. J. H. (1975). A survey of asthma mortality in patients between ages 35 and 64 in the Greater London hospitals in 1971. *Thorax* **30**, 300–5.

Cohen, S. I. (1971). Psychological factors in asthma: a review of their aetiological and therapeutic significance. *Postgrad. med. J.* **47**, 533–9.

Connolly, C. K. Asthma – expiratory dyspnoea? *Br. med. J.* **284**, 1632.

Cook, N. J., Crompton, G. K., and Grant, I. W. B. (1979). Observations on the management of acute severe asthma. *Br. J. Dis. Chest* **73**, 157–63.

Fletcher, C. M. and Peto, R. (1977). The natural history of chronic airflow obstruction. *Br. med. J.* **i**, 1645–8.

Grant, I. W. B. (1982). Are corticosteroids necessary in the treatment of severe acute asthma? *Br. J. Dis. Chest* **76**, 125–9.

Gregg, I. (1982). Misplaced confidence in nebulised bronchodilators in severe asthmatic attacks. *Br. med. J.* **284**, 46–7.

Grimwood, K., Johnson-Barrett, J. J., and Taylor, B. (1981). Salbutamol: tablets, inhaled powder, or nebulizer? *Br. med. J.* **282**, 105–6.

Hetzel, M. R. and Clark, T. J. H. (1980). Comparison of normal and asthmatic circadian rhythms in peak expiratory flow rate. *Thorax* **35**, 732–8.

Hetzel, M. R., Clark, T. J. H., and Branthwaite, M. A. (1977). Asthma: analysis of sudden deaths and ventilatory arrests in hospital. *Br. med. J.* **i**, 808–11.

Howarth, N. J. and Gadsby, R. (1980). Nebulised salbutamol in general practice. *Lancet* **ii**, 1202.

Kerrebijn, K. F., Fioole, A. C., and van Bentveld, R. D. W. (1978). Lung function in asthmatic children after year or more without symptoms or treatment. *Br. med. J.* **i**, 886–8.

Knowles, G. K. and Clark, T. J. H. (1973). Pulsus paradoxus as a valuable sign indicating severity of asthma. *Lancet* **ii**, 1356–9.

Lenney, W. (1978). Nebulised salbutamol in treatment of acute asthma in children. (Letter.) *Lancet* i, 440–1.

—— and Milner, A. D. (1978). Recurrent wheezing in the preschool child. *Archs dis. Child.* 53, 468–73.

Macdonald, J. B., Macdonald, E. T., Seaton, A., and Williams, D. A. Asthma deaths in Cardiff 1963–74: 53 deaths in hospital. *Br. med. J.* ii, 721–3.

—— Seaton, A., and Williams, D. A. (1976). Asthma deaths in Cardiff 1963–74: 90 deaths outside hospital. *Br. med. J.* i, 1493–5.

McFadden, E. R. (1975). The chronicity of acute attacks of asthma – mechanical and therapeutic implications. *J. Allerg clin. Immunol.* 56, 18–26.

McKenzie, S. A., Edmunds, A. T., and Godfrey, S. (1979). Status asthmaticus in children. A one year study. *Archs Dis. Child.* 54, 581–6.

McNicol, K. N. and Williams, H. B. (1973). Spectrum of asthma in children – 1, clinical and physiological components. *Br. med. J.* iv, 7–11.

Martin, A. J., Landan, L. I., and Phelan, P. D. (1982). Asthma from childhood at age 21: the patient and his disease. *Br. med. J.* 284, 380–2.

—— McLennan, L., Landon, L. I., and Phelan, P. D. (1980). The natural history of childhood asthma to adult life. *Br. med. J.* 280, 1397–400.

Miller, K. (1982). Sensitivity to tartrazine. *Br. med. J.* 285, 1597.

Milner, A. D. (1981). Bronchodilator drugs in childhood asthma. *Archs Dis. Childh.* 56, 84–5.

—— (1982). Childhood asthma: treatment and severity. *Br. med. J.* 285, 155–6.

Morris, M. J. (1981). Asthma – expiratory dyspnoea? *Br. med. J.* 283, 838–9.

Ormerod, L. P. and Stableforth, D. E. Asthma mortality in Birmingham 1975–7: 53 deaths. *Br. med. J.* 280, 687–90.

Rubinfield, A. R. and Pain, M. L. F. (1976). Perception of asthma. *Lancet* i, 882–4.

Seaton, A. (1978). Asthma – contrasts in care. *Thorax* 33, 1–2.

Shim, C. and Williams, H. M. (1978). Pulsus paradoxus in asthma. *Lancet* i, 530–1.

Speight, A. N. P. (1978). Is childhood asthma being underdiagnosed and undertreated? *Br. med. J.* ii, 331–2.

Turner-Warwick, M. (1977). On observing patterns of airflow obstruction in chronic asthma. *Br. J. Dis. Chest* 71, 73–86.

Warner, J. O., Prue, J. F., Soothill,, J. F., and Hey, E. N. (1978). Controlled trial of desensitisation to dermatophagoides pteronyssimus in children with asthma. *Lancet* ii, 912–5.

Williams, J. and McNicol, K. N. (1969). Prevalence, natural history, and relationship of wheezy bronchitis and asthma in children. An epidemiological study. *Br. med. J.* iv, 321–5.

Wilson, N. and Silverman, M. (1982). Controlled trial of slow-release aminophylline in childhood asthma: are short-term trials valid? *Br. med. J.* 284, 863–6.

Wright, B. (1978). A miniature Wright Peak-flow meter. *Br. med. J.* ii, 1627–8.

6 Chronic bronchitis

Robert Gilchrist

Chronic bronchitis has been defined as a 'chronic productive cough for more than three months in the year, for two successive years' (Medical Research Council), and this is probably the most useful definition for general practice. There are three points arising out of this:

1. There is no mention of breathlessness in the definition, although the problems which arise from chronic bronchitis are almost all associated with shortness of breath.

2. This is a retrospective definition since two years must elapse before it is fulfilled, and this may have implications if the possibility of screening for early disease is considered.

3. This is essentially an epidemiological definition and is not a clinical or pathological diagnosis, and it should be regarded as a rag-bag of conditions, some well worked out, and with known pathology, and others as yet only vaguely understood. Perhaps some day all the conditions will be properly differentiated, but at present the terminology is still very confused.

INCIDENCE AND PREVALENCE

It has been estimated that 8 per cent of males and 3 per cent of females fall into this category. 8500 deaths per annum are registered in the United Kingdom as being due to chronic bronchitis before retiring age, and 30 000 in all, and the loss of working days has been estimated at thirty million per year. However, since this is a condition which increases in incidence and severity with age, there may be as many as 25 per cent of the male population between 50 and 59 who fall into this category. It is also well established that it is not evenly spread throughout the population. It is much more prevalent in: (i) urban than in rural communities; (ii) the North of the country, than the South (even when allowance is made for urbanization); Classes V and IV than in Classes I and II.

Therefore the impact of the condition on any one practice will depend very much on its geographical location and the class structure of the patients. For what its worth, an average practice of 2500 patients will contain about 300 sufferers of whom 90 will see their general practitioner each year at some time, and ten will be respiratory invalides.

DIAGNOSIS

When presented with a case of chronic bronchitis, the first problem facing the doctor is to weed out those conditions which are clearly identifiable. These fall into several categories, the first two (and two which should never be out of mind) are tuberculosis and carcinoma since both these conditions can occur in association with other forms of chronic bronchitis.

Tuberculosis

Of those patients still dying today of pulmonary tubersulosis most are old people who have been currently labelled as having 'chronic bronchitis', and who have 'lit up' an old tuberculosis focus, and deteriorated without the cause ever being suspected. The diagnosis depends on suspicion, X-ray, and sputum culture. It is of course eminently treatable. Occasionally the breakdown of a TB focus is also due to one of the following.

Carcinoma

Again this often supervenes on other causes of chronic bronchitis. Unfortunately it is often of merely academic interest as, if there is any substantial loss of lung function, it will mean that the condition is necessarily inoperable; but it has a very different prognosis. Examination of the chest and supraclavicular fossa may arouse suspicion which can be confirmed by X-ray or bronchoscopy; or it may present as a secondary deposit, sometimes cerebral, or with inappropriate endocrine secretion.

Sarcoidosis

This rarely presents in the chronic bronchitis group but can usually be diagnosed on X-ray and by Kveim test. This is a field for specialist physician.

Bronchiectasis

This usually has a much longer history dating back to childhood and the diagnosis is confirmed by bronchogram. The prognosis, with adequate management, in particular postural drainage, is usually much better than that for the usual 'chronic bronchitis'.

Cystic fibrosis

This invariably presents in childhood, but the disability and progression make it similar in its course to 'chronic bronchitis'.

Late-onset (intrinsic) asthma

This condition is also known as reversible airways obstruction (see Chapter 5). A trial of steroids may be necessary to exclude this diagnosis with certainty.

Various allergic conditions

These are important to distinguish because they require different treatment.
They are:

(a) Allergic alveolitis

(i) Farmers lung – the diagnosis is usually clear from the history.

(ii) Bird fanciers' lung – more easily overlooked since a coal miner who smokes may race pigeons in his spare time.

(b) various industrial allergic diseases e.g. mushroom workers' lung; malt workers' lung; workers with biological detergents; workers with electrical solders, etc.

Although some of these are well documented, general practitioners should always be on the look out for new examples which will occur as new industrial processes are discovered. The diagnosis can usually be made from the history and can be confirmed by immunological tests. Removal of the patient from the antigen may result in dramatic improvement, but this is not always possible as some of the antigens are always present in the air.

(c) allergic aspergillosis – the diagnosis is usually made by X-ray and confirmed by immunology. Removal from the antigen is not possible as the fungus is ubiquitous, and indeed may be grown from the plugs coughed up by the patient, or be seen as a mycetoma on the X-ray.

Industrial lung diseases of non-allergic nature

(a) Those due to dust:

Coal miners' pneumoconiosis

Silicosis

Asbestosis, etc.

These are important because the patient may be entitles to industrial compensation, and also they should be preventable. It is not clear whether coal miners' lung in itself causes deterioration of lung function, or whether this is caused by other causes of chronic bronchitis (particularly silicosis from the rock strata or from tobacco smoke, or the fumes from plentiful coal fires inhaled by the miner away from work). However, compensation is paid largely on the extent of the X-ray changes and mediated through the pneunoconiosis panel.

(b) those due to toxic fumes – these are usually clear from the work history and are not usually progressive once the patient is removed from the source or irritation.

Fibrosing aveolitis, lung fibrosis without obvious cause, and drug-induced lung diseases

These are properly the province of the chest physician.

Congestive cardiac failure

This is often a concomitant of chronic bronchitis (cor pulmonale) and may make the state of the patient worse. Treatment may make a worthwhile improvement.

There is also the large amorphus group of chronic bronchitis proper.

CHRONIC BRONCHITIS

This group contains by far the largest number of patients, but the terminology is very confused and often represents hypotheses about the disease processes rather than a description of the disease entities.

Emphysema is essentially a morbid anatomical pathological diagnosis which is little help in the management during life. In many cases 'emphysema' on a chest X-ray report simply mean hyper-inflation. It is useful to discuss X-ray reports of this nature with the radiologist if at all possible or the reports may be misleading. There is a rare pathological cause of emphysema due to alpha-1-antitrypsin deficiency, which is important as it is inherited as a Mendellian recessive.

Chronic obstructive airways disease, or chronic irreversible airways obstruction. The importance of this definition is to remind one that the obstruction may be reversible.

Chronic mucus hypersecretion which is another way of saying chronic productive cough.

The 'disease' in the whole group is undoubtedly related to smoking habits, and has been shown repeatedly to be so. There is some evidence that it is also related to atmospheric pollution, and there have certainly been many more hospital admissions due to exacerbations when this has been at a very high level (e.g. London smog). However, this is now hardly a problem in this country owing to the Clean Air regulations.

The regional variations between the North and South have not been satisfactorily explained. There may be some hereditary factor, or differences in social habits or differences in environment, or possible some of all three. The disease (if it is a single disease) takes a steadily, but individually variable, progressive course with increasing interference in respiratory function punctuated by acute exacerbations of 'bronchitis'. It has been shown that stopping smoking will reduce the rate of deterioration of lung function to that of the non-smoker, and reduce the number of acute attacks.

Management

As far as the general practitioner is concerned, the management of chronic bronchitis can be divided into:

1. The treatment of acute exacerbations.
2. Long-term management.
3. Prevention.

Treatment of the acute exacerbations

Since chronic bronchitis has an insidious onset, the acute exacerbation is the way that it is usually brought to the GPs attention. Early in the disease the exacerbations can usually be managed at home, or even in the surgery, but later if respiratory failure threatens, hospital admission may be necessary.

The first priority when dealing with any exacerbation is to review the diagnosis. This does not mean a formal full medical examination and investigations, but a mental check: (i) have the more identifiable diseases been excluded, particularly allergic disease? (ii) has some other disease supervened: tuberculosis; carcinoma; pneumothorax; pneumonia; cardiac failure? At some stage in the episode a chest X-ray may well be valuable. For treatment, the therapeutic possibilities are:

Antibiotics

Sputum culture is rarely helpful or necessary. One of the broad-spectrum antibiotics: ampicillin or amoxicillin, co-trimoxazole, or tetracycline probably being the drugs of choice. They should be continued in adequate doses for ten days. Early treatment with antibiotics often shortens the attack, and there is a good case for giving the patient a supply to keep at home for use should he feel an attack of 'bronchitis' coming on. This will also save unecessary urgent visiting. There is no evidence that long-term antibiotics are of any help either in the prevention of attacks of bronchitis or in halting the deterioration of respiratory function.

Bronchodilators

Although chronic bronchitis is theoretically associated with irreversible airways obstruction, during the acute episode bronchodilators often appear to be helpful. The drugs available are salbutamol (Ventolin); terbutaline (Bricanyl); rimiterol (Pulmadil) and fenoterol (Berotec), and there is probably little to choose between them. The preferred route of administration is by inhalation, either as a metered pressure aerosol, or in a rota-haler, or perhaps in a home nebulizer. They can also, of course, be given by mouth or by injection, but the dose required to be effective in the lungs often produces side-effects. The theophyllines, particularly the newer long-acting preparations Phyllocontin and Nuelin SA are sometimes found to be helpful but are often associated with gastrointestinal side-effects. The atropine analogue ipratropium bromide is said to be of some help in the long-term management of 'chronic bronchitis'.

Mucolytics, e.g. bromhexine (Bisolvon)

These are also sometimes helpful.

Oxygen

Conventionally 'chronic bronchitics' have been divided into two groups: (i) the 'pink and puffing' and (ii) the 'blue and bloated'. The former have a good respiratory drive and the latter have a poor respiratory drive mainly dependent on hypoxia. In an individual patient these categories are often not clear cut, and in practice those who are on oxygen on a long-term basis (see below) will use it during an acute attack, and those who are not should probably be admitted to hospital where there is a facility for monitoring blood gases. In any case oxygen should always be administered through a ventilation mask which delivers 24 per cent oxygen, unless the respiratory drive is known to be good. Ambulance men should be discouraged from giving 100 per cent oxygen to patients with chronic bronchitis and respiratory distress on their way to hospital since this may abolish their respiratory drive. They can safely administer 24 per cent oxygen through a ventilation mask and the doctor ordering the ambulance should be careful to specify this. Patients and their relatives should be warned of the extreme danger of smoking in the presence of oxygen.

Steroids

Generally these should not be used in an acute exacerbation unless there is good evidence that there is bronchospasm, and they should always be covered by antibiotics. There is a considerable place for a trial of steroids during a period of remission (see below).

Cough mixtures

There is little objective evidence that these do any good, and many of them contain sedative antihistamines (e.g. benylin and actifed) which may be dangerous in a patient in whom the respiratory drive is already threatened. For an unproductive cough Codeine linctus may be appropriate, but for the same reason should be used with great care. If a cough mixture must be given as a placebo, it should probably be cheap and there is much to recommend the olde-tyme remedies: Mist expect (ammon ipecac), Miss tuss nig (Mist morph et ipecac), Mist tuss sed (ammon chlor et morph). All these are cheaper than the charge to the patient.

Diuretics

These may be very helpful if there is associated cardiac failure.

Beta-blockers

'Chronic bronchitis' is often associated with cardiac conditions, particularly angina and hypertension, but it should be remembered that all the beta-blockers cause bronchoconstriction even those which are 'cardio-selective', and their use should be reviewed if respiratory function is impaired.

Long-term management

This usually arises after the short-term treatment of acute episodes when it is necessary to review in tranquility the pattern of the disease. The provision of antibiotics for the patient at home has already been mentioned, but this may lead to a danger of self-treatment so that the patient does not present to the doctor at all and the number of episodes is therefore under reported. Frequently the presentation will be in order to get a certificate or repeat prescription, and there is a grave danger that at busy times (e.g. in winter when attacks are usually more common) both these may be issued without the necessary thought.

So there is a need to review these patients at intervals, perhaps annually or bi-annually, particularly being sure that other diseases have been excluded, notably asthma. As mentioned above, it may be appropriate to try a course of prednisolone with careful measurement of respiratory function, e.g. 30 mg a day for ten days, with peak expiratory flow measured three times a day on a mini peak-flow meter lent to the patient (Figs. 6.1 and 6.2). This is much more

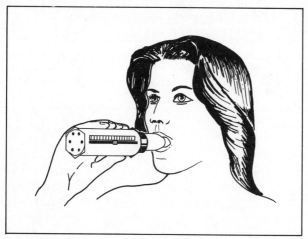

Fig. 6.1. The mini-Wright Peak Flow Meter. (After Partridge, M. *Chronic bronchitis and chronic airflow limitation.* Update. Postgraduate Centre Series (1981) with permission of the manufacturers, Clement Clarke International, Ltd.)

reliable than casual measurements in the surgery where an improved patient may be measured on a bad day, and appear to be worse than an unimproved patient on a good day. In particular the diurnal variation of airways obstruction characteristically seen in late-onset asthma is abolished by the use of steroids. A course of ten days can usually be stopped without trouble. Steroids should only be continued if there is objective evidence of improvement since they give a sense of euphoria which may not be borne out by objective measurements.

It may well be appropriate to seek a consultant chest physician's opinion if the diagnosis is not certain.

Respiratory function tests

It is worth considering doing a measurement of FEV_1 and FVC on a Vitalograph (Figs. 6.3 and 6.4) as this is a better way of determining long-term changes in pulmonary function than using the peak flow meter alone.

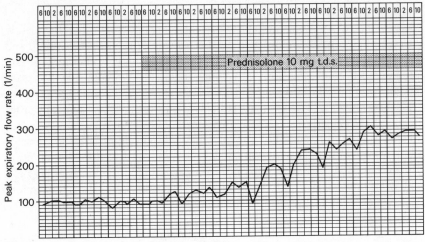

Fig. 6.2. Domiciliary mini-Wright peak flow recordings taken at four hourly intervals before and during a trial of prednisolone in a 70-year-old man. (From Partridge, M. *Chronic bronchitis* (2nd edn). Update Postgraduate Centre Series (1981).)

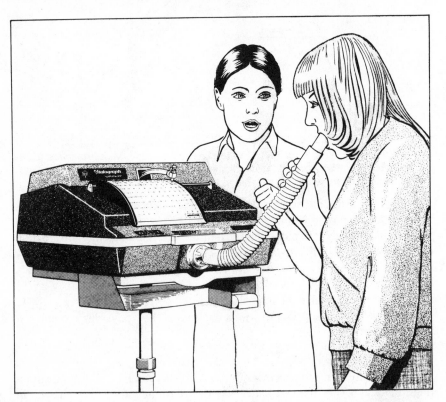

Fig. 6.3. Vitalograph used for measuring forced expiratory volume and vital capacity. (After Partridge, M. *Chronic bronchitis and chronic airflow limitation*. Update Postgraduate Centre Series (1981) with permission of the manufacturers, Vitalograph, Ltd.)

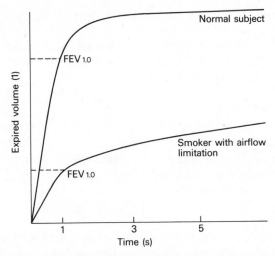

Fig. 6.4. Spirogram for a normal subject and a smoker with airflow limitation. (From Partridge, M. *Chronic bronchitis* (2nd edn). Update Postgraduate Centre Series (1981).)

Exercise tolerance test

Various tests have been suggested, e.g. the distance a patient can walk in 12 minutes, but it may be more helpful to have a subjective points scale, e.g. (i) normal; (ii) able to walk with normal people of his own age and sex on the level but unable to keep up on hills and stairs; (iii) unable to keep up with normal people on the level but can walk long distances at his own pace; (iv) unable to walk more than 100 metres on the level before being stopped by breathlessness; (v) unable to walk more than a few steps without dyspnoea, and becomes breathless on washing and dressing.

Patients probably do not need an annual chest X-ray but there is much to be said for doing an X-ray when an acute exacerbation has settled down, and if there has been no X-ray for two years it may be appropriate to consider one.

Consider long-term oxygen therapy

It has been shown that long-term oxygen therapy can improve survival time in some patients with severe airways obstruction, but it needs to be given about 15 hours a day, and this is obviously expensive. The choice is between oxygen cylinders or an oxygen concentrator which separates oxygen from ordinary air. At present, oxygen in cylinders can be obtained on prescription and therefore comes from an unlimited budget, whereas an oxygen concentrator, which would be cheaper in the long run, relies on capital expenditure which comes from a limited budget. The recent RCP working party suggested that this anomaly should be investigated.

A small portable oxygen set is sometimes helpful for patients with severe distress in helping them to climb stairs, but it clearly must be very light or the patient will lose in carrying the extra weight what he gains in improved respiratory function. Oxygen therapy at home at present implies an able-bodied relative who is able to hump cylinders and undo stiff taps. The effort required is usually too much for a disabled chronic bronchitic. There is no indication for oxygen therapy in any patient who continues to smoke.

Review of smoking habits

For the less disabled or early chronic bronchitic who is showing deterioration this is clearly the most important element of the review. The assistance provided by nicotine containing chewing gum is at present under critical analysis, but it may well become prescribable in the future on the NHS. The patient's weight could be reviewed at the same time.

Influenza

Influenza innoculation has not been convincingly shown to be effective in protecting the bronchitic from acute exacerbations, but it is clearly undesirable that he should have a full-blown attack of influenza, and annual recall for innoculation may well be appropriate.

Review of employment

The amount of time lost from work, the ability to do the job, and the actual conditions of work if they irritate the bronchial tree should be considered. The possibility of change to more appropriate employment before it is forced upon the patient by deterioration in lung function can be discussed. Unfortunately, the preponderance of sufferers in Class V with little skills and often little motivation to change their habits, often makes this rather difficult.

Referral to the disablement resettlement officer should be considered as well as registration as disabled and the provision of a disabled badge for the motor car to assist in parking when shopping and at work.

Lastly it is well to consider whether the patient should obtain a pre-payment certificate for his prescriptions. The cost of these are for ever escalating, but in general terms if a patient requires more than two items per month, it will be in his interests to purchase such a certificate.

Prevention

The two major effects are by reducing atmospheric pollution and stopping smoking. Atmospheric pollution has been so much improved by the Clean Air Act that the overall problem is not very great, but the atmospheric pollution in domestic situations due to the smoking habits of others should not be forgotten.

Smoking

Clearly a major impact could be made on the incidence, and disability caused by 'chronic bronchitics' if smoking were abolished. The RCP working party suggested that the tax on cigarettes should be doubled, but the argument against effective action are formidable. In a written answer to a question in the House of Commons in 1981 the Health Minister stated that the revenue from cigarettes was four times the cost of treating smoking related diseases.

It is probably unrealistic to expect much effective action from the Government, but there is no excuse for individual doctors not supporting both national and local campaigns against smoking (see the earlier section on smoking – p. 000).

So it will be left to individual GPs in practice to do what he can to improve the health of his practice population. There are three ways in which this can be approached:

1. By example: no smoking should be allowed on the surgery premises by any of the staff or the doctors, and no ashtrays should be provided.

2. Campaigns and advertising: this is probably best done in short sharp bursts rather than becoming part of the surgery wall-paper. Posters and leaflets can be obtained from the anti-smoking lobby (ASH), and more opportunities should be given to the propagation of statistics which, for instance, suggests that 30 per cent of smokers die from smoking related diseases.

3. Opportunistic health education, particulary at Child Health clinics, school health education sessions, and advice during pregnancy. The health visitors and midwives can clearly make a large contribution here.

PRACTICE IMPLICATIONS

Equipment

Every doctor should possess a mini peak flow meter, and there should be several spare in the surgery for loaning out to patients for diagnostic purposes.

Surgeries might consider having a vitalograph for the more accurate assessment of respiratory disorder, particularly in long-term care, and the practice should possess a portable nebulizer.

Records

1. Each episode of bronchitis should be recorded, otherwise there is a danger that the severity of the disease will be overlooked.

2. The summary of patient's record should contain a work history and hobbies, as well as the response to a trial of steroids if this has been done.

3. A repeat prescription system should ensure that all prescriptions issued are entered in the notes and that the patient is recalled after a predetermined number of times.

4. There should be a disease index for bronchitis with a recall system for assessment and influenza innoculation.

Screening for the early signs of deterioration of lung function might be considered as it would then be possible to concentrate propaganda efforts, particularly about smoking, where it is most needed. This might usefully be done by screening for peak respiratory flow rate, and if it is much below the expected value for age and height to investigate further.

Although 'chronic bronchitis' is often seen as a hopelessly progressive disease, much can be done by the general practitioner both to arrest its development and to alleviate the suffering and disability caused. Perhaps each time a patient with bronchitis presents himself, the GP should have flit through his mind four balloons labelled SMOKING, ASTHMA, TB, CARCINOMA.

PATIENT ASSOCIATION AND SELF-HELP GROUPS

National Society of Non-Smokers,
Information and Advice Centre,
Latimer House,
40–48 Hanson Street,
London W1P 7DE

ASH,
5–11 Mortimer Street,
London W1N 7RH

Chest, Heart and Stroke Association,
Tavistock House North,
Tavistock Square,
London WC1H 9JE

Health Education Council,
78 New Oxford Street,
London WC1A 1AH

These organizations produce patient books and leaflets.

PERFORMANCE REVIEW CHECK LIST

General

1. Can the practice identify all its chronic bronchitic patients?
2. Does the practice have a policy for the general management of chronic bronchitis?
3. Can the practice identify all patients who would benefit from influenza vaccination?

Patients on treatment

1. How many of the following were recorded at initial assessment: allergies, smoking habits, and social consequences?
2. How many of the following have been recorded at initial and subsequent assessments: chest X-ray result, peak flow or vitalograph measurements, exercise tolerance test measurements?

3. Is there any record of the patient's ideas or the information given to the patient?
4. Are the current drugs and dosage clearly recorded?

Acute exacerbations

1. Is there a practice policy for the management of acute exacerbations?
2. Is there a record of patient instructions for action when the breathing· deteriorates?

REFERENCES

British Medical Journal (1976). Twelve minute walking test for assessing disability in chronic bronchitis. *Br. med. J.* i, 822–3.
—— (1977). The natural history of chronic airflow obstruction. *Br. med. J.* i, 1645–8.
—— (1979). Effect of general practitioners' advice against smoking. *Br. med. J.* ii, 231–5.
Medical Research Council Working Party (1981). Long-term domiciliary oxygen therapy in chronic hypoxic cor pulmonale complicating chronic bronchitis and emphysema. *Lancet* i, 681–6.
Royal College of Physicians Committee on Thoracic Medicine (1981). Disabling chest disease: prevention and cure. *Jl. R. Coll. Physns* 15, 69–87.

FURTHER READING

Flenley, D. C. (1981). *Respiratory medicine.* Baillière Tindall, London.
Pantridge, M. R. (1981). *Chronic bronchitis and chronic airflow limitation.* Update, London.

7 Diabetes mellitus

Tom Stewart

The term diabetes mellitus should not be considered a diagnosis, but rather a description of a state of chronic hyperglycaemia of two braod types, insulin-dependent and non-insulin-dependent, accompanied by certain other metabolic abnormalities and characterized by a variety of clinical features. The condition is associated with an absolute or relative deficiency of insulin activity and may lead to a distressing series of complications.

PREVALENCE

Diabetes is not rare, there are approximately half a million known sufferers in the United Kingdom, and probably as many again are unrecognized, comprising between 1 and 2 per cent of the population: 20 per cent are insulin dependent, 75 per cent are non-insulin dependent, and 5 per cent are of various other types. A general practitioner with a list of about 2500 patients will have at least 30 known diabetics in his practice, but by looking for them he would identify another 20 or more. Between six and ten of his patients will require insulin.

INCIDENCE

The annual incidence of insulin dependent (Type 1) diabetes is between 8 and 13 per 100000 population, whereas that of the non-insulin dependent (Type 2) variety is about 70 per 100000 population. Type 1 diabetes reaches a peak of incidence at about 15 years of age and then falls. Type 2 diabetes reaches its peak incidence at about age 70 and then levels out.

CLASSIFICATION

The terms juvenile onset and maturity onset should no longer be used because they are inaccurate and not truly descriptive. A better classification is one based on the need for exogenous insulin. It so happens that it is the younger patient who has this type of diabetes, whereas the older one usually does not need insulin injections. In some respects, even this classification is too restrictive, but insulin-dependent diabetes mellitus (IDDM or Type 1) and non-insulin-dependent diabetes mellitus (NIDDM or Type 2) are now the generally accepted terms in wide use. Type 2 diabetes is further subdivided into the obese and the non-obese type.

The term 'impaired glucose tolerance' describes the equivocal area between normality and true clinical diabetes and replaces the bewildering collection of labels such as 'chemical', 'borderline', or 'early' diabetes applied to asymptomatic individuals. The importance of impaired glucose tolerance is that it recognizes patients who have biochemical abnormalities, but are spared the label 'diabetic' with all the disadvantages and restrictions that this implies. The chance of this group developing microvascular disease, such as retinopathy, is negligible, but the risk of developing large vessel disease, such as coronary heart disease, is as high as the clinical diabetic. Some patients return to normal glucose tolerance; 2–4 per cent of individuals with this condition will develop clinical diabetes.

Table 7.1. *Comparison of IDDM and NIDDM*

	IDDM	NIDDM
Age	Usually children and young adults	Middle aged and elderly
Sex	Male ≥ female	Male > female
Onset	Usually weeks	Months or years
Symptoms	Present	Often absent
Nutrition	Normal	Often obese
Weight loss	Marked	Often absent
Ketosis and coma	Common	Rarer
Response to insulin	Sensitive	Relatively insensitive
Plasma insulin	Absent or low	Usually normal
Response to oral agents	None	Usually good
Predominant vascular disease	Microangiopathy	Atherosclerosis

The importance in recognizing the two types is in the prognosis and type of treatment. A considerable proportion of patients may not readily be placed in either category at the time of diagnosis.

AETIOLOGY

The causes of both types of diabetes are far from completely known but there is increasing evidence that heredity and environment play an important part. Their roles, together with other factors, vary in the two types.

In IDDM (Type 1) only about 25 per cent of the offspring of two diabetic parents are likely to develop the condition, assuming average life expectancy. If one identical twin under the age of 45 develops IDDM, there is only a 50 per cent chance of the other developing the disease. A diabetes-susceptibility gene has recently been discovered associated with HLA genes. The immune response is almost certainly a component in the aetiology as it has been shown that circulating islet cell antibodies are present for some time before the disease develops. Viral infection seems to be the link between genetic susceptibility and the immune response which ultimately damages the β-cell. A significant environmental component must also exist, so the clinical importance of identifying susceptible people becomes evident as a means of protecting them from the diabetes-producing elements in their environment.

In NIDDM (Type 2) diabetes genetic susceptibility plays a more definite part. If an identical twin over 45 develops NIDDM the other will always develop it, for example. Family history is stronger in the non-obese type of patient. Environmental factors are important as evidenced by a sometimes huge increase in diabetes when a population changes habitat. Natural ageing with resultant loss of β-cell responsiveness is a cause. Obesity, both in degree and duration, is an important trigger in the already susceptible individual: 60–80 per cent non-insulin-dependent diabetics are obese.

PATHOLOGY

In IDDM there is failure of the β-cells of the islets of Langerhans to produce insulin and there is also loss of the cells themselves. In NIDDM the pathology is different. The insulin response is reduced or inappropriate or both. In addition there is loss of sensitivity of the peripheral tissues to the action of circulating insulin. Where there is genetic weakness of the β-cells, persistent demand for excess insulin exhausts them, leading to hyperglycaemia. Weight reduction of itself reduces the demand and the β-cells may then cope.

NATURAL HISTORY

Diabetes can become a distressing condition. Diabetic retinopathy is the commonest single cause of blindness in the middle-aged. Myocardial infarction and cerebrovascular accidents are much more severe and occur twice as often in the diabetic, especially the diabetic woman, as in the general population. Gangrene of the foot is more frequent and can occur at an early age. Renal disease and neuropathy may become chronic sources of particular misery for many diabetics. The effect of improved medical care on the long-term prognosis remains uncertain, although there is some suggestion that microvascular disease, leading to retinopathy, neuropathy, and nephropathy, is related to the duration and level of hyperglycaemia. The answer to this last point will not be found until a much closer approach to physiological normality can be found in the diabetic. Large vessel disease may be partly an accompaniment, influenced by such factors as smoking and blood lipid levels, rather than a direct consequence of the disease. It is much less common in populations normally taking a diet high in unrefined carbohydrate and low in total fat, although still slightly more often found in diabetics in that population.

CLINICAL FEATURES

Diabetes is not abrupt in onset. It takes many weeks to develop in the younger patient and may be asymptomatic in the older patient for many months and even years. Almost 20 per cent of patients present with symptoms of complications. In children and young adults the symptoms are thirst, polyuria, weight loss, and lethargy. Only in about one-third of patients are these symptoms severe enough to be termed 'classical'. Secondary nocturnal enuresis in children is an important presentation. All the symptoms are progressive and persistent if left untreated.

In middle-aged adults the symptoms are less intense and often intermittent, precipitated by overeating and relative inactivity. They are as for younger diabetics, but additionally, weight loss in isolation, pruritis vulvae in women and occasional balanitis in men, changes in visual acuity, paraesthesiae, aching calves and muscle cramps may occur.

There may be no abnormal physical signs or the patient may look ill and wasted and may have vulvitis or balanitis. Obesity may be an obvious sign in the older patient, or the only signs may be those due to complications. It is worth remembering that diabetes has replaced syphilis as the great mimic.

DIAGNOSIS

The diagnosis of diabetes is usually simple in a suspect and is based on the clinical features, the presence of glycosuria and the finding of hyperglycaemia. The first two findings may, however, be absent, leaving hyperglycaemia as the constant diagnostic characteristic.

Urine testing with Diastix, which is specific for glucose, will reveal significant glycosuria if the plasma glucose is above about 9 or 10 mmol/l. Diastix is easier to use than Clinitest. Ketodiastix will detect the presence of ketones in the urine also. In the young, glycosuria may be due to a lowered renal threshold for sugar in a non-diabetic. This is rare in the older patient because the renal threshold rises with age, therefore hyperglycaemia without glycosuria can be a diagnostic and management pitfall. Postprandial rather than fasting urines should be the ones tested in older patients. In all patients, even with significant glycosuria, the diagnosis of diabetes should always be confirmed by a blood test. In a symptomatic patient a random plasma glucose above 11 mmol/l or a truly fasting plasma glucose above 8 mmol/l are diagnostic of unequivocal diabetes. In the asymptomatic patient it is vital to obtain two abnormal values before making the diagnosis, with its far reaching implications, as laboratory errors are by no means unknown.

A random plasma glucose of 8 mmol/l or below or a fasting plasma glucose of 6 mmol/l or below can be taken as normal. Only if the findings are equivocal, if the pregnant patient develops glycosuria or in the exclusion or follow up of impaired glucose tolerance need an oral glucose tolerance test (OGTT) be carried out.

In the simplified version of the test 75 g of glucose is given to the non-fasting patient and the plasma glucose is measured two hours later. If the value is 6.1 mmol/l or below, the patient is normal. If the figure is above 11.9 mmol/l the diagnosis is unequivocal. If the figures fall between the values, the standard OGTT is required. For this, 75 g of glucose is given to the overnight fasting patient, who will have taken his normal diet for the preceding few days, and blood is taken fasting and two hours after the load. The figures for venous plasma are quoted in Table 7.2 and Fig. 7.1, those for whole venous blood and capillary blood are about 15 per cent lower.

Table 7.2. *Standard oral glucose tolerance test*

	Diabetes	IGT	Normal
Fasting	> 8 mmol/l	< 8 mmol/l	< 6 mmol/l
After two hours	> 11 mmol/l	8–11 mmol/l	< 7 mmol/l

After Keen (1981).

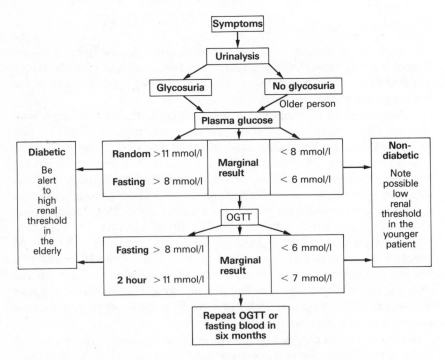

Fig. 7.1. Suggested diagnostic flow chart. (After Brown (1978).)

If the OGTT suggests impaired glucose tolerance it should be repeated in six months and at intervals thereafter, as there is an increased likelihood of the eventual development of diabetes in such a patient (the more so the higher the plasma glucose is above 8 mmol/l), although monitoring the fasting plasma levels in such a patient may be a cheaper and easier alternative in general practice.

COMPLICATIONS

1. Infection – there is an increased incidence of infection, especially of the skin, mainly candidal, and, possibly, staphylococcal.

2. Obliterative arterial disease – this presents in the lower limbs with intermittent claudication, cold feet, absent pulses, sepsis, and ulceration.

3. Neuropathy – damage to peripheral nerves is common in diabetes. Symptomatic neuropathy occurs in about one in eight diabetics. The common findings are numbness and tingling in the feet. If in the hands, carpal tunnel syndrome, which is common in diabetics, should be suspected. Pressure ulcers on the soles of the feet may occur, as well as muscular weakness and wasting, patchy loss of sensation, absent ankle jerks, loss of vibration sense, painless bone destruction ('Charcot joint') in the feet, and erectile impotence in men.

4. Retinopathy and cataract – 14 per cent of all new blind registrations are due to diabetic retinopathy, whose features include: (i) background retinopathy involving all the elements of the vascular tree – the arteries, veins and capillaries: it is seen as micro-aneurysms, venous dilatation, haemorrhages, soft and hard exudates; (ii) proliferative retinopathy, which is a later manifestation – new vessel formation is often followed by retinitis proliferans.

5. Renal disease – diabetes damages glomerular capillaries and arterioles, giving rise to proteinuria, impaired renal function and hypertension. The microvascular lesions produce renal ischaemia which, combined with neuropathic damage to bladder and ureters, predispose to lower and upper urinary tract infection.

6. Coronary and cerebral arterial disease – this is due to increased atherosclerosis accompanying diabetes, thus producing a higher risk of coronary and cerebral infarction. The coronary risks, particularly in women, are significantly increased. Myocardial infarction may well be painless, as a result of neuropathic changes, and will upset diabetic control. The achievement of normoglycaemia seems to have little effect on the coronary risk.

7. Hyperlipidaemia – many diabetics have raised triglyceride but average cholesterol levels are only slightly higher than in non-diabetics. It is probably contributory to increased atherosclerosis and usually responds as IDDM comes under control, but not necessarily in NIDDM.

8. Large babies and increased fetal mortality – the dangers to the fetus are in the last few weeks of pregnancy, when it may become large and plethoric, and shortly after birth. Neonatal deaths are due more to metabolic disturbance and

congenital abnormality, rather than hyaline membrane disease, which is now much less common as a result of better diabetic care.

9. Comas in diabetes
(a) Hypoglycaemia
(b) Hyperglycaemia – there are three types, ketoacidosis, hyperosmolar, and lactic acidosis. Hyperosmolar coma is uncommon, is characterized by very high plasma glucose in the absence of ketosis and tends to occur in the older patient, who may have impaired renal function and be taking diuretics or be given sweet drinks. Lactic acidosis is clinically important in patients taking biguanides, especially phenformin. Additional factors are renal and hepatic impairment, trauma, or severe illness. The plasma glucose may be normal. There is no effective treatment and the mortality is 50 per cent. The distinction between hypoglycaemia and the commonest of the hyperglycaemic comas, ketoacidosis (with a mortality of 5–25 per cent), is vital (see Table 7.3).

PROGNOSIS

The prognosis depends very much on complications, but on average, life expectancy may be reduced, the amount being dependent on the age at onset. The younger the age at onset, the greater the reduction in life expectancy. Later years may be clouded by failing vision or the other degenerative changes already described, but before the advent of insulin treatment, the outlook for children could be measured in weeks and months. Diabetic women usually have healthy children. In older patients, diabetes increases the dangers of myocardial infarction and arterial insufficiency. The major risk in the elderly is vascular disease, but maculopathy and cataract are also prominent. Even mild diabetics,

Table 7.3. *Comas in diabetes*

	Hypoglycaemia	Ketoacidosis
Onset	Previously well, sudden	Gradual: thirst, polyuria, vomiting, infection
Skin	Warm, normal or moist	Dry and cold
Tongue	Moist	Dry and shrivelled
Pulse	Normal or bounding	Thin and rapid
Blood pressure	Normal	Usually low
Breathing	Normal	Deep and sighing – 'Kussmaul'
Breath	Normal	Smells of acetone
Urine	Sugar – little or none	Sugar – + +
	Acetone – absent	Acetone – + + +
Blood glucose*	< 2 mmol/l	> 13 mmol/l
Treatment	i.v. dextrose	i.v. saline and electrolytes
	i.m. glucagon	Insulin
	Sugar by mouth	Always in hospital
	Usually at home	

*Using Dextrostix with or without meter, or BM-Glycemie 20–800 strips.

or those 'well controlled', are not always spared the ravages of severe degenerative disease.

IMPACT OF DIABETES

The reaction of the patient on being told he has diabetes is fear, bred by
ignorance. From their different standpoints, all those involved, parents,
teachers, employers, insurance companies, and even doctors, view the illness
with apprehension. Patients are usually afraid of the effect diabetes will have
on their everyday lives, such as employment, recreation, travel, food, having
children, going into a coma, developing gangrene, and becoming blind. Family
doctors often tend to reinforce the patient's sense of being 'abnormal' by
hastily abdicating the routine care of such individuals to the hospital.

The parents of the diabetic child, when first told the diagnosis, are often
appalled at the prospects for their child and the implications for them managing
the illness, the diet, the insulin injections and the task of achieving control. All
too often they are given confusing advice and conflicting goals making it well
nigh impossible for them to cope. The child, feeling himself to be 'different'
may find it very hard to accept the dietary restrictions, the insulin injections
and the urine testing, leading to difficulties at school and play.

Unless carefully handled the emotionally vulnerable adolescent may present
many problems. He feels prevented by his illness from merging with his peer
group, from abandoning regular, calculated meals and from eating 'teenage'
foods. His concern about his body and image, his delayed physical maturity
and his constant reminders that he is 'defective' in some way or another,
increase his resentment at being examined, having blood tests and, worse still,
urine tests. His desire to deny the disease or use it to manipulate his emotional
environment often results in poor control and repeated hospital admissions,
which tend to disrupt the patient's daily life, schooling, and employment.
Childhood fears of injections may be behind him or her, but new fears about
the future, sex and contraception open up, usually inadequately dealt with by
an unfamiliar overworked junior doctor at the clinic. The medical emergency in
these patients is often a cry for help, a social emergency in disguise.

The diabetic adult also has to cope with many restrictions. He has to pay a
higher life insurance premium, he has to spend significantly more on his diet,
although his drugs and equipment are free of charge. His choice of job is limited,
especially if taking insulin. He is barred from flying aircraft, active service in
the Armed Forces, or driving public service vehicles, and heavy goods vehicle
licences are only obtained with the greatest difficulty. Jobs involving heights
and shift work are inadvisable. Loss of visual acuity in later life may lead to
pressure for premature retirement. Every diabetic driver has to inform the
Driver and Vehicle Licensing Centre and his insurers as soon as he is diagnosed.
Failure to do so constitutes an offence and invalidates his insurance policy.
Even those sufferers not taking insulin or oral hypoglycaemic agents are

included. Driving licences will be issued for limited periods at a time only. Impotence is the man's great fear, and, once established, difficult to overcome. Fear of passing on the disease may inhibit couples from embarking upon having a family. Oral contraception may require an increase in insulin requirements.

Diabetes is a chronic illness in which appropriate and proper treatment may well improve the quality of life. Clearly, this involves general practitioners, specialist nurses, health visitors, district nurses as well as hospital doctors and paramedical staff. Above all, it must involve the co-operation and understanding of the patient and his family.

Society's attitude to the diabetic is still negative. Too little is done to enable him to lead a normal life, too many restrictions are imposed beyond the need to protect him and others from the consequences of a hypoglycaemic attack. In terms of driving, employment, recreation, and travel each case should be assessed on its merits.

General practice with the primary care team provides the ideal environment for the management, supervision, and counselling of the diabetic. The average general practitioner with his 30 or so diabetics often needs to make a conscious decision to overcome his misgivings about his competence to cope. The temptation to hand over the patient to the impersonal, busy, and harassed hospital diabetic clinic is great.

Every Health District should have a phsyician with a special interest and training in diabetes, providing a service to the hospital and the community. The hospital clinic which he supervises should be the focus for specialist treatment of diabetes and a centre for the education of staff and patients. Certain categories of patient must be referred for an initial assessment, but few should continue to attend for follow up. As well as the consultant, the clinic staff comprises junior doctors, nurses, dietician, chiropodist, technician, and diabetic liaison nurse or health visitor who work with the patient at home and reinforce the lessons learnt. The services of the dietician and the chiropodist are being incorporated in health centres and surgeries in some localities.

UNDERSTANDING THE DISEASE

At the time of diagnosis the patient is often in no fit state to take in the flood of information given him on diet, urine testing, tablets, and injections. He is still bewildered by his fears and if he is to take the necessary major part in managing his disease, he must be painstakingly educated to improve his confidence and raise his morale. In a proportion of patients this process begins in the hospital clinic or ward and is continued by the primary care team at home. The majority of newly diagnosed diabetics will be entirely managed by the general practitioner and his team. Many of these patients will have relatively few symptoms and will deem the limitations of the disease unjustified. They probably need more encouragement and explanation to achieve co-operation in management than the patients with more marked symptoms.

The British Diabetic Association was founded in 1934 to provide mutual aid and assistance and to promote the study, the diffusion of knowledge and the proper treatment of diabetics. It has over 150 branches and clubs and membership is open to anyone interested in supporting the Association's aims. It publishes a bimonthly journal, advisory leaflets and books on cookery and diets. In addition it provides advice on diet, employment, insurance, travel, holiday, and diabetic aids. Branches organize social, fund-raising, and welfare events. The Association organizes supervized holidays and camps for diabetic children. It promotes the education of the general public, diabetics themselves and professionals, as well as supporting medical, scientific, and social research. All patients, and those doctors concerned with diabetes should join the Association.

MANAGEMENT

General principles

The aims of long term management are:
1. To establish and maintain normoglycaemia.
2. To achieve and maintain the patient's well being.
3. To minimize the severity and delay the onset of complications.
4. To increase the patient's understanding of his illness and participation in its management.

Most patients with diabetes can be managed entirely by their general practitioners, with the exception of the unstable Type 1 (IDDM) patient, children, pregnant women. Only the pregnant woman will need entirely specialist supervision, whereas in the other two groups it may effectively be shared. Integrated care has become quite highly developed in several places abroad and in one or two centres in this country. Good communications and uniform objectives are crucial to the success of such a scheme. A specially trained diabetic liaison nurse or health visitor, together with the use of some sort of co-operation card, can forge strong links between the primary care team, the patient and his family, and the hospital.

The general practitioner needs to be aware of the anxieties, the ignorance and the emotional problems of the diabetic patient and to use all his skills, together with those of the other members of the primary care team, to handle them. Awareness of the resources available to the patient and the health care teams, such as free prescriptions, supplementary benefit, local hospital services (including chiropody and the dietician), social services and voluntary agencies, is most important.

DIET

Diets must be simple, acceptable, and tailored to the patient's needs and preferences. Artificial sweeteners such as saccharin are helpful, but 'diabetic' foods containing sorbitol can cause gastro-intestinal disturbances and weight gain, are expensive and divert attention from dietary goals.

Type 1 diabetics should have enough food to maintain growth, weight, and energy appropriate to their age, height, sex, and degree of physical activity. The carbohydrate in the food should be as unrefined as possible, with a high proportion of fibre, and must be eaten throughout the day in relation to insulin treatment to prevent hypoglycaemic attacks. There is no justification for the so-called 'free diet' which makes control in adult life more difficult. Animal fats should be replaced with appropriate vegetable oils.

Type 2 diabetics ought to have a regime with an energy (calorie) intake designed to achieve and maintain the desired weight for their height. Of this, the carbohydrate content, in unrefined form with a high proportion of fibre, should be over 60 per cent, which implies a significantly proportionate reduction in the energy derived from fat.

DRUGS

Insulin

This is required in patients who produce no endogenous insulin, in children and young adults, those who have significant ketosis at any age, those who fail to respond to oral agents (albeit temporarily) and those who are pregnant and not controlled by diet alone. Insulin is prepared commercially from beef and pork. The former is more antigenic, interfering with its effectiveness. The differences in insulin are length of action, acidity, and animal source. All preparations were available in two strengths, 40 units per millilitre and 80 units per millilitre and are supplied in 10 ml containers. Soluble insulin BP is also available as 20 units per millilitre and 320 units per millilitre. In March 1983 the

Table 7.4. *Common types of insulin available*

Action	Duration	Insulin	Brand
Early- and short-acting	½–8 h (peak 2–4 h)	Insulin BP Neutral insulin BP	Soluble Actrapid MC Velosulin Neusulin
Medium-acting	1–20 h (peak 6–12 h)	Isophane insulin BP Globin Zinc BP Biphasic insulin BP	Neuphane Globin Rapitard MC Mixtard 30/70 Initard 50/50
Long-acting with delayed onset	4–30 h (peak 10–20 h)	Insulin zinc suspension BP	Neulente Insulatard Monotard MC Ultratard MC
		Protamine zinc insulin BP	PZI

replacement of these insulins by highly purified 100 units per millilitre strength began, the purpose being to reduce the confusion and dangers accompanying the previous practice of having two insulin strengths administered from a syringe originally designed for neither. Insulin 100 units per millilitre (U100) has been successfully in use in various parts of the world. Specially manufactured 0.5 millilitre and 1.0 millilitre syringes (holding a maximum of 50 units and 100 units of U100 respectively) are available. The smaller syringe has a graduation line for each unit, the larger for every two units. The conversion and patient instruction process will be concentrated mainly on hospital diabetic clinics, but many general practitioners will have been involved and may be so for several months to come, particularly in persuading stable diabetics to change to a new regime.

The newly diagnosed diabetic, when well enough, will need to be taught carefully and patiently the skills of self-administration of insulin and the importance of looking after the equipment.

The design of insulin regimes varies from clinic to clinic and awareness of local policy is important to avoid conflict. The majority of insulins fall into one of the three main groups, depending on their action – early and short-acting, medium-acting, and long-acting with delayed onset. There is a very wide selection available and the doctor should become familiar with a few in each group. Better control is achieved with twice daily insulin and is especially important in children, where long-term good control promotes normal growth and development and reduces the risks of degenerative changes, also in pregnancy, where it improves the chances of a healthy baby and in unstable, ketosis-prone patients. If two injections of short-acting insulin (one before breakfast and one before the evening meal) lead to uneven control, then part of the dose may be replaced by using a medium-acting preparation. Alternatively a long-acting insulin given later in the day and a short-acting preparation super-imposed twice daily may be used. It is important to tailor every patient's regime individually to control the plasma glucose and to avoid hypoglycaemis attacks, but, broadly speaking, two-thirds of the daily dose is given in the morning. Single-dose regimes have a place in those on less than 32 units of insulin daily, in the elderly and in those who would not comply with more frequent injections. Some non-insulin-dependent diabetics, in whom diet and full doses of oral agents have failed to achieve optimum control, may be helped by a small daily dose of a very long acting insulin. This helps the β-cells to recover partially and cope with the intermittent demand made by meals.

Highly purified (HP) and monocomponent (MC) insulins are produced by a process of ultra-refining pork insulin to isolate a pure product. Insulin antibodies barely develop and local allergic reactions are uncommon. Patients who are well controlled and have few side-effects should not be changed from the older type of insulin to a highly purified preparation needlessly, but if this is con-templated great care must be taken to prevent serious hypoglycaemia. The new requirements will be at least 20 per cent less generally to begin with, and may well continue to fall in ensuing weeks as the antibody levels fall. This is the more so, the higher the initial dose of insulin.

It is probably better to admit to hospital any patient starting insulin, where more intensive education, including how to cope with a hypoglycaemic attack, can be provided.

Progress is being made towards producing means of injecting insulin in a more physiological way by the use of continuous drive syringes which respond to alterations in the plasma glucose. The problems in the manufacture of these and in synthetic transplantation have yet to be overcome. This should not deflect attention and effort from the available methods of improving control.

Oral hypoglycaemic agents

These are indicated in the Type 2 diabetic, in the absence of significant ketosis, who fails to respond to diet alone. There are two main types: (i) **Sulphonylureas** – which stimulate insulin production and enhance its effects on lowering plasma glucose. They are ineffective in the absence of endogenous insulin (IDDM). They may cause hypoglycaemia and weight gain but are, in general, well tolerated. The longer-acting preparations may cause devastating hypoglycaemic attacks which are difficult to correct and should therefore be avoided in the elderly or those who may miss or delay meals. They may need to be used quite early in the non-obese patient whose weight continues to fall.(ii) **Biguanides** –

Table 7.5. *Some oral hypoglycaemic agents*

Group	Name	Daily dosage
Sulphonylureas	Tolbutamide	1.5–3 g daily in three divided doses
	Chlorpropamide	100–750 mg once daily
	Glibenclamide	5–25 mg daily in one or two doses
Biguanides	Metformin	500 mg–3 g daily in divided doses

which delay absorption of glucose from the bowel, inhibit hepatic gluconeo-genesis and increase peripheral uptake of glucose. They may cause gastro-intestinal disturbance and irreversible lactic acidosis. The latter is especially true of phenformin, in the elderly and in patients with impaired renal function. There is often a useful decrease in weight.

FACTORS INFLUENCING MANAGEMENT

1. Weight – this must be brought to the desirable level for the patient's age and height.

2. Infections and illness – these must be prevented wherever possible and treated vigorously. Influenza vaccination should be encouraged. Medication may need to be temporarily increased, and those Type 2 patients only just controlled on full doses of oral agents may need to have insulin temporarily if

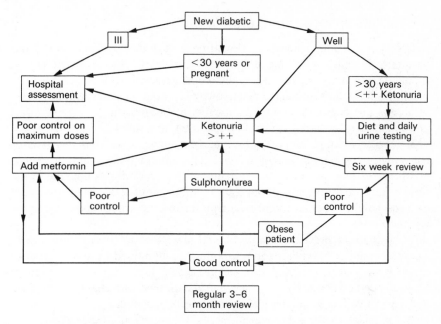

Fig. 7.2. Management plan flow-chart for diabetics. (After Brown (1978).)

seriously ill. Insulin must never be reduced if an ill patient is not eating properly or is vomiting. The carbohydrate intake must be maintained in palatable form such as high-carbohydrate drinks, etc.

3. Effects of certain drugs and alcohol – the latter, together with β-adrenergic blockers and monoamine oxidase inhibitors may cause hypoglycaemia. Corticosteroids and diuretics, especially thiazides, may cause hyperglycaemia.

4. Omitting or delaying meals and inadequate dietary adjustment for increased physical activity may cause hypoglycaemia in patients on insulin or sulphonylureas.

5. Monitoring control – with the advent of relatively cheap home glucose monitoring meters the Type 1 diabetic has a more readily accurate means of improving control without the constant and understandable fear of hypoglycaemic attacks.

The sporadic measurement of plasma glucose by the clinic or the general practitioner is a poor index of long-term control. In some centres haemoglobin A_1c estimations are available and give helpful indications of the level of control over the preceding two months or so. Hyperglycaemia modifies haemoglobin A at a constant rate during the lifetime of the red blood cell, with the formulation of haemoglobin A_1c. This normally accounts for only 3–6 per cent of total haemoglobin, but is increased three- or fourfold in poorly controlled diabetics.

MANAGEMENT OF COMPLICATIONS

1. Hypoglycaemia – oral sugar should be used in the conscious patient but intramuscular glucagon 1 mg or intravenous dextrose 50 mg, given slowly, should be used in the inconscious or unco-operative patient. Patients should be taught to avoid hypoglycaemic reactions by knowing the early warning signs, by always carrying sugar and taking it early, by not delaying or missing meals and by taking extra carbohydrate if unduly exerting themselves.

2. Hyperglycaemic coma of any type (see above) – to avoid this type of coma, patients should be taught to increase the amount of insulin, if necessary, and never to omit an injection, to maintain their carbohydrate intake in the form of glucose drinks (e.g. about eight fluid ounces of 'Lucozade' contain 50 g glucose) and to obtain prompt treatment for infections and illness. Vomiting is a danger sign.

3. Pregnancy – pregnant women should always be referred to hospital as early as possible. Meticulous control, preferably monitored by a home glucose meter, is vital, using insulin, but never oral agents, if diet alone is not enough. Close co-operation between the obstetrician and the physician must be maintained and the baby will need initial care in a special care baby unit.

4. Vascular disease – the patient needs to be asked about intermittent claudication and smoking. The feet must be examined regularly, the points to look for being the shape of the feet and ankles, the texture and colour of the skin (which may be pale and hairless over the legs), the presence or absence of the peripheral pulses, excess callosities and ulceration. There are three phases of management. The first is the prophylactic phase when the patient is carefully educated in a regime of care and strongly advised to stop smoking. He should inspect his feet daily and report any inflammation or ulceration at once. He must ensure the cleanliness of his feet, socks or stockings and wear soft socks and well-fitting shoes which should be inspected daily for pebbles or protruding nails, etc. Extremes of heat and cold should be avoided and he should never walk barefoot. He should be seen regularly by an experienced chiropodist who will treat any callosities. The Society of Chriropodists produce a useful leaflet for patients 'Care of the feet for diabetics'. The second, conservative, phase involves rest, relief of pressure, antibiotics, adequate analgesia, careful explanation, and surgical footwear for any fixed deformities of the feet. Referral to a vascular surgeon in resistant cases may be appropriate at this point in case the third, operative, phase, involving drainage procedures or amputation, becomes necessary. In all cases blood lipids should be checked regularly and, if raised, be reduced and controlled.

5. Diabetic renal disease – is more common in the Type 1 diabetic. The presence of oedema should be looked for and the urine should be checked for protein at each visit. Urea and creatinine should be checked regularly. Treatment is symptomatic and comprises diuretics for oedema, reduced protein intake and extra care with drugs if renal function is significantly impaired, hypotensives for hypertension and chemotherapy for urinary tract infection.

6. Diabetic neuropathy – which leads to widespread disorders of limbs and viscera. Features to look for include pain and paraesthesiae, numbness, and tenderness in the feet, aching calves with wasting, loss of sensation, painless trophic ulcers on the soles of the feet, absent or diminished reflexes, sudden monoeuropathies (e.g. squints or diplopia with rapid recovery), stasis of urine in the bladder, delayed stomach emptying (vomiting), nocturnal diarrhoea, and, in men, loss of erectile potency. Good control of diabetes often leads to an improvement in symptoms. Particularly careful and sympathetic counselling is needed with the impotent patient.

7. Diabetic retinopathy – photocoagulation in the form of the xenon arc and the argon laser has revolutionized the outlook for the sight of these patients. Vitrectomy may restore some sight to previously virtually blind patients. Nevertheless, early diagnosis and treatment are vital if improved results are to be achieved. Visual acuity (using Snellen's type and maybe a pin-hole) and the fundi (with the pupils dilated by a short-acting preparation, such as tropicamide 0.5–1 per cent) should be checked regularly. Patients must be warned about the effects of the drops on their vision and told to wear dark glasses for the next few hours. The management plan should embody the following principles: (i) 30 years or younger at diagnosis – refer to hospital; (ii) 30–40 years at diagnosis with IDDM – refer to hospital; (iii) 40 years or older at diagnosis – see Table 7.6

Table 7.6. *The eye in the diabetic*

Retinopathy	Visual acuity	Action	Follow up
Absent	6/6–6/9	Nil	Check visual acuity annually, when reduced, check fundi, – if no retinopathy ⟶ optician – if retinopathy → ophthalmologist Check fundi five yearly
Absent	Worse than 6/9	Send to optician, if no better → ophthalmologist	Examine fundi five yearly
Present but mild or minimal	6/6–6/9	Nil	Check visual acuity and fundi after six months – if both worse ⟶ ophthalmologist – if visual acuity same and retinopathy no worse ⟶ check annually retinopathy same ⟶ ophthalmologist
Proliferative or preproliferative	6/6–6/9	Send to ophthalmologist	At hospital eye department
Present (mild or severe)	Worse than 6/9	Send to ophthalmologist	At hospital eye department

After British Diabetic Association guidelines.

ORGANIZATION AND DELIVERY OF CARE

The satisfactory organization of care must involve the entire practice team – doctors, nurses, health visitors, reception staff, and, if at all possible, the dietician.

The first step is to identify the diabetics in the practice – often a difficult job and done by memory (the least accurate), flagging the records using the age/sex register, using a diagnostic register and a computer. The size of the problem can now be assessed. The next step is to determine the nature of the problem, in terms of accuracy and completeness of data in the patient's record. At this stage it has to be gone through and compared with the following checklist – length of history, diet and type of treatment, measurements of weight, urine and plasma glucose, and evidence of checks for complications and appropriate action. Armed with this information regarding his current practice, the doctor knows what needs improving in the organization.

A carefully planned **diabetic clinic** in general practice provides the advantages of the hospital yet avoids most pitfalls. It brings together all personnel involved in the familiar environment of the consulting room, and at a time when the unpredictable pressures of general practice are less likely to influence the standard of follow up needed. At every follow up visit a suitably trained nurse sees the patient initially, asks about general health and symptoms, carries out the tests and measurements and much of the examination, leaving the doctor to do only the more specialized tasks and thus allow him more time with the patient. At annual review she would prepare the patient for fuller examination and tests. A meter for measuring plasma glucose on the premises, enabling immediate changes in management to be made, is highly desirable. Further follow up appointments are usually made before the patient leaves, enabling easier identification and recall of defaulters. Diabetes is a chronic illness requiring entries in the ordinary medical record spread over many pages, militating against their effectiveness. Despite adding further to the number of sheets in the notes, a **flow chart** is most helpful. This contains details of the illness from the beginning on one, two or, at the most, three consecutive pages. Initial data recorded would include complete identification of the patient, occupation, marital state, whether or not a smoker, age or year of onset, presenting complaint, dietary history, current and past medication, changes in weight and visual acuity, symptoms of angina, claudication, paraesthesiae, or feet problems. A family history would be sought. The initial examination would include height, weight, blood pressure, visual acuity, the fundi, signs of heart failure or renal damage, the state of the skin and peripheral circulation and a neurological assessment. Initial investigations might include an OGTT (if appropriate), full blood count, plasma glucose, urea and creatinine, lipid profile, urine analysis for sugar, protein, ketosis and infection, chest X-ray, and, in a patient with suspected angina, an electrocardiogram. At this point an outline management plan should be recorded. The remainder of the flow chart will contain follow up data, recorded at each visit, such as the date, time, weight, plasma glucose, urine sugar, protein and ketones, dietary changes, medication changes, general comments, and interval to next appointment. Periodic, usually annual, review details such as blood pressure, state of the peripheral pulses, reflexes, condition of the feet and fundi, visual acuity, urea and cholesterol are also entered. The target weight recorded in a prominent place and a short action check list (such as referral to the health visitor, dietician and chiropodist, advice regarding entitlements, influenza vaccination, and information about the British Diabetic Association) are useful prompts, facilitating audit.

MEASURING THE QUALITY OF CARE

In deciding what to measure, one returns to the general principles stated earlier. The difficulty lies in defining what is 'good' or 'acceptable' care and needs to be done in personal, biochemical, and social terms. One practice (Kratky 1977) looked at the regularity of follow up and at the objectives of each consultation under four headings – provision of adequate symptom relief, provision of adequate biochemical control, detection of complications and advice about diet, dentistry, chiropody, and joining the British Diabetic Association. Improvement was found to be needed in regularity of follow up, in the tendency for the Type 1 diabetics to be looked after by the hospital, in advice to patients, in detecting complications, in ensuring regular biochemical monitoring and in recording information regularly in an easily discernible way. The proposed changes included designing an effective recall system, designing an effective follow up chart and combining the efforts of the primary care team to provide more effective examination, measurement and recording procedures and advice to the patient. The process described seems to be an acceptable audit protocol and worthy of general adoption.

'Diabetes mellitus is an ideal condition for the general practitioner to manage. It is often seen, very easily diagnosed, and has a lifelong course that affects several systems; its management is rational and rewarding and usually within the competence of the GP' (Ruben 1976).

PERFORMANCE REVIEW CHECK LIST

General

1. Can the practice identify all its diabetic patients?
2. Does the practice have a policy for the detection and general management of diabetes?
3. Can the practice identify all patients scheduled for influenza immunisation?

Patients on treatment

1. Is it clear from the records on what basis the diagnosis was made?
2. How many of the following were recorded at initial assessment: smoking habits, presenting symptoms, family history?
3. How many of the following have been recorded at initial or subsequent assessments: fasting plasma glucose, blood pressure, dietary details, weight,

visual acuity, fundal appearances, examination of feet, reflexes, urinanalysis (for protein, sugar and ketones), influenza immunization.
4. Is there any record of the patient's ideas or the information given to the patient?
5. Are the current drugs and dosage clearly recorded?
6. What proportion of patients on treatment have fasting plasma glucose levels above 6 mmol/l or random levels above 11 mmol/l?
7. How many patients are members of the British Diabetic Association?

Emergencies

1. Does the practice have a policy for the management of hyperglycaemic or hypoglycaemic coma?
2. Is there a record of patient instructions on what may make their diabetes go out of control and what to do?

PATIENTS' ASSOCIATION

The British Diabetic Association,
10 Queen Anne Street,
London W1M 0BD,
Telephone: 01-323-1531.

BOOKS AND LEAFLETS

Balance published by BDA
Dietary exchange leaflets (BDA)
Cookery books (BDA)
Urine testing book (BDA and Ames Laboratories)
Care of the feet for diabetics published by
Society of Chriopodists,
8 Wimpole Street,
London W1M 8BX
Telephone: 01-580-3228

REFERENCES

Brown, K. G. E. (1978). Diabetes – clinical and biochemical characteristics. *Update* **16**, 55–63.
Brown, K. G. E. (1978). Diabetes – management. *Update*, **16**, 343–6.
Garvie, D. G. (1981). Diabetes mellitus: care in general practice. *Geriatric Medicine* (May) 46–51.
Ireland, J. T., Thomson, W. S. T., and Williamson, J. (1980). *Diabetes today.* H. M. +M., Publishers Ltd., Aylesbury.
Jackson, M. (1981). Diabetes mellitus: the health visitor's role. *Geriatric Medicine* (June), 42–7.
Jarrett, J. and Keen, H. (1981). Management of diabetes. Medicine International, **1**, 330–3.

Keen, H. (1981). The nature of the diabetes syndrome. *Medicine International,* 1, 327–9.
Kratky, A. P. (1977). An audit of the care of diabetics in one general practice. *J. R. Coll. gen. Practrs,* 27, 536-43.
Ruben, L. A. (1976). Diabetes and the general practitioner. *Br. J. hosp. Med.* 241–5.
Simpson, J. E. P. and Levitt, R. (1981). *Going home.* Churchill Livingstone, Edinburgh.

8 Epilepsy

Martin Lawrence

Epilepsy is a condition which has traditionally been treated by most general practitioners by a combination of referral and neglect. But since it is a condition for which both the disease itself and the treatment are liable to produce morbidity, continuing supervision must be essential.

WHY SHOULD WE REVIEW OUR PATIENTS WITH EPILEPSY?

If most GPs were to carry out such a review they would find that many patients had not been seen for several years, and few of them would have had a systematic review of their disease and management. The main problems resulting from this are likely to be:

Polypharmacy – many patients will be on several drugs when one might do.

Drug toxicity – due to incorrect dosage or too many drugs.

Inadequate control of seizures.

Long-term side-effects of drug treatment.

The patient's lack of understanding of his disease – which results in unnecessary unhappiness and often inappropriate behaviour.

Inadequate help and counselling over social problems, for instance work, marriage, and schooling.

INCIDENCE AND PREVALENCE

The size of the task for each general practitioner is not large. The incidence is approximately 5 per 10 000 per year (Hauser and Kurland 1975), so a general practitioner is likely to see only one or two new cases each year. The prevalence is approximately 7 per 1000 in children under 16, and 3.5 per 1000 in adults, so there will only be about four children and seven adults on his list at any one time. When this number is compared to the number of patients with conditions like hypertension or diabetes it can be seen that the task involved in the regular supervision of patients with epilepsy is not a large one.

On the other hand, a difficulty arising from the small number per doctor is that he obtains less experience in managing the condition. This is particularly true of the rarer forms of epilepsy. Most of the general remarks about continuing care made in this chapter will apply to adults with grand mal epilepsy.

DEFINITION

In common with many other chronic 'diseases' – for example diabetes or hypertension – it has become apparent that the label of epilepsy is one which cannot be applied in a simplistic way. We can say that an *epileptic seizure is an abnormal paroxysmal discharge of cerebral neurones* and that *epilepsy is a continuing tendency to epileptic seizures.* (The requirement for 'continuing' tendency is to avoid the label being applied on the basis of a single seizure.) But whether someone who has has two seizures at ten year intervals is 'an epileptic', or when a patient who had many seizures as an adolescent but none since ceases to be 'an epileptic' is a matter of semantics. Indeed anyone can have a seizure if sufficiently provoked, but some people have lower thresholds than others. What is important, especially because of the social penalties with regard to motor driving, is that the label of epilepsy should not be applied loosely.

DIAGNOSIS

A diagnosis of 'epilepsy' cannot be regarded as adequate. First, it is a term which covers a heterogenous range of seizure disorders and so it is important to make the diagnosis much more precise, because the different types of epilepsy are often best managed by different types of treatment. Secondly, the severity of the disease and the degree to which it affects the patient's life may be variable even in patients with the same seizure pattern. A man who has had a grand mal attack every ten years has quite a different problem from one who has several attacks a week despite treatment. A travelling salesman who develops nocturnal epilepsy is affected very differently from a housewife with similar fits.

Epilepsy is indeed a condition which needs to be diagnosed in 'clinical, psychological, and social terms'. It is better to use not a diagnosis, but a diagnostic description, which should include:

1. Type of seizure.
2. Onset, severity, and family history.
3. Present frequency of seizures, on present treatment.
4. Associated disabilities.
5. Precipitating factors.
6. Psychological effects and the patient's understanding of his disease.
7. Social position.

For example, not Mr A. L. is epileptic, but Mr A. L. began having epilepsy at age 51. All his attacks have been when asleep and he had three before being put on treatment. His EEG shows a focal discharge in the right parietal area. He has had no fits for a year while taking phenytoin. He works as a pest control officer and is having great difficulty in managing without his driving licence.

CLASSIFICATION

There have been many advances in the understanding of epilepsy during the past decade, and the classification of the seizure types has become much more logical. The International Classification of Epilepsy as adopted by the WHO is extremely complicated, and such detail need not concern us here. The current view is that seizures should be divided into two main groups. *Generalized* – those with no evidence of focal onset – and *partial* – those which start with one group of neurones. This is a useful division because it helps management – partial seizures are investigated and treated differently from generalized seizures as will be seen below. Partial seizures may evolve to tonic-clonic seizures (sometimes called secondarily generalized seizures), but these are better classified as partial seizures because they are managed in that way.

Generalized seizures	**Partial seizures**
1. Absences (petit mal)	1. Simple partial – no impairment of consciousness
2. Tonic-clonic seizures (grand mal)	2. Complex partial – consciousness impaired, focus (usually) in temporal lobe
3. Less common seizures especially in children (e.g. myoclonic seizures as in infantile spasms)	3. Partial seizures progressing to generalized tonic-clonic convulsions – evidence for focal origin may be clinical (aura) or EEG

Absences—petit mal

This is a condition, almost invariably of children, which usually remits by early adult life, but progresses to grand mal epilepsy in 30 per cent of cases. It is characterized by sudden short 'absences', sometimes associated with 3 per second movements especially of the eyelids. The EEG shows a characteristic 3 per second spike and wave pattern. Petit mal is specific condition and *not* a term for mild epilepsy. It is relatively uncommon, and many cases of suspected petit mal are either due to temporal lobe epilepsy or not due to epilepsy at all. The distinction between petit mal and temporal lobe epilepsy is important. Petit mal absences are short (usually less than 10 seconds) but may be frequent, start and end suddenly, remit in adulthood and are usually easy to treat. Temporal lobe seizures last over 30 seconds, start and end gradually and are often difficult to treat.

Tonic-clonic seizures—grand mal

Grand mal seizures begin with generalized muscular contraction during which the tongue may be bitten and urine passed. Breathing movements cease leading to cyanosis. This is followed by 2–3 minutes of generalized clonic movement, a period of stillness, the resumption of breathing, and return of consciousness with postictal confusion.

Partial seizures

The symptoms depend on the site of the group of neurones in which the seizure originates. Thus the symptoms may be motor (producing a Jacksonian fit), sensory, aphasic, illusional, olfactory, etc. Seizures which do not affect consciousness are called *simple*, but if awareness of reality is impaired the seizure is termed *complex*. Since the focus of a complex partial seizure is usually in the temporal lobe, 'temporal lobe epilepsy' and 'complex partial seizures' are almost synonymous.

Partial seizures progressing to tonic-clonic seizures

The focal discharge of a partial seizure may become generalized and then the patient suffers a tonic-clonic fit preceded by an aura – the aura being the partial seizure. Sometimes the partial seizure may be so brief that the initial symptom is not reported, and the focal origin may be revealed only by EEG. Because of the management and therapeutic implications it is important to identify a focal origin, by description or investigation, in order to distinguish between a seizure which is generalized from the outset and one which has a focal origin.

Treatment will be discussed below, but a simple guide would be:

Generalized seizures
1. Petit mal. Ethosuximide or
      Sodium Valproate
2. Tonic-clonic. Carbamazepine,
      Sodium Valproate,
      or Phenytoin
3. Children's seizures. Usually
      Carmazepine or
      Valproate

Partial seizures
All types. First-choice Carbamazepine
      Second-choice Phenytoin

DIFFERENTIAL DIAGNOSIS

Jeavons (1975) surveyed 470 patients at epilepsy clinics and decided that 20 per cent of them did not suffer from epilepsy. The mistaken diagnosis was most frequently made in cases of vaso vagal syncope and episodes of psychological origin. Other conditions which must be differentiated are cardiac dysrhythmias or Stokes Adams attacks, migraine, and hyperventilation. In children breath-holding attacks and night terrors cause confusion and absences must be distinguished from day-dreaming and masturbation.

Almost all these differentiations can be made on the history alone, and *a history given by the patient or a witness is by far the most important piece of clinical evidence in the diagnosis of epilepsy*. In general the characteristic features of epileptic seizures are:

(i)   *paroxysmal* – sudden onset unrelated to circumstances;
(ii)   *stereotyped* – same sequence of events;
(iii) *precipitating cause* – e.g. time of day, flickering lights, time in menstrual cycle, hypoglycaemia;
(iv)   *out of character*;
(v)   *unease* or *insomnia* prior to an attack;
(vi)   *injury* or *incontinence* during an attack;
(vii) *drowsiness, confusion,* or *amnesia* after an attack.

Despite the apparent distinct differences the differentiation can be difficult, not least becuase anoxia produced by vasovagal syncope, cardiac dysrhythmia or breath holding can induce a convulsion. But a combination of history – in the case of syncope the patient is invariably upright – and if necessary EEG and/or ECG monitoring can elucidate many problems.

INVESTIGATIONS

On the basis of the history, epilepsy may be suspected, or even diagnosed with certainty. The doctor then must decide how much further he need go to confirm the diagnosis or establish a cause.

Certainly the patient needs a full clinical examination. In the majority of cases there will be no physical signs, but occasionally neurological abnormality may be found – usually either some deficit in the same area as the site of focal onset, or evidence of associated retardation. In any such case further investigation will be directed towards the area of neurological deficit.

The two main tools for investigation are EEG and CT scanning. The EEG is probably not as useful as is widely believed. It is useful for identifying a seizure type or confirming a suspected focus. But it is normal between seizures in many cases of epilepsy – about 30 per cent – and abnormal in many patients who do not have seizures. Patients frequently believe that the EEG recording can tell the doctor all he needs to know about their possible fits, and it must be explained to them, preferably before the test is done, that it is not definitive. With the coming of long-term EEG recording systems, (so that the EEG is continually monitored and the patient or observer can record by pressing a button the times when there is an 'event') the value of the EEG has greatly increased, especially in the diagnosis of childrens' absences.

CT scanning is now widely available and a very useful and non-invasive test in the elucidation or exclusion of structural lesions.

In most centres EEG recording and CT scanning are only available on specialist referral – correctly so since they must be expertly interpreted in conjunction with all other clinical evidence. So the general practitioner's decision must be whether his patient requires such referral. Investigations available to the general practitioner, such as blood tests and plain skull X-ray are rarely of value in the diagnosis of adult epilepsy.

It cannot be repeated often enough that the patient's history or the eyewitness account is the most important evidence of all.

MANAGEMENT OF THE NEWLY SUSPECTED OR DIAGNOSED CASE

The Reid report (1970) stated that 'the family doctor will undoubtedly wish to refer the majority of his patients with epilepsy', and the evidence is that most patients presenting with epilepsy are indeed referred. But the evidence is also that many referrals are unnecessary, and that resulting follow-up is erratic.

The reasons for referral must be:

1. To exclude underlying neurological disease or identify a focal cause for the seizures.
2. To reassure the patient.
3. Because the case is difficult to control without specialist help.
4. For team management of a patient with social or multiple disabilities.

It has usually been held that a single non-focal fit in a child or young adult without neurological signs is not an indication for either investigation or treatment. But a high proportion of young adults go on to have further fits and non-invasive tests such as skull X-ray and CT scanning are now available which reassure both doctor and patient that there is at least no intracranial danger.

Neonates can usually be treated by treatment of the cause of the convulsions if that is hypoglycaemia or hypocalcaemia, and no further action is required. Febrile convulsions are usually handled in practice without referral, as described later.

Children with epilepsy usually require referral both for elucidation of seizure type, and to ensure that the disease and treatment interfere as little as possible with their personal development and learning ability. Epilepsy can cause severe learning handicap, as can anticonvulsants, so the paediatric neurology team including an educational psychologist is often invaluable.

Adult-onset epilepsy requires investigation particularly in the case of partial seizures, when a focal lesion must be excluded. Hopkins and Scambler (1977) showed that in a survey of adult epileptics on 17 doctors' lists, 50 per cent had clinical evidence of partial seizures, and 12 per cent more had EEG evidence of focal onset. It seems that fewer and fewer cases of epilepsy will be diagnosed as 'idiopathic' unless they have developed out of child-onset petit mal, and that investigation of all adult-onset epilepsy for a focal cause must be carried out.

Patients who develop epilepsy following a CVA comprise one group of people which will surely become larger and for whom referral is not usually necessary. Although malignancies are commoner in the elderly it is reasonable to assume that the onset of epilepsy in a patient who has recovered from a major stroke is due to infarction scarring. I have no fewer than four on my list, all of whom have responded well to anticonvulsants.

DRUG TREATMENT OF EPILEPSY

This is another area where modern management has made things easier for the general practitioner. Most cases can be well controlled if a few simple guidelines are followed:

1. Treatment should not be started until the diagnosis is beyond doubt, and only exceptionally after a single fit.
2. Only a small range of drugs need be considered.
3. Only one drug should be used if possible – 90 per cent of epileptics can be controlled with one drug, usually carbamazepine or phenytoin.
4. One drug should be introduced at a time, and blood levels monitored.
5. The dosage should be simple – daily or twice daily.
6. Patients must be watched for side-effects and drug toxicity.
7. Drug interactions should be remembered in all prescribing for patients taking anticonvulsants.

These rules are important, and each will be considered in more detail.

Treatment should not be started until the diagnosis is beyond doubt, and only exceptionally after a single fit

It is extremely difficult to remove a chronic disease label once it has been attached. The patient becomes reconciled to his 'label' and is liable to adopt the role, with all the advantages and disadvantages: to question it later may upset an equilibrium. The doctor will become fearful of unmasking convulsions if he were to withdraw treatment, with all the social consequences that may result. The commencement of anticonvulsant treatment is a long-term decision and not to be begun casually: if there is any doubt the patient should be referred before treatment is begun. In particular it is important that a patient is not called epileptic and treated on the basis of a single fit (even though investigation may be begun in some cases) because of the legal and social consequences.

Only a small range of drugs need be considered

Most patients with epilepsy will be controlled on phenytoin, carbamazepine, or sodium valproate. Ethosuximide is still the drug of first choice in petit mal, but such cases will almost certainly have been referred for specialist care.

Carbamazepine

This is a drug which was for a long time avoided for first time use because it was thought to be a frequent cause of bone-marrow dyscrasia. Recent work has shown that this is not so, and indeed that marrow damage is extremely rare. It has few other side-effects, the commonest being dizziness and ataxia, and in particular it is free of serious sedative properties. It is now the first choice of treatment for focal epilepsy in adults and children.

Phenytoin

This is still the usual first choice of treatment for generalized epilepsy. It has the major advantages of a very long half-life which enables it to be prescribed as a single daily dose and it is free of sedation. The major problems with phenytoin are the long-term ones of disfigurement due to gum hyperplasia, hirsutes, and the coarsening of facial features. These side-effects are usually acceptable to adults, particularly in men, but would be best avoided in children if there were an alternative drug. Phenytoin has been suspected of teratogenicity in rare cases. The foetal abnormality rate for epileptic mothers is three times that of the general population (7.5 per cent to 2.7 per cent) but most abnormalities are minor, and the Committee on Safety of Medicine (1973) stated that 'the risk appears to be low and does not justify stopping anticonvulsants where they are necessary for the control of epilepsy'. The other main problem with phenytoin is ataxia due to overdosage, but this is reversible if the dose is reduced immediately.

Phenobarbitone

This is becoming rapidly superseded as an anticonvulsant because of its side-effects of sedation and, especially in children, irritability, hyperactivity, and learning problems. It is also a danger in cases of drug abuse and overdose. If used it can be given as a single night-time dose.

Sodium valproate

For several years after its introduction there were high hopes of valproate being an ideal anticonvulsant. Its relatively short half-life meant rapid attainment of therapeutic drug levels: it is highly effective in all forms of epilepsy, particularly generalized epilepsy, petit mal epilepsy, and febrile convulsion prophylaxis. The only problems which occurred with any frequency were gastric intolerance and alopecia. But it has recently been reported that transaminase levels are (usually transiently) raised in a large number of patients on sodium valproate (*The Lancet* 1980), and over 40 deaths from hepatic failure have been reported during the first six months of treatment (*Drug and Therapeutic Bulletin* 1981). Many of these deaths were in children on multiple therapy and those with severe epilepsy and brain damage are most at risk. Valproate is widely prescribed and such fatal damage is a rare complication of an otherwise fairly non-toxic drug. The manufacturers now recommend routine monitoring of liver function, but it is probably more important to try and avoid the drug in patients with liver disease, monitor those at high risk, and in particular suspect hepatotoxicity in patients who become ill while taking the drug. There are also reports of haemostatic defects, so coagulation tests should be performed prior to dental extractions. The possibility of teratogenicity is not yet resolved.

Only one drug should be used if possible

The usual reason for failure of control of seizures is that the anticonvulsant is not being used in an adequate dose. If one drug is being given in inadequate dose, then the addition of another will not help to control the seizures, but may cause further side-effects.

Moreover many anticonvulsants interact with each other, and the effect of adding a second or third anticonvulsant may be to alter the effect of the first. In particular, phenytoin and carbamazepine reduce the plasma levels of each other: valproate has a variable and unpredictable effect on phenytoin levels, but increases carbamazepine and phenobarbitone levels: and if sulthiame is used it may greatly increase phenytoin levels to the point of toxicity.

With these possible hazards, and the knowledge that over 90 per cent of cases can be controlled with one drug alone it is important to try and achieve that. The facility to measure drug levels gives the physician much greater confidence in prescribing each drug in adequate doses.

One drug should be introduced at a time and blood levels monitored

When treatment is begun the drug of choice should be introduced and the doctor should monitor its effect on the seizure rate. It is important not to regard the blood levels as absolute or in isolation, but it is extremely useful to know the level as an aid to management (see Table 8.1). If seizures are well

Table 8.1. *Properties of anticonvulsants*

	Average maintenance dose (mg)	Therapeutic range (μmol/l)	Usual dosage
Phenytoin	300–400	40–100	Once daily
Phenobarbitone	120	65–170	Once daily
Carbamazepine	600	17–42	Twice daily
Sodium valproate	1800	350–700	Twice daily
Ethosuximide	1000	285–850	Once daily

From Hopkins (1980).

controlled with a level apparently below the therapeutic range there is no reason to change (although one might reconsider the diagnosis). If the patient shows signs of toxicity or intolerance with the drug level in the therapeutic range then a change should be made. But if seizures continue, then, in the absence of side-effects, a drug should not be rejected until levels well into the therapeutic range have been achieved.

Plasma level monitoring is particularly important in the case of phenytoin because its pharmacokinetics are such that, as the dose is increased, the blood

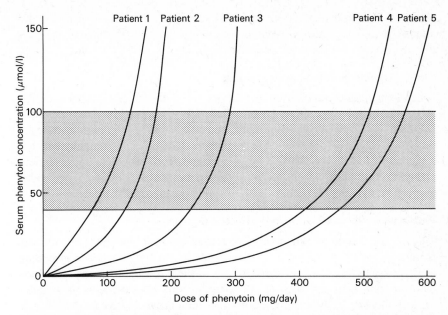

Fig. 8.1. Serum phenytoin levels in five epileptic patients taking various doses of the drug. Note the steeper relationship between serum level and dose as the latter increases. The shaded area indicates the therape range. (From Richens and Dunlop (1975).)

levels rise disproportionately fast. Work done by Richens and Dunlop (1975) shows that in some patients an increase of less than 100 mg can take a patient from subtherapeutic to toxic blood levels (see Fig. 8.1).

Plasma level monitoring can be carried out at any time with phenytoin, carbamazepine, or phenobarbitone; but valproate has a short half-life and blood levels have little meaning except when timed in relation to dose. In any case there is evidence that the anticonvulsant effect of valproate is not directly related to the plasma level – hence its widespread use on a twice-daily basis despite its short half-life.

If control is unsatisfactory on one drug used at a therapeutically satisfactory dose, then a second drug should be substituted. The best way to carry out this procedure is to introduce the second drug while the patient continues to take the first. When satisfactory blood levels have been achieved with the second drug, or when control has been established, then the first drug should be withdrawn – watching all the time for side-effects due to drug interaction (for instance if carbamazepine were being substituted for phenytoin, the carbamazepine level would rise when phenytoin was withdrawn).

It is particularly important to withdraw phenobarbitone slowly, as rapid withdrawal can precipitate seizures. If control cannot be established on one drug, and certainly if it cannot be established on two drugs, then referral is indicated. No patient should be subjected to polypharmacy without a specialist attempt to achieve a simple regime, for the usual results of polypharmacy are toxicity, non-compliance, and so worse control.

The dosage regime should be kept simple

All anticonvulsants can be given in daily or twice-daily dosage. The only possible exception to this is valproate whose half-life is short – but it appears that valproate is effective given twice daily. The disadvantages of a midday dose are that it is frequently forgotten and it may have to be taken in company which is sometimes socially embarrassing, especially for schoolchildren. Indeed phenytoin and phenobarbitone can be taken as a once-daily dose – preferably at night, so that any transient side-effects will take place during sleep.

Patients must be watched for side-effects and toxicity

This appears obvious. But many side-effects are insidious and patients with epilepsy often do not complain – they either regard the effects as a necessary evil or cease to take the treatment. It is up to the physician to produce the least harmful regime. In particular drug toxicity must be considered as the possible cause of any strange psychiatric disturbance until proved otherwise.

Drug interactions should be remembered in all prescribing

This works both ways. Anticonvulsants can alter blood levels of other drugs, mainly by lowering them due to hepatic enzyme induction. And other medicines can affect the levels of anticonvulsants. Of particular importance in practice are the effects on anticoagulants, where anticonvulsant withdrawal may increase anticoagulant levels so producing a risk of dangerous bleeding. As to the effect on the contraceptive pill, it is more difficult to be specific. There have been reports of pregnancies in patients who have been taking anticonvulsants and the contraceptive pill but these are few. It is probably advisable for patients taking anticonvulsants to use 50 μg pills rather than those of lower dose.

GENERAL COUNSELLING

The diagnosis and drug control of epilepsy are only the beginning of the management required of the general practitioner. He must also counsel and support his patient in coming to terms with the condition and coping with its consequences.

The patient diagnosed as 'epileptic' has just received a piece of information which he and his fellow human beings may not understand, and which will have major consequences maybe for the rest of his life. He and his family will need extensive explanation and support. It may well be that this will be offered by the hospital, especially in the case of children referred to specialist units. But many patients are not referred – and in the long run most are discharged to the general practitioner's ongoing care, so it is good to build a relationship with the patient and family from the outset.

There is a long history of epilepsy being regarded as a nasty, almost evil affliction. In 'King Lear' the Duke of Kent begins by insulting Oswald as 'A knave, a rascal, an eater of broken meat; a base, shallow beggarly, three suited, hundred pound, filthy, worsted suited knave; a lily livered whoreson . . .' and ends up by invoking 'a plague on your epileptic visage'. Some of the ideas which patients have of their illness remain intensely threatening today. They may believe that epilepsy is a brain illness which is debilitating and will eventually lead to madness: that they are likely to die in an attack: that rough games are a danger: or even that they should not marry and have children. Many patients also believe that an abnormal EEG means that there is something seriously wrong with the brain. The only way to prevent the persistence of such beliefs is to try to find out what they are, so that the counselling can be meaningful.

The most helpful explanation is usually in terms of electricity. 'The nerves in the brain are like a collection of wires carrying electricity. If the insulations on the wires are weak, the electricity short-circuits and you get too much electricity in one place, which produces a convulsion. It is as if taking medicines makes the insulation on the wires better, and the electricity stays in the right place.'

It should be explained that epilepsy is not an illness that is 'caught' and can be 'cured', but rather a predisposition to fits which has to be *controlled* and for which very long-term treatment will be required, maybe lifelong. So the need to take medicines consistently should then make sense, and it can be explained that any changes should be made in consultation with the doctor. Many patients worry that long-term treatment may mean that the drug effects 'wear off' so that they do not work any more, that the drugs will have long-term bad effects on them or that they may become addicted. So they need counselling and reassurance that they will be regularly seen by their GP so that any problems which arise can be sorted out.

SPECIFIC COUNSELLING

There are certain specific topics which counselling must include.

Driving

The regulations concerning driving by epileptics are clearly and explicitly laid down in the Government handbook *Medical aspects of fitness to drive* and there is no substitute for the doctor reading that pamphlet and if necessary showing it to the patient. In brief the rules are that nobody who has been diagnosed as suffering from epilepsy may drive who has had a seizure while awake within the past three years, and that if seizures are only experienced while asleep they must have been going on for at least three years before driving is allowed. The holding of a PSV or HGV licence is banned to anyone ever diagnosed as having seizures after the age of three years. Other less well known points are that driving should be stopped for a period if the anticonvulsant regime is altered – a powerful argument for inactivity; and that it is recommended that a patient should not drive after a single fit prior to investigation, and then not for 6–12 months if the cause remains undetermined.

Work

There are certain inevitable restrictions on a person with epilepsy when it comes to looking for work, mainly concerned with danger which might be caused either to himself or to others. For example he should not become a surgeon or an air traffic controller, nor work with high-speed machinery or electric power cables. The Armed Forces and Police will not accept people subject to continuing seizures. Driving restrictions make certain jobs inappropriate. It is advisable for parents of children with epilepsy to find out whether there will be problems with careers in which they show interest, while taking care not to over protect or to damp enthusiasm unless absolutely necessary.

Activities

It is always preferable to insist on as few constraints as possible, and on the whole there is more danger from overprotection by parents and families than from the results of seizures. A few precautions are sensible. Those with frequent seizures should not swim alone, climb trees or ropes, or take up mountaineering. Mothers should not bathe their babies when alone, and fires need guarding. But bicycle riding is usually an acceptable risk, and there need be little restriction on school activities and games.

Genetic

Parents or prospective parents with epilepsy usually worry whether the condition will pass on to their children. The precise nature of inheritance is complicated, but in broad terms the position is that if the parents suffer from *focal* epilepsy the risk of having children affected is hardly greater than for the general population. If a parent has *generalized* epilepsy the risk is much higher, but even so epilepsy is likely to be a significant problem in less than 5 per cent of the children.

There is a higher incidence of congenital malformations in babies born to epileptic mothers – 7.5 per cent against 2.7 per cent for the general population – but the malformations are frequently mild.

There is therefore rarely reason to advise against marriage and children on genetic grounds, except possibly if the woman were to have uncontrollable fits so that she might not be able to cope with a baby, or if the husband could not maintain a family.

SUPPORT FOR THE FAMILY

First aid

It is important that the family of a person with epilepsy knows what to do by way of first aid. When a seizure develops they are frightened, fearing that the sufferer will damage himself or even die and they feel helpless. A few simple instructions enable them to look after the person having the seizure, and in the process make them more confident.

1. They should restrain the patient enough to prevent him from hurting himself. If it is possible to lie him down in the lateral position (to prevent swallowing of the tongue or vomit) so much the better, but this may well have to wait until after the tonic-clonic phase is over.

2. They should not try to force objects between the teeth. The tongue is bitten in the initial tonic phase so it can do no good and may do damage.

3. The doctor should be called if the seizures are repeated, or if it goes on for longer than usual – say more than two or three minutes.

4. In the early stages of the disease they should feel free to call the doctor after a seizure, partly for reassurance, and partly so that the doctor gets to know the situation and can alter treatment or procedures if necessary. But some families quickly get used to coping with occasional seizures.

Emotional support

Families need the support of the doctor to help them come to terms with this illness in one of them. This is particulary true of parents of children with epilepsy. There are parallels with the process of bereavement and many of the same psychiatric processes go on in people who are bereaved of good health, or parents who are bereaved of their healthy child. There is the same searching for a 'cause', guilt feelings of responsibility, anger at 'life' and often at the medical profession, rejection of the diagnosis, and sometimes deep sadness or depression. It is important to be aware of these possibilities because each can make it more difficult to cope with the disease – anger can cause rejection of the diagnosis and treatment, and so interfere with compliance: guilt can result in parents being grossly overprotective and so depriving the child of a full life.

Families must realize that a person on antiepileptic treatment must be regarded as normally as possible, and that the more they regard the sufferer as 'normal' the more will their friends and workmates. One way in which doctors can help this process is by their own attitude and language. We often refer to patients by their disease category (such as diabetics, primigravidae), and so call these patients 'epileptics'. But the term 'people with epilepsy' emphasizes that they are indeed people and not a category apart, and in the case of a condition which for many years has carried a social slur, perhaps a special effort should be made. Finally, they must be assured of easy access to their GP, especially soon after the diagnosis is made, to give maximum opportunity for education, to increase their confidence, and reduce the inevitable anxiety.

FOLLOW-UP

Once the diagnosis is made and treatment established, visits to the doctor may become infrequent, with medicines obtained on repeat prescription. It is advisable for the patient to be seen occasionally to confirm that no ill effects are coming from disease or treatment, and that there are no other deficiencies which can be remedied.

As an *aide mémoire* for the doctor, it is helpful to have a check list of topics which may be covered at review, and this could be kept to hand by the GP, or better, be included in the notes in the form of a 'flow card' which would also serve as a clinical record. For example the card shown in Fig. 8.2 (adapted from Ian Tait's work (1977)) could be kept with EC7 size cards.

DATE	Nov '78	Jun '79	Sept '79	Apr '80	Apr '81	Apr '82	
MEDICINES	Epanutin 200:200	Epanutin 200:200	Epanutin 200:200 →		Epanutin 200:100 →		
		Tegretol 400:200	Tegretol 200:200 →		Tegretol 400:400 →		
COMPLIANCE	Good	Good		Good			
BLOOD LEVELS	105	EP 40	80	80		75	
		TEG 27	20	25		35	
SIDE EFFECTS	None						
FIT RATE	1/month	1/month	1/3 months		2 this year	None for 9/12	
OTHER BLOOD TESTS		FBC ✓	Urea 6.6			FBC ESR 50	
		LFT ↑				Urea 8.5	
FAMILY/JOB/ SCHOOL							
PROBLEMS	CVA1977					Weaker	
	Hemiplegia					Cardiac failure	
						R Digoxin Diuretics	
DRIVING LICENCE	NONE						
EPILEPSY ASSOC.	NO						

(Left margin labels: FLOW SHEET D.O.B. EPILEPSY R.T. CONDITION: NAME:)

Fig. 8.2.

With A4 records more information can be recorded, and there would also be space to include the basic information at time of diagnosis, instead of having to refer back to the general records.

One or two points regularly crop up under these headings.

Medicines

The patient is not always taking what the doctor believes he is. It is a good idea to ask the patient to bring the tablets, and ask whether they are taken regularly –

though even that is not a reliable evidence. Non-compliance must always be considered in cases of uncontrolled fits, and blood levels may give some guidance.

Consideration must always be given to simplifying or withdrawing treatment. Prevalence rates for epilepsy are only 10 times higher than incidence, so that an average duration of the disease of 10 years would be a good estimate. In the absence of predisposing factors or a long previous history of fits, gradual withdrawal of drugs after two or three years free of convulsions may well be an appropriate trial.

But it is *essential* that any change in dose should be discussed with the patient. This is particularly the case with car drivers. An epileptic should not drive for six months after a change of drug regime (Medical Committee on Accident Prevention 1978), and medical evidence is that one in three adults relapse if medication is withdrawn after a three-year period free of seizures. If a change of treatment were to increase the chance of a fit with socially disastrous consequences, the patient may, rightly, prefer to leave alone.

Blood levels

Blood levels should not be measured on a routine basis. In the absence of seizures or side-effects it is unecessary to alter the dose or measure the blood level regularly. It is much more important to assess the state of health of the patient, and measure blood levels only if a change on dosage is envisaged, or possibly to ensure high dosage in a driver who is desperate to avoid a single fit.

Seizure rate

It is difficult to know when seizures are adequately controlled until the next one occurs. The EEG on treatment is no help – seizure control is a clinical exercise. The degree of control must be agreed between patient and doctor. The eradication of all seizures must be the ideal, but the patient may agree that an occasional seizure – especially if partial or nocturnal – is a reasonable price to pay for less medication and fewer side-effects. It is the right of the patient and not of the doctor to decide on the degree of control he wishes.

If unsatisfactory control is being achieved then the doctor should consider the following possible causes:

(i) the wrong anticonvulsant is being used;
(ii) the correct drug is being used but in too low or too high a dose;
(iii) the patient is not taking the medication;
(iv) there is progressive pathology;
(v) there is a psychological precipitating factor.

Other blood tests

Although plasma folate or calcium may be reduced in patients on anticonvulsants, and their is an occasional case of marrow suppression, it is not necessary to carry out routine checks unless there are other clinical indications.

Social problems

These problems must be enquired about as they are often not volunteered. Problems at work or at home may be embarrassing to comment on even to the doctor. It may help if the patient comes with his wife – and it is even more important in the cases of children that they should attend with their parents. In particular school problems must be enquired after, and any hint of poor attendance, learning problems or social difficulties should be looked into, if necessary with other members of the health team.

It may be sensible to recommend membership of the British Epilepsy Association. The address is at the end of the chapter.

METHODS FOR FOLLOW-UP

With such small numbers the keeping of a practice register of epileptics, and extraction of the records each year to check attendance, is simple and adequate.

FEBRILE CONVULSIONS

Febrile convulsions, although falling within the definition of epilepsy, are rather different. They are common, occurring in 3 per cent of all children: they always occur with fever: and rarely occur after the age of six. There is a strong genetic factor, the incidence being 25 per cent in the sibs of a child who has such a convulsion, and 80 per cent in the case of identical twins. Convulsions seem to be more closely related to a rise of temperature than the level of the temperature, and indeed a convulsion in some children may be the first symptom of a febrile illness.

On each occasion every effort should be made to stop the convulsions as rapidly as possible and to prevent their recurrence. Parents of children at risk should be taught to dress the child lightly when it has a fever: to sponge it with tepid water (not ice cold water which can cause cutaneous vasoconstriction and so increase core temperature), and to give aspirin 60 mg per year of age every four hours. If convulsions occur or persist despite this care then the drug of choice is diazepam given intravenously or rectally. The doctor can administer 0.2–0.3 mg/kg intravenously if the child is still convulsing when he arrives, or for children at high risk the parents can be left a syringe and diazepam with instructions to administer 5 mg rectally (and clear instructions to remove the needle from the syringe before introducing it into the rectum!). If the child has already received diazepam then a further dose by the doctor carries the risk of apnoea, and paraldehyde 0.2 ml/kg intramuscularly, preferably with hyaduronidase, would be the best treatment.

Once the seizure is controlled consideration must be given to ruling out a serious underlying cause, particularly meningitis. Many texts recommend that the child should be admitted to hospital for lumbar puncture especially following a first fit, but this is not always necessary provided that the child is carefully observed at home and the parents know to call their doctor if there are any adverse signs, such as confusion or headache. In any case of doubt the child should be admitted.

There is then the long-term problem of whether to administer prophylactic medication, and to this question there is at present no universally agreed answer. It is agreed that a child who has a febrile convulsion has a 30–40 per cent chance of having another, and during each convulsion there is a small chance of the child injuring himself, or, if the convulsion were very prolonged, that it may produce cerebral anoxia and neurological damage. It is also accepted that a child who has febrile convulsions has a higher than average chance of developing epilepsy in later life, but that significant risk factors separate children at high risk of developing later epilepsy from those at low risk. The high risk group are those who have:

1. Seizures with focal features, or which last for over 15 minutes.
2. Pre-existing neurological or developmental abnormalities.
3. A family history of seizures.
4. Onset before the age of 12 months.

If children have none of the above features then the chance of their developing late epilepsy is about 2–3 per cent – some four times as high as that of the general population. If they fall into the high risk group the·risk rises to over 10 per cent (Nelson and Ellenberg 1976). In the face of these risks it would seem sensible to prescribe prophylactic medication to children at risk, but the situation is not straightforward. First, there is no evidence that prolonged therapy with anticonvulsants prevents the development of later epilepsy or significant neuro-logical defects (NIH 1980). Secondly, the medicines have significant side-effects. Phenobarbitone, 5 mg/kg per day, is recommended by many, but 40–50 per cent of children develop problems such as irritability, hyperactivity or rash, and treatment has to be stopped in about 20 per cent. Sodium valproate, 20–30 mg/kg per day, is highly effective but carries the risk of liver damage as mentioned above. Phenytoin is not effective.

Current practice is to recommend no drug treatment for children who do not fall into the high-risk group, but prophylactic treatment with phenobarbitone or sodium valproate for those who do, until two years after the last seizure. Some doctors compromise by giving prophylaxis only when the child has a fever. This method often fails because the convulsions may be the first sign of fever; and if the method is used then a rapidly acting medicine (valproate or rectal diazepam) should be employed. The giving of phenobarbitone at first sign of fever is of no value, because it takes several days to reach therapeutic levels.

Finally, the parents will need clear explanation and counselling – both regarding the convulsions themselves and the prognosis.

PERFORMANCE REVIEW CHECK LIST

General

1. Can the practice identify all its patients with epilepsy?
2. Does the practice have a policy for the general management of epilepsy?

Patients on treatment

1. Is it clear from the records on what basis the diagnosis was made?
2. How many of the following have been recorded at initial and subsequent assessment: seizure frequency, social consequences, drug side-effects, anticonvulsant blood levels?
3. Is there any record of the patient's ideas or the information given to the patient?
4. Are the current drugs and dosage clearly recorded?
5. Is advice about driving licences recorded?

Emergencies

1. Is there a practice policy on the management of convulsions?
2. Is there a record of patient's and relatives' instructions on what to do in the event of a convulsion?

PATIENT ASSOCIATIONS AND SELF-HELP GROUPS

British Epilepsy Association,
Crowthorne House,
New Wokingham Road,
Wokingham,
Berks RG11 3AY

Scottish Epilepsy Association,
48 Govan Road,
Glasgow G51 1JL

PATIENT BOOKS AND LEAFLETS

British Epilepsy Association literature.
Laidlaw, M. V. and Laidlaw, J. (1980). *Epilepsy explained.* Churchill Livingstone, Edinburgh. An excellent book, intelligible to most patients.
Hopkins, A. (1981) *Epilepsy: the facts.* Oxford University Press. A more complicated book, for intelligent patients or parents and also excellent for doctors.

REFERENCES

Drug and Therapeutics Bulletin (1981). Sodium valproate reassessed. *Drug Ther. Bull.* **19**, 93–5.
Hauser, W. A. and Kurland, L. T. (1975). The epidemiology of epilepsy in Rochester, Minnesota, 1935 to 1967. *Epilepsia* **16**, 1–66.

Hopkins, A. (1980). Epilepsy in adults. *Medicine* 32, 1632–40.

—— and Scrambler, G. (1977). How doctors deal with epilepsy. *Lancet* i, 183.

Jeavons, P. M. (1975). The practical management of epilepsy. *Update* 10, 269–80.

The Lancet (1980). Leader. *Lancet* ii, 1119–20.

Medical Committee on Accident Prevention (1978). *Medical aspects of fitness to drive.* London.

National Institutes of Health (1980). *Consensus Conference on febrile seizures.* Bethesda, Maryland.

Nelson, K. B. and Ellenberg, J. H. (1976). Predictions of epilepsy in children who have experienced febrile convulsions. *New Engl. J. Med.* 295, 1029–33.

Reid Report (1970). *People with epilepsy.* HMSO, London.

Richens, A. and Dunlop, A. (1975). Serum-phenytoin levels in management of epilepsy. *Lancet* ii, 247.

Tait, I. G. (1977). The clinical record in British general practice. *Br. med. J.* ii, 683–8.

FURTHER READING

Laidlaw, J. and Richens, A. (1976). *Textbook of epilepsy.* Churchill Livingstone, Edinburgh.

Richens, A. (1976). *Drug treatment of epilepsy.* Kimpton, London.

9 Hypertension

Theo Schofield

INTRODUCTION

High blood pressure is important. It is a major risk factor for arterial disease, particularly ischaemic heart disease and stroke, which causes half of all premature deaths in people between the ages of 45 and 65. 20 per cent of all these deaths and 50 per cent of all strokes could be prevented by adequate control of high blood pressure.

Managing patients with high blood pressure is already the commonest reason for patients attending their general practitioner for continuing care, and yet there is considerable evidence for the 'rule of halves'; that within our practice populations half the severe hypertensives are unknown, half of those known are not treated, and half of those treated are not controlled.

Dr Julian Tudor Hart in his general practice in Glyncorrwg wrote:

It is one of the first major areas in medicine to be invaded by numeracy and logic on a strategic, rather than a purely individual, tactical scale, integrating the management of individuals with a planned care of whole populations, and imposing on general practice the same disciplines of follow-up and teamwork long familiar in hospitals (Hart 1980).

It is these challenges that this chapter seeks to explore, first by reviewing some of the evidence about high blood pressure in the population, it's risks and the benefits of treatment, and then considering how this can be applied in practice.

BLOOD PRESSURE IN THE POPULATION

Different people have different levels of diastolic and systolic blood pressure, and there have been a number of studies which show the distribution of these levels in the population. One of the most important of these has been conducted by Dr W. E. Miall in the Rhondda Fach and Vale of Glamorgan between 1954 and 1971 (Miall and Oldham 1955, 1958; Miall and Chinn 1974).

This and other studies have shown:

1. Both systolic and diastolic blood pressures are distributed in the population according to a curve which has a slight positive skew. It has been argued that this positive skew is due to two separate populations. One normal and the other

diseased, but there is no evidence in these population studies of any natural dividing line into two populations at any level.

2. The mean blood pressure of the population increases with age, but it tends to rise faster in some individuals than in others. Miall and Lovell (1967) showed that the rate of rise of blood pressure that they observed over a 10-year period was positively correlated with the initial level of blood pressure. Age appears to play a part solely because blood pressure changes on average are positive and increase with higher pressures.

3. 30 per cent of men and women between 35 and 65 will have diastolic blood pressures 90–109 mm Hg and 3.9 per cent of men and 5.5 per cent of women will have diastolic blood pressures in excess of 110 mm HG.

SIGNIFICANCE OF HIGH BLOOD PRESSURE

The significance of high blood pressure lies in its association with increased mortality and morbidity from cardiovascular, cerebrovascular, and renal disease. It is important, however, to distinguish between significance for the individual and significance for the population.

The data about the risk for the individual have been gathered from actuarial studies by insurance companies, and from prospective studies in the population, notably the Rhondda Fach and Vale of Glamorgan Study already mentioned, and also the Framingham Study (Kannel and Dawber 1974). The important facts to emerge from these studies are:

1. The risk of subsequent death in otherwise healthy subjects increases with blood pressure. This curve again does not show any division into two populations normal and abnormal, but shows the risks steadily and progressively increasing from low levels of pressure.

2. The association between raised blood pressure and subsequent acute or chronic heart failure or cerebrovascular accident is twice as great as it is for coronary or peripheral artery disease.

3. The risk of any given level of blood pressure at this same age is twice as great overall for men than for women. The risk, however, of cerebrovascular disease at any given level of blood pressure is the same for both sexes.

4. Raised blood pressure is only one risk factor in the development of coronary artery disease. In the Framingham Study it ranked third after age and cigarette smoking. The risk of an elevated blood pressure was greatly increased in subjects who smoked or had high plasma cholesterols. There was a similar additive effect with diabetes.

5. Systolic pressure is as important a predictor of coronary artery disease as diastolic blood pressure and is more important as a risk factor for stroke. This risk does not diminish with age (Kannel and Dawber 1981).

These risks to different groups with varying levels of blood pressure can be expressed in a number of ways; for example, as the number of morbid events in each group per thousand patient years, or the ratio between the mortality in each sub-group and the mortality of the whole group. Both these ignore the size of the group, and there are many more people with mild elevations of their blood pressure and therefore mildly increased risks, than there are with severe elevations and at severe risk.

To overcome this one may calculate the number of deaths attributable to different levels of raised pressure. Rose (1981) calculated that two-thirds of the attributable coronary deaths and three-quarters of the attributable deaths from stroke occur in men with diastolic pressures below 110 mm Hg, and about half attributable coronary deaths and a quarter of the attributable deaths from stroke occur below 100 mm Hg. (Table 9.1).

Table 9.1. *Mortality attributable to blood pressure*

Diastolic BP	Cumulative % of excess deaths attributable to hypertension	
	Coronary heart disease	Stroke
< 80	(0)	(0)
< 90	21	14
< 100	47	25
< 110	67	73
≥ 110	100	100

From Rose (1981).

THE PATHOLOGICAL CONSEQUENCES OF RAISED ARTERIAL PRESSURE

The increased mortality and morbidity associated with raised arterial pressure is caused by its damaging effect on the arterial tree and on the heart. Some of these effects are closely related to high blood pressure, and do not occur in its absence, while in others high blood pressure is only one contributory factor.

Large arteries can develop atheroma and while raised arterial pressure is only one of the factors in the development of coronary artery disease it is more closely associated with cerebrovascular atherosclerosis and ischaemic stroke.

Smaller arteries can develop hypertrophy of the muscular layer and thickening of the intima which in turn produces ischaemic changes in the kidney and brain.

The small *intracerebral arteries* can also develop microaneurysms which were first described by Charcot and Bouchard. These are probably the chief cause of intracerebral haemorrhage associated with high blood pressure.

The *heart* is not only effected by coronary artery disease but also develops left ventricular hypertrophy. This may in turn lead to progressive congestive cardiac failure or acute left ventricular failure.

The onset of *malignant or accelerated hypertension* is closely related to the height of the blood pressure and its rate of rise. The underlying pathology is a fibrinoid necrosis of the arterioles which in turn can cause cerebral oedema, hypertensive encephalopathy, and renal failure.

Renal failure as a consequence of raised blood pressure is now rare in the absence of the malignant phase. Impairment of renal function may occur due to an underlying renal disease and uncontrolled high blood pressure may significantly accelerate the onset of renal failure.

THE CAUSES OF HIGH BLOOD PRESSURE

If we investigate those individuals whose blood pressures are at the higher end of the distribution in the population, in the vast majority no specific abnormality causing a raised blood pressure can be found. A number of physiological differences can be detected, including increased blood volume, cardiac output, and peripheral resistance and in some cases altered renal physiology. These may be the mechanisms whereby the higher blood pressure is maintained, but are not its cause. They will not be discussed further, as they do not advance the argument about how to manage high blood pressure in general practice.

It follows therefore that if different levels of blood pressure are distributed in the population then it is to the population that we must look for the factors that are associated with higher pressures.

The single most important factor that was identified by Miall and Oldham (1955, 1958) was *genetic*. The conclusion was that levels of blood pressure were subject to polygenic inheritance in a similar manner as height and that the resemblance between relatives was the same at all levels of pressure. Siblings resembled one another more closely than they resembled their parents. These genetic factors depend on environmental variables for their expression. The factors which have been identified as contributory include:

1. **Obesity** – despite difficulties with measurement of blood pressure in obese subjects the Framingham Study showed that fat young adults are more likely to develop raised blood pressures. They also showed that young adults with higher pressures were more likely to become fat, suggesting that some underlying common mechanism influences both weight and blood pressure.

2. **Salt** – comparisons between whole populations show a correlation between average daily salt intake with the prevalence of high blood pressure. On the other hand within-population studies including those of Miall, and the Framingham Study, were unable to show any link between individual salt intake and individual blood pressure. It has been suggested (Freis 1976) that reducing salt in our diet would be an important public health measure to prevent high blood pressure.

3. **Stress** – the belief that stress is a cause of high blood pressure demonstrates the power of words 'High blood pressure is the disease of high-pressure society' is so attractive as to appear self-evident. Ostfeld and Shekelle (1967) reviewed the literature on the subject and came to two conclusions: (i) it is established

beyond reasonable doubt that acute physiological stress may initiate sudden and transient elevations of blood pressure in some persons; (ii) it is not established that repetitive and continued psychological stress leads to the sustained elevation of blood pressure in anyone.

4. **Alcohol** – there is evidence from a large population study (Klatsky *et al.* 1977) that there is only an association between high levels of alcohol intake and raised blood pressure, and that moderate drinking not only has no effect on blood pressure, but can also reduce the risk of coronary heart disease.

5. **Smoking** – smokers tend to have slightly lower pressures than non-smokers, probably because they are less obese. The other risks of smoking are well known, and greatly outweigh any benefit from this effect.

In a small number of patients it is possible to find a definable cause for their high blood pressure. The causes of **secondary hypertension** are shown in Table 9.2).

Table 9.2. *Causes of secondary hypertension*

(a)	**Iatrogenic**
	Oral contraceptives
	Carbenoxolone
	Steroids
	Sodium-retaining anti-inflammatory drugs. (e.g. Phenylbutazone)
	Sympathomimetics
	Mono-aminoxidase inhibitors and cheese
(b)	**Diseases of the kidneys and urinary tract**
	Glomerulonephritis
	Chronic pyelonephritis
	Renal artery stenosis
	Polycystic kidneys
	Collagen diseases
(c)	**Coarctation of the aorta**
(d)	**Primary aldosteronism**
(e)	**Cushing's syndrome**
(f)	**Phaeochromocytoma**
(g)	**Pre-eclamptic toxaemia**

One estimate of the incident of secondary hypertension in the population was provided by the survey of middle-aged men in Göteborg (Bergelund *et al.* 1976). Out of 7455 men aged 45 to 54 screened in the Community 689 (9 per cent) had pressures 175/115 mm Hg or more on two visits a fortnight apart. A specific cause for hypertension was detected with reasonable certainty in 40 (6 per cent) of which 25 were renal parenchymal disorders and four renovascular. Only one of the latter was previously unknown and the screening procedure led to surgery in only two patients, one with renal artery stenosis and one hydronephrosis, both of whom subsequently required less antihypertensive therapy. The screening procedures in this study included either isotope renogram or intravenous pylogram. Similar results have been found in other studies of patients attending hypertension clinics.

As essential hypertension usually represents a more or less gradual rise in pressure with age, young subjects with high blood pressures are much more likely to have some form of secondary hypertension. In addition a rapid rise of pressure over a short period makes a secondary cause more likely.

THE DEFINITION OF HYPERTENSION

When we use the term 'a disease' we may refer to a described and recognizable combination of symptoms and signs, a phenomenon associated with a specific disorder of structure or function, or a phenomenon due to a specific cause or causes. The common concept is that diseases exist, each causing a particular sort of illness. Is there a disease that we can call 'hypertension'?

It should be clear from the previous sections that with the exception of the few cases of secondary hypertension it is impossible to define two subgroups within the population, one with 'normotension' and the other with 'hypertension', either by finding a definable cause or definable consequences which occur in one group and not the other. As Sir George Pickering (1968) wrote:

However we look at high arterial pressure, whether at its causes or its consequences we find a relationship that is quantitative. If then we choose to call essential hypertension a disease, it is a disease a kind hitherto unrecognised by medicine, a disease characterized by a quantitative deviation from the norm.

The most helpful definition of hypertension is that offered by Peart (1978) as 'The level of pressure at which the decision to investigate or treat is taken because the doctor believes it would be harmful to ignore'. This definition implies a balanced judgement between the risks of particular blood pressure and the potential cost and benefits of treatment. This judgement depends on, and may vary with, the evidence available at the time, but is essentially a clinical decision.

Pickering in 1968 proposed that the level of arterial pressure that alone justified therapy should confer a mortality two and a half times the normal. The figures he suggested were for diastolic pressure:

	Male	**Female**
Under 40	100	110
40 and over	105	115

More recent evidence has suggested that there may be benefits of treating milder elevations of blood pressure. This evidence will now be reviewed.

PHASE 4 OR PHASE 5

When measuring arterial pressure with a sphygmomanometer diastolic blood pressure can be taken either as the point where the sounds become softer or muffled (phase 4) or when the sounds disappear (phase 5). Phase 4 seems to compare best with intra-arterial recordings taking simultaneously, but is more difficult to determine in practice. Diastolic blood pressure phase 5 is between 5–10 mm Hg lower than phase 4, but this difference varies from patient to patient.

Most early British studies used phase 4, as did the Framingham Study, while more recent studies used the fifth phase. The most helpful practice is to indicate which definition is being used, and this will be adopted wherever possible in this discussion.

THE BENEFITS OF TREATING HIGH BLOOD PRESSURE

Severe hypertension

The benefits of treating patients with severely elevated blood pressures have long been established. Hamilton *et al.* (1964) conducted a trial with 61 patients under 60 years of age who were symptom free, had no signs of end organ damage, and all had diastolic (IV) blood pressures exceeding 110 mm Hg. They were allocated at random into treatment and no treatment groups. There were 10 treated males whose blood pressures were held below 110 mm Hg and of whom none suffered any cardiovascular events. Of the 12 untreated cases four suffered a stroke and one a myocardial infarction. The results in the women were less clear cut. Only one treated case with good or fair control suffered any cardiovascular event compared with three strokes and two infarcts in the controls, and two strokes and one infarct in the patients who were poorly controlled. The mean pre-treatment pressures were 229/132, and the follow-up period was between two and four years.

The Veterans Administration in the United States conducted a randomized control trial in men aged 30–75 divided into two groups, those with diastolics (V) 90–114 mm Hg and 115–129 mm Hg. These readings were taken while they were up and about in hospital, and patients who did not show the ability to comply with medication by taking a placebo for a two-month period were excluded from starting the trial.

The diastolic 115–129 group was studied for only three years because the difference between the treated cases and the controls was so great that it was unethical to continue (Veterans Administration Study Group 1967).

Patients in the lower diastolic range 90–114 mm Hg continued the trial for the full five years and the estimated risk of developing a morbid event was reduced from 55 to 18 per cent by treatment. Treatment was more effective in preventing congestive heart failure and stroke than in preventing the complications of coronary artery disease. These findings have been criticized because the starting levels of pressure in hospital were probably lower than usual, and the rate of complication in the control group was much higher than would be expected for mild hypertension (Veterans Administration Study Group 1970).

A more recent study conducted in Goteborg (Berglund *et al.* 1978) treating 1026 men aged 47 to 54 with pressures in excess of 175/115 (V) showed that both the total, and the cardiovascular mortality was about half as great in the treatment group as in the untreated controls.

The conclusion from these trials is that people with moderately severely elevated blood pressure similar to those levels recommended by Pickering are at substantial risk from their blood pressure; and that this risk can be reduced considerably by effective treatment. This is highly significant for any patient with such a blood pressure, but as has already been discussed this group are only approximately 3 per cent of the population and only account for one-third of the deaths from coronary artery disease and a quarter of the deaths from stroke that can be attributed to high blood pressure. It is therefore of crucial importance to obtain evidence about whether treatment will benefit patients with mildly elevated blood pressure.

Mild hypertension

Four major trials have recently been reported and a fifth, the Medical Research Council Trial, is still in progress. These have recently been analysed fully (WHO/ISH Mild Hypertension Liaison Committee 1982). This chapter will attempt to draw some of the conclusions that may effect our management in practice.

The Australian National Blood Pressure Study (1980) was a randomized placebo controlled trial with 3427 subjects aged 30–69 with diastolic pressures in the 95–109 mm Hg range. Active therapy was Chlorothiazide with second- and third-order drugs added if necessary. Patients with diastolic pressures (V) over 100 mm Hg who adhered to treatment had a mortality one-third of that observed in the controlled group. This was due to a reduction in fatal myocardial infarct and strokes while non-fatal ischaemic heart disease occurred in similar numbers in the treated and controlled groups. No benefit from treatment was found in patients with diastolic pressures between 95 and 100 mm Hg.

They also observed (1982) that in the untreated group mean pressures fell from 158/102 mm Hg at the first reading to 144/91 mm Hg three years later. At that time 32 per cent of pressures had remained within the mild hypertension range while 12 per cent had risen above, and 48 per cent had fallen below it. They speculated that this might have been due to adaptation to the procedures of blood pressure measurement or in part to the phenomenon of regression to the mean. They concluded that patients suspected of having mild hypertension required repeated evaluation before beginning drug therapy.

The trial conducted by the Hypertension Detection and Follow-up Program Co-operative group in the United States (1979) compared the effects on five-year mortality of a systematic antihypertensive treatment programme provided in special clinics (stepped care) with that with the treatment provided by the patients normal sources of medical care (referred care). The trial involved 10 940 men and women aged 30–69 who were recruited by population screening. They were divided into three strata according to their base-line diastolic (V) blood pressure 90–104 mm Hg, 105–114 mm Hg, and 115 + mm Hg.

In the stepped-care treatment regime medication was increased step wise to bring patients to or below their goal diastolic blood pressure, defined as 90 mm Hg for those entering with diastolic blood pressures of 100 mm Hg or greater, and a 10 mm Hg decrease for those entering with a diastolic blood pressure of 90–99 mm Hg. The initial treatment was Chlorthalidone 25–100 mg a day with additional drugs as necessary. Over the five years of the study more than two-thirds of the stepped-care participants continued to receive medication and more than 50 per cent achieved blood pressure levels within the normotensive range. Control of blood pressure was consistently better for the stepped-care than for the referred-care group.

Stepped-care participants, however, were also offered free medication and transport to the clinic if necessary, waiting times were minimized and appointments were made at convenient hours. Patients who were markedly overweight, hypercholesterolaemic, or heavy smokers were also offered counselling with regards to controlling these risk factors. In all counselling, however, the primary emphasis was on the drug therapy to achieve blood pressure control.

Five-year mortality from all causes was 7.70 per cent in the referred care group and 6.37 per cent in the stepped-care group, a 17 per cent reduction. This is impressive as the referred group were also receiving treatment.

This trial has been criticized because it is difficult to be certain which components in care of the stepped care contributed to its effectiveness. Preliminary analysis, however, indicated that it was not due to reductions in plasma lipids, cigarette smoking, or weight as these were similar in both groups. The conclusion of the authors that 'The systematic effective management of hypertension has a great potential of reducing mortality in the large numbers of people with high blood pressure in the population including those with "mild" hypertension' has major, inescapable implications for general practice.

The Medical Research Council Trial of Treatment for Mild Hypertension (1977) is a multicentred trial based largely on general practices in the United Kingdom. It involved screening over half a million people, and there are 17 359 patients participating in the trial. The criteria for entry were diastolic (V) pressures between 90–109 mm Hg and systolic pressures below 200 mm Hg. The patients were randomly allocated at entry to one of four treatment groups, Bendofluazide, Propranolol, or two identical placebos. There was also a small group assigned to a regime of observation only.

No conclusions about the benefit treatment have yet been published despite 38 000 patient years of observation, but a number of preliminary observations have been made that are particularly relevant to general practice. They made a similar observation to the Australian trial that the mean blood pressure in the placebo group fell and there was also a similar fall in the 'observation only' group. They have been able to compare the effectiveness and side effects of the two active drugs and found Propranolol was less effective in older than in younger patients. The five-year cumulative percentages of men withdrawing from randomly allocated treatment because of adverse reactions was 17 per cent on Bendrofluazide and 16 per cent on Propranolol. Corresponding figures for women were 13 and 18 per cent (1981).

The results of this screening programme provide an estimate of the prevalence of hypertension in the middle-aged population of Britain, and the size of the population who potentially could be treated for mild hypertension. Of the people who attended the screening (74 per cent of those invited) 1 per cent were previously undiagnosed hypertensives with diastolic pressures of 110 mm Hg or more. A further 5.7 per cent were patients already on antihypetensive therapy, 9.2 per cent were mildly hypertensive. Extrapolation to the whole population of England, Scotland, and Wales suggests that about 10 per cent of the 35–65-year-old population may have undiagnosed blood pressure at a level which may require either continued observation or treatment. This would amount to 1.8 million people, and this figure does not include those already having therapy, or the elderly.

The organization of the MRC trial also has important implications for general practice and these will be considered later in this chapter.

These trials all highlight the central dilemma of balancing the risks of mildly elevated blood pressure against the potential costs and benefits of treatment, both to the individual and the community. The mortality in the untreated groups in the trials described range from 0.5 to 1.5 per cent per annum, and while the reductions in this mortality with treatment was statistically significant their clinical significance for the individual is less certain. For the community the potential gain of the reduction in premature death, and disability must be balanced against all the implications of treating up to 10 per cent of the population.

Hypertension in the elderly

The evidence of the risks and the benefits of treating high blood pressure in older patients is less clear cut. The Framingham Study (Kannel and Dawber 1981) of a cohort of patients showed that systolic pressure rose faster with age than diastolic pressure, that systolic pressure was an important predictor of the risk of stroke, and that this risk did not diminish with age. On the other hand Anderson and Cowan (1976) in a prospective study of apparently healthy people aged 70–89 found that neither systolic nor diastolic pressure had any predictive value for survival.

There is no good controlled evidence of the benefits of initiating treatment for high blood pressure in patients aged over 70 or of the effects of stopping treatment which had been started in younger patients. Two trials are currently in progress, one in Europe and the other conducted by the Medical Research Council which are seeking to answer these questions.

Multiple risk factor interventions

A number of studies have attempted to reduce the risk of coronary artery disease by simultaneously seeking to control cigarette smoking, hypertension, and hypercholesterolaemia (Puska *et al.* 1979; Hjermann *et al.* 1981; Multiple Risk Factor Intervention Trial 1982). All three trials produced marked reductions in cigarettes smoking and high blood pressure, and less marked reductions in cholesterol by dietary advice. The American and Finnish Trials, however, did not show a significant difference in mortality between the treated and controlled groups. It has been suggested (Oliver 1982) that this was due to parallel changes in the control groups who also reduced their cigarette consumption and the incidence of coronary artery disease, and also possibly the fact that the 'incubation' period of coronary atherosclerosis was far longer than the duration of the trials.

THE COSTS OF TREATING HIGH BLOOD PRESSURE

The costs to the community of treating high blood pressure are impossible to estimate accurately, but include not only the costs of the drugs, currently approaching £100 million per annum in the United Kingdom, but also all the medical and nursing time involved.

We must also be concerned for the cost to the individual of detecting and treating their raised blood pressure. These include not only the side-effects of hypotensive drugs if they are prescribed, but also the psychological and social effects. Mann (1977) found that patients who had been screened and treated in the MRC Trial had fewer neurotic symptoms, for example anxiety and depression, than untreated controls and suggested that this might be due to the reassuring effects of treatment in the clinic. On the other hand Jachuck *et al.* (1982) found that while patients started on treatment and their doctors could see little change in their quality of life, their close companions reported that the large majority of patients had experienced adverse changes including undue preoccupation with sickness, decline in energy, general activity, and sexual activity, and irritability.

Haynes *et al.* (1978) found that the labelling of patients as hypertensives resulted in an 80 per cent increase in absenteeism from work. This was related to the patients becoming aware of their condition, and was not related either to the degree of high blood pressure, or whether the worker was started on therapy or not.

The major reflection, however, of the patient's view of the costs and benefits of treatment of high blood pressure, is that a substantial proportion cease to continue to take treatment as prescribed. This problem of treatment adherence or comliance has been extensively studied, and recently reviewed by Blackwell (1976), and the NHLBI Working Group (1982). It has been estimated that up to 50 per cent of patients started on treatment for high blood pressure do not continue it.

A number of factors have been identified that can influence this rate of compliance. These include a regime which is simple, free of side-effects, and tailored to the patient's own daily life: minimizing the inconvenience and waiting time in surgeries and clinics: and increased personal continuing care from either a doctor or a nurse. Using this close contact to impart knowledge about the disease does not produce any lasting effect if the close supervision is withdrawn. O'Brien and Hodes (1979) also found that the level of knowledge about high blood pressure was not related to the rate of uptake of an offer of screening for blood pressure.

Alternative approaches that may be more effective at improving treatment adherence will be considered later in the chapter.

MANAGEMENT IN PRACTICE

Assessment of the patient

The purpose of assessing a patient with suspected raised blood pressure is to decide whether the patient should be recommended to have treatment, and if so which treatment, and secondly to decide what level of blood pressure control and what follow-up is appropriate, whether the patient is treated or not. The questions that need to be answered are:

1. Is this patient's blood pressure actually raised, or is the apparent elevation due to faulty technique or the anxiety of measurement?

2. Is there a definable cause for this patient's blood pressure that could be treated (see Table 9.2)?

3. Are there any other factors that put this patient at particular risk from their high blood pressure; for example, smoking, raised cholesterol, impaired glucose tolerance, or a bad family history of premature cardiovascular disease?

4. Is there any evidence that high blood pressure has already damaged this patient's heart, circulation, or renal function?

5. Are there any physical or psychological factors that influence the choice of treatment in this particular patient, for example, obesity as an indication for for weight reduction, or raised uric acid or glucose intolerance as a contra-indication to diuretics. The choice of treatment will be considered in more detail later in the chapter.

The assessment of the patient should therefore include:

Accurate measurement of the blood pressure

This apparently simple measurement is sibject to a number of errors, including:

(i) **Mechanical faults** – The standard mercury sphygmomanometer gives incorrect readings if the air vent is blocked, if the tube is dirty, or if the mercury does not fall to zero when the machine is deflated. Aneroid or electrical sphygmomanometers are more prone to error and need to be checked frequently against a mercury machine.

(ii) **Cuff size** – Narrow cuffs give falsely high readings when applied to large overweight arms.

(iii) **Observer error** – Allowing the pressure to fall too qickly, particularly with slow pulse rates can introduce errors of up to 10 mm Hg. Errors can also be caused by the observer having a preference to certain digits, usually those ending in 0 or 5, and lastly by bias, when the doctor has a preconceived idea of what the patient's pressure either will or should be.

Repeated measurements of blood pressure

Patients found to have a raised blood pressure on one occasion usually have lower pressures at follow-up visits. Hartley *et al.* (1983) found that with repeated visits the systolic pressure dropped appreciably in the intervals between the first and the second visits, and again between the second and third visits, while the diastolic pressure fell appreciably only between the first and second visits. They therefore recommend that patients with newly identified blood pressures that are mildly raised should be seen at two further visits before a decision about treatment is made.

History

It is well established that high blood pressure does not cause patients any symptoms, and any association with such things as headaches and dizziness is because these patients are more likely to attend their doctor and have their blood pressure taken (Robinson 1969).

The history however should include:

(i) **Significant past history** including renal disease, toxaemia of pregnancy, gout, asthma, or depression.

(ii) **Current symptoms** including angina, claudication, shortness of breath, or transient disturbances of consciousness.

(iv) **Present or past therapy,** both for high blood pressure and other conditions.

(v) **Social factors** including occupation, driving, exercise, smoking habit, and alcohol consumption.

Physical examination

This should include:

(i) **General examination** including weight.

(ii) **Examination of the cardiovascular system** for cardiac enlargement, heart failure, and peripheral arterial disease.

(iii) **Palpation** to detect enlarged kidneys, and auscultation to detect abdominal or femoral bruits.

(iv) **Examination of the fundi.** The changes in the retinal arterioles are related both to the degree and the duration of raised blood pressure. Pickering classified these changes into two types. The first was arteriosclerotic retinopathy which included variation in the calibre of the retinal arterioles, and arteriovenous nipping. As the arterioles become thickened they also develop increased light reflex, and become generally narrower. In association with these changes there may be hard-edged white exudates, usually grouped around the terminations of the retinal vessels. The second type of retinopathy Pickering called hypertensive neuroretinopathy associated with accellerated hypertension. The stigmata of this include soft exudates due to retinal oedema surrounding the disc (macular star), retinal haemorrhages, and papilloedema.

Investigations

Routine investigations of hypertensive patients should include serum potassium (fresh or centrifuged specimen), cholesterol, blood glucose (fasting or two hours postprandial), uric acid, urine microscopy, ECG, and chest X-ray.

More invasive and expensive investigations, for example, IVP or VMA, are only indicated in patients with accelerated or resistant hypertension, patients under the age of 30, or those with a history of renal disease or phaechromocytoma.

When to start treatment

The doctor making the decision to recommend treatment to lower blood pressure of an individual patient must take into account not only all the evidence from the clinical trials that have already been reviewed, but also all the evidence and knowledge that he possesses about the individual patient. He will be seeking to balance the potential benefits of treatment against its possible costs, but because these benefits and costs are almost entirely the costs and benefits to the patient it is essential that the patient is involved at the time in making the decision. Not only does this approach answer the rhetorical question 'Whose life is it anyhow?', but it is also more effective. If the patient is not involved in making the decision to take treatment in the consulting room they are much more likely to make the decision not to take it when they leave.

The factors that the doctor will be taking into account in formulating his advice include:

The age of the patient

In the absence of any complicating factor patients over the age of 65 and certainly over the age of 70 should not be started on antihypertensive therapy as the risks probably outweigh the proven benefits. Patients under 35 with moderately raised blood pressures are more likely to have a secondary cause, and probably warrant initial investigation in a hospital clinic.

Level of blood pressure

In the light of the available evidence all patients with diastolic (V) blood pressures greater than 105 mm Hg should be offered treatment aimed at lowering their blood pressure. In view of the evidence of the equal risk of stroke with a given blood pressure in both sexes and also its preventability with treatment it is probably no longer appropriate to recommend tolerating higher blood pressures in females than in males.

At the present time it seems appropriate to recommend that patients with diastolic (V) blood pressures 90–105, who have no associated risk factors should not be started on treatment, but should be observed at regular intervals and those patients whose blood pressure subsequently rises should then be recommended treatment.

This opinion differs from the recent WHO/ISH guidelines for the treatment of mild hypertension (1983) which recommend that when an individual was found on one occasion to have a diastolic blood pressure above 90 mm Hg this measurement should be repeated on at least two further occasions over a period of four weeks. If it remained above 100 mm Hg treatment should then be instituted. If it had fallen below this level observation should be continued for a period of three months, and a decision to begin treatment should be made if at the end of that period the diastolic pressure continued to exceed 95 mm Hg. They recommended that patients whose blood pressure had fallen below 95 mm Hg should continue to be observed.

The reasons for proposing a more conservative policy are that the actual risk to any one individual from mildly raised blood pressure is in absolute terms small, and over a more prolonged period of observation a substantial proportion of patients' blood pressures will fall. The benefits of treatment to the individual are therefore a small reduction in an already small risk which must be balanced against the physical and psychological costs of initiating treatment.

An additional consideration which will be discussed in more detail later in the chapter is that at the present time the quality of care and blood pressure control that we are providing for patients with more severe hypertension who are at greater risk is far from optimal and it would be more appropriate to concentrate our resources on detecting and treating these patients adequately.

Target organ damage

Any evidence of damage to the heart, retinal vessels, circulation, or renal function due to high blood pressure places the patient at substantially greater risk and is an indication for recommending treatment when diastolic blood pressure is greater than 90 mm Hg.

Associated risk factors

The presence of associated risk factors including a raised systolic as well as diastolic pressure, smoking, raised blood cholesterol, and impaired glucose tolerance all increase the risk of a particular level of raised pressure. Their presence is therefore an indication, both for management in their own right, and also for treatment when the diastolic (V) pressure exceeds 90 mm Hg.

Family history

It is common practice to be more ready to treat patients who have a family history of premature cardiovascular disease as they are at greater risk of cardiovascular disease themselves. Whether this is due to inheritance of factors other than high blood pressure which places them at greater risk, or whether treatment is just more acceptable, both to doctor and patient, is not certain.

Management

The aim of management of patients with high blood pressure is to reduce their risk of complications as far as possible while interfering with their quality of life as little as possible. While the mainstay of treatment is drugs other aspects of management are equally if not more important.

Risk factor reduction

As a raised blood pressure places a patient at greater risk of developing arterial disease, and as the presence of other risk factors greatly increases that risk, it is essential that all patients with raised blood pressures, whether thay are going to be treated by other methods as well or not, should receive advice aimed at reducing the other risks. This advice should give particular emphasis to smoking, diet, and exercise.

As Tudor Hart (1980) pointed out 'Antihypertensive medication accompanied by continued smoking is a common absurdity'. Stopping smoking is important for all hypertensives and with mild hypertensives reduced the risks more effectively than treating blood pressure itself.

Dietary advice should have two aims. First to eliminate obesity which may in itself be sufficient treatment to lower the blood pressure to normal, and secondly the reduction of the proportion of total calories taken as fat, particularly saturated fats. Patients with hypercholesterolaemia should receive stricter advice.

Advising patients to take regular exercise may not only have a protective effect on their coronary arteries, but also increase their wellbeing and counteract any belief that high blood pressure is an illness.

Non-pharmacological control of blood pressure

The other non-pharmacological approach is to aim not just to reduce associated risk factors, but also to reduce the blood pressure itself. Weight reduction is well established as an effective method, but recently more interest has been shown in other methods. Andrews *et al.* (1982) reviewed 37 reports of the treatment of hypertension by non-pharmacological means and compared them with the results of treatment by standard drug regimes. Treatment of drugs produced the greatest lowering of blood pressure while treatment by weight reduction or muscle relaxation produced smaller but appreciable changes. The effects of meditation, exercise training, biofeedback and salt restriction were inferior to those of the other regimes, and were not significantly different to the effects of placebo treatment. Other trials, however, for example, Beard *et al.* (1982) have shown that no added salt diets can significantly lower the blood pressure and reduce the need for other medication. Two-thirds of the patients said that they would be happy to continue with that sort of diet, and it may be that this should be an option that should be placed before our patients with mild hypertension.

Anti-hypertensive drugs

The decision to start anti-hypertensive drug therapy is a major one. All available drugs carry some risks and some side-effects and the treatment may need to be continued for many years. The decision therefore should not be taken without an adequate period of observation of blood pressure before treatment, without clear indications, and without a definite target for blood pressure reduction. Once patients are started on treatment this target should be a diastolic pressure below 90 mm Hg, or if the pressure was under 100 mm Hg at the time of starting therapy then the aim should be to produce a fall of at least 10 mm Hg.

Over 70 per cent of patients will be satisfactorily controlled with either a diuretic, or a beta-blocker, or a combination of both. In the absence of specific contra-indications to either group of drugs the choice of which to start with is often a matter of personal choice. The experience of the MRC trial, however, would tend to favour a diuretic for women and a beta-blocker for men.

There are a large number of thiazide diuretics which are effective as anti-hypertensives. Chlorthalidone has a long course of action suitable for once daily dosage while Bendrofluazide is cheapest. Larger doses are no more effective at controlling blood pressure, but increase the risk of side-effects particularly raising serum uric acid and impairing glucose tolerance. It is only necessary to add potassium supplements in patients taking Digoxin or in elderly patients.

Beta-blockers are effective when used alone in about the same percentage of patients as diuretics. Again there are a large number available and doctors should become familiar with one or two of them. Atenolol and Metoprolol have the advantages of being relatively cardio-selective, of having a flat dose-response curve, and of being effective in once-daily dosage.

Increasing the dosage of either group of drugs beyond that recommended for the treatment of hypertension will not increase their antihypertensive effect and only increase the risk of side-effects. If treatment with a single drug fails to achieve the target blood pressure the next step is to add one of the other groups of drugs. Because the doses are fairly standard, preparations that combine diuretic drugs and beta-blockers may be more convenient and help to maintain patients' compliance.

In a small group of patients whose blood pressure is not adequately controlled by a combination of diuretic and beta-blocker, and in those patients with contra-indications, other drugs must be considered. Available drugs now include:

Vasodilators – for example Hydralazine and Prazosin;
Centrally acting drugs – for example Methyldopa;

Angiotensin converting enzyme inhibitors – for example Captopril;
Slow calcium channel blockers – for example Nifedipine.

These drugs will not be considered in detail because the information is available elsewhere and new drugs continue to become available. It is essential, however, for doctors prescribing these drugs to know their pharmacology, indications, and possible side-effects, and only to use those preparations with which they are familiar.

Patient education

Health education is frequently criticized as being more concerned with persuading patients to behave in ways that doctors think are good for them than in educating patients to make their own fully informed choices. This is valid because many of our suggested managements are not appropriate to our patients' needs, and because we do not seek to achieve a truly shared understanding about the nature of the problem and its management with our patients.

Giving information to the patients is not the same as sharing understanding. This includes not only whether the patients remember what the doctor has said on a particular occasion, but also whether they understand what the decision means, why and how the doctor has reached the decision, and lastly how the information relates the patients' own pre-existing theories and ideas about the problem.

There is overwhelming evidence (Tuckett 1982) that the explanation and information given to patients in consultations is not of a kind likely to help them make informed decisions or to integrate their own ideas with those of their doctors. There are a number of reasons for this, including the time that we are either able or prepared to allocate to this, an erroneous belief that patients are unable to remember important information given to them, and our readiness to make assumptions about, rather than to actually explore, our patients' own ideas and values. There is also an assumption shared by many doctors and patients that it disturbs the relationship if the patient questions the doctor and his management.

All our efforts in general practice at detecting, investigating, and managing our patients with high blood pressure are fatally undermined if half our patients do not adhere to that management. Unfortunately, all the evidence indicates that this is indeed what happens, and it is therefore crucially important that we not only seek to achieve a shared understanding of the nature of the problem with our patients, but also help to establish their motivation to adhere to treatment.

Simple attempts to induce fear, for example of a stroke, will not be effective if the patients see it as a remote and distant possibility. It can also be counterproductive if taking tablets is a constant reminder of a risk that they would prefer to deny.

Another ineffective strategy is to link the management to symptoms. This may happen if the patients' raised blood pressure is an incidental finding when they present with other symptoms and when the symptoms resolve they are likely to stop the treatment.

Patients' health beliefs (Becker 1974) include not only the overall interest in their own health, but also beliefs about their own vulnerability and the seriousness of any potential problem. They also have a view about the costs and benefits of any change in behaviour and may be prompted into change by a variety of cues. It is these beliefs which predict whether patients will adhere to their treatment and it is these beliefs which need to be explored with each patient.

Motivation not only needs to be created at the outset but also must be maintained. This can be helped by involving the patient in setting goals, and providing positive feedback about the degree of achievement of those goals, for example weight reduction or blood pressure control. Some patients will be happy with their doctor supervising their progress, while others seeking to reject a sick role may prefer an active involvement in managing their own health and monitoring their own pressure.

Follow-up

Planned follow-up is an essential part of the management of patients with raised pressure which in most patients will continue over many years. Follow-up has a number of purposes:

1. To achieve and to maintain the targets for blood pressure control

This is important whether the methods of treatment include drugs or not. If antihypertensive therapy is started the patients will need to be seen at fairly frequent intervals (1–2 weeks) to adjust the dosage and to add additional drugs if required. Once the pressure is satisfactorily controlled follow-up can be much less frequent (3–6 months). If a patient who has previously been well controlled again develops a raised pressure, it is essential to enquire whether the patient is continuing to take their treatment, and if so, repeat the reading in 1–2 weeks, and then to adjust the therapy as required. It is too easy to coast along accepting only partial control, particularly if the target for good control is not clearly stated.

The results of the Hypertension Detection and Follow-up Program emphasized the importance of tight blood pressure control. A recent survey in this country however (DHSS Hypertension Care Computing project 1982) comparing patients managed in hypertension clinics with patients managed in general practice found that while the pretreatment blood pressures were higher in hospital patients, the treated diastolic pressures at 18–24 months were lower in the hospital than the general practice group (156/97 v. 150/92 mm Hg). The hospital patients did not receive a greater variety of drugs, but were prescribed them in higher doses. Blood pressure control, however, was considered to be inadequate in many patients in both groups. At 18–24 months 26 per cent of the general practice group had diastolic pressures of 105 mm Hg or more as had 13 per cent of the patients followed up in hospital clinics.

2. Reporting of side-effects

All forms of drug therapy may have side-effects which are much more likely to be reported if they are sought at the time the patient is seen. If they are not dealt with and discussed the patient is much more likely to stop the therapy themselves.

3. Encouraging compliance

The difficulty of maintaining the compliance and the importance of continued personal care and positive feedback has already been emphasized.

4. Risk factor reduction

The patient is likely to judge the importance the doctor places on giving up smoking, weight reduction, and a healthy diet, on whether the doctor enquires about these factors at follow-up. The achievement of these changes in behaviour all require continued, positive reinforcement.

5. To detect and monitor target organ damage

If any target organ damage has been detected then its progress should be carefully monitored. This is particularly essential if there has been any impairment of renal function as poor blood pressure control can cause its continued deterioration. Patients on diuretics should have serum potassium, uric acid, creatinine, and glucose re-estimated three months after beginning treatment, and repeated subsequently every one to two years.

All patients should be reviewed every one to two years. This should include: (i) enquiry for any new symptoms; (ii) examination of the fundi; (iii) serum creatinine; (iv) examination of the urine.

Referral

It is rarely necessary to refer patients with high blood pressure for specialist advice. The indications that may arise are:

1. Accelerated or malignant hypertension.
2. Significantly raised blood pressure in a patient under 35.
3. Evidence of a treatable secondary cause for raised blood pressure.
4. Failure to control blood pressure with patients who are taking full doses of therapy. The purpose of these referrals is to obtain both further advice and possibly further investigation.

ORGANIZATION OF CARE IN GENERAL PRACTICE

In the first section of this book we have discussed the need to provide a high standard of continuing care in general practice for patients with chronic conditions, and some of the implications of this for the organization of general practice. In this section we will discuss the particular arrangements that need to be made for the detection and management of high blood pressure in practice.

Policy for the detection of raised blood pressure in the practice population

Hypertension fulfils all the criteria that Wilson and Jungner (1968) proposed should be fulfilled before embarking on screening for any condition. It is a major health problem both for the community and for the individual. It can be totally asymptomatic, but detectable by a simple and acceptable test. Its natural history and the benefits and costs of treatment are all well established.

Patients at risk can be detected by mass screening programmes, but if these are conducted by outside agencies without arrangement for continued share they are both costly and ineffective (D'Souza *et al.* 1976; Christie 1979).

The alternative is to take advantage of the opportunity we have in British general practice of providing continuing care for a defined population of patients, 90 per cent of whom attend our surgeries within five years. It is therefore possible to ensure that a large majority of our adult patients have had their blood pressure taken (Hart 1970).

To achieve this in practice a special effort has to be made, preferably by agreement with the whole practice. There needs to be a policy about the age group to be screened, the levels of blood pressure which if sustained will be treated, and the levels below which the patient will be regarded as definitely normal. It is particularly important to have a policy for those patients whose blood pressures are mildly raised and therefore fall between these two limits, both to assess them to detect factors which may place them at special risk, and to ensure that they are followed up adequately.

Records for case finding

Unless we are to take every patient's blood pressure every time they attend it must be clear from the records when, if ever, the patient last had their blood pressure taken. This can be done by a variety of methods. Entries of blood pressure can be highlighted in the ordinary continuation record or a space can be allocated on a summary card for the entry of blood presures. Again it is particularly important to highlight mildly elevated readings so that the doctor is made aware that they need repeating. Two recent surveys have emphasized the need for this type of effort. Fleming and Lawrence (1981) in a survey of randomly sampled records from 38 Thames Valley general practitioners found that the average proportion of men aged 40 to 69 in the practice population who had had their blood pressure taken in the previous five years was 51 per cent, though the range was from 24–95 per cent. Ritchie and Currie (1983) in a survey in practices in north-east Scotland of the records of men aged 20 and over found that only 34 per cent had had their blood pressure taken in the previous 10 years and that only 56 per cent of raised blood pressures (DBP > 100 mm Hg) had had a recorded follow-up blood pressure.

Registers for detection

It is possible to use an age/sex register to monitor whether patients have had their blood pressure taken or not. This involves transfering a large amount of data from the records to the register, and as a large proportion of the blood pressures will be normal this is probably only possible in obsessional practices or those with computer facilities. Maintaining a register of those patients whose blood pressure have been found to be raised is much more cost-effective. The register can be used to identify patients who have not been followed up and as a means of monitoring the success of the detection programme.

Records of treated patients

The advantages of flow charts in the records of patients with chronic conditions were discussed in Chapter 4. They are particularly suitable for the management of high blood pressure as they allow changes and trends in control to be seen clearly, and can encourage an organized and structured approach to the assessment and management of the patient. The provision of spaces for items of information helps to ensure that information is collected and recorded.

At its simplest a flow chart could consist of a table or graph of the patients blood pressure, pulse, and weight with space for symptoms and changes in management. A more comprehensive record would include:

1. The data base with pretreatment blood pressures, significant history, initial examination, and the results of investigations.

2. A plan for management including targets for blood pressure and weight, risk factor reduction, and patient education.

3. Record of regular attendance with blood pressure, pulse, weight, symptoms, and changes of management.

4. Episodic review with repeat examination and investigation.

The items that should be included under each of these headings have been discussed in the preceding sections of this chapter.

An additional advantage of using a structured record of this sort is that it makes the records much more suitable for audit.

Team care

The Medical Research Council Trial of Treatment for Mild Hypertension has shown that it is possible in general practice to provide adequate supervision of patients, control of blood pressure, and compliance, in clinics largely run by nurses. The clinic nurses have taken the screening blood pressures, performed the initial investigation, and continued the follow-up adjusting doses of treatment when required. Doctors initially assess the patients and see them for examination and review once a year, but are available at other times at the request of the nurse. The ingredients that have made this possible are:

1. A clear protocol setting out the policy of the trial and giving clear instructions to the nurse including the limits of their responsibility.

2. A structured record that reflects the protocol.

3. A willingness on the part of the doctors to work in partnership with nurses and to recognize their ability to organize clinics, make decisions and provide care for patients.

4. Shared experience and support from a nurse who has set up the run clinics in other practices.

Many of the practices involved in the trial are now using the same methods for managing their other hypertensive patients.

The importance in management of patient education and reducing other risk factors such as smoking, and weight, have already been discussed. Other members of the team, particularly health visitors, may have greater expertise in these areas which can be used, both with individuals and groups of patients.

Performance review

An integral part of organizing the care of patients with high blood pressure in practice must be to incorporate methods of reviewing and providing feedback about our levels of performance. Without this it is difficult to maintain motivation or performance, and impossible to alter policies or practices in the light of experience. Information can be obtained from:

(i) records of patients being treated for hypertension, identified either when they are seen or receive a repeat prescription;

(ii) records of a sample of the practice population drawn at random;

(iii) records of patients who can be identified as ever having been treated or observed for high blood pressure; this requires a practice register.

Donabedian (1966) divided the areas for evaulation of medical care into structure, process, and outcome. It is impossible in an individual practice to evaluate such outcomes as the prevention of heart disease or stroke, as the numbers are so small. However, as these outcomes are so clearly related to the quality of control of high blood pressure and associated risk factors it is sufficient to evaluate these items in the process of care.

For performance review to be of value it needs to be related to criteria of a good practice which are based on the available evidence and are agreed and accepted by our peers. This chapter has attempted to argue such an approach to the management of high blood pressure in practice.

PERFORMANCE REVIEW CHECK LIST

General

1. Does the practice have a policy for the detection of raised blood pressure, whom to follow-up and whom to treat?
2. Can the practice identify: (i) patients who have ever been started on therapy?
   (ii) patients whose blood pressures have been observed to be raised?

Random sample of records

1. What percentage of patients aged 35 to 65 have:
   (i) ever had their blood pressure taken?
   (ii) had their blood pressure taken in the last five years.
2. Of those with a recorded diastolic blood pressure:
   (i) > 90 mm Hg.
   (ii) > 105 mm Hg.
   What proportion have either been followed up or treated?

   What proportion of these patients also have records of weight or smoking habit?

Patients on treatment

1. How many raised blood pressures were recorded before treatment was started?
2. Is there a record of assessment before treatment?
3. Is the patient's weight and smoking history recorded?
4. Is there any record of patient's ideas or of the information given to the patient?
5. What proportion of treated patients have diastolic blood pressures less than 90 mm Hg?

Patients ever started on treatment

1. What proportion of patients started on treatment are no longer receiving it?
2. Can the reasons for stopping treatment be identified from the records?

PATIENT ASSOCIATION

The Chest, heart and Stroke Association,
Tavistock House North,
Tavistock Square,
London WC1H 9JE

PATIENT BOOKS AND LEAFLETS

Facts about high blood pressure. The Chest, Heart and Stroke Association, London.
Lewis, P. J. (1981). *High blood pressure.* Churchill Livingstone, Edinburgh.

REFERENCES

Anderson, F. and Cowan, N. T. (1976). Survival of health older people. *Br. J. prevent. soc. Med.* **30**, 231.
Andrews, G., MacMahon, S. W., Austin, A., and Byrne, D. G. (1982). Hypertension: comparison of drug and non-drug treatments. *Br. med. J.* **284**, 1523–6.
Australian National Blood Pressure Study Management Committee (1980). The Australian Therapeutic Trial in Mild Hypertension. *Lancet* **i**, 1261–7.
—— (1982). Untreated mild hypertension. *Lancet* **i**, 185–91.

Beard, T. C., Cooke, H. M., Gray, W. R., and Barge, R. (1982). Randomised controlled trial of a no-added-sodium diet for mild hypertension. *Lancet* ii, 455.

Becker, M. H. (1974). The health belief model and personal health behaviour. *Hlth Educat. Monogr.* 2, 236.

Berglund, E., Anderson, D., and Wilhelmsen, L. (1976). Prevalence of primary and secondary hypertension: studies in a random population sample. *Br. med. J.* ii, 554–6.

Berglund, G., Wilhelmsen, L., Cannersedt, R., Hansson, L., Anderson, O., Swertsson, R., Wedel, H., and Wikstrand, J. (1978). Coronary heart-disease after treatment of hypertension. *Lancet* i, 1–5.

Blackwell, B. (1976). Treatment adherence in hypertension. *Am. J. Pharm.* 148, 75–85.

Christie, D. (1979). Screening for hypertension – some practical problems. *J. R. Coll. gen. Practrs* 29, 597–601.

DHSS Hypertension Care Computing Project (1982). A comparison of blood pressure control in hypertensive patients treated in hospital clinics and in general practice. *J. R. Coll. gen. Practrs* 32, 98–102.

Donabadian, A. (1966). Evaluating the quality of medical care. *Millbank Mem. Fund Q.* 44, 166–206.

D'Souza, M. F., Swan, A. V., and Shannon, D. J. (1976). A long-term controlled trial of screening for hypertension in general practice. *Lancet* i, 1228–31.

Fleming, D. M. and Lawrence, M. S. T. A. (1981). An evaluation of recorded information about preventive measures in 38 practices. *J. R. Coll. gen. Practrs* 31, 615–20.

Freis, E. D. (1976). The prevention of hypertension. *Circulation* 53, 589.

Glifford, R. W. (1969). Evaluation of the hypertensive patient with emphasis on detecting curable causes. *Millbank Mem. Fund Q.* 47, 170.

Hamilton, M. *et al.* (1964). The role of blood pressure control in preventing complications of hypertension. *Lancet* i, 235.

Hart, J. T. (1970). Semicontinuous screening of a whole community for hypertension. *Lancet* ii, 223.

—— (1980). *Hypertension*. Churchill Livingstone, Edinburgh.

Hartley, R. M., Velez, R., Morris, R. W., D'Souza, M. E. and Heller, R. F. (1982). Confirming the diagnosis of mild hypertension. *Br. med. J.* 286, 287–9.

Haynes, R. B., Sackett, D. L., Taylor, D. W., Gibson, E. S., and Johnson, A. L. (1978). Increased absenteeism from work after detection and labeling of hypertensive patients. *New Engl. J. Med.* 299, 741–4.

Hjermann, I., Byre, K. V., Holme, I., and Leren, P. (1981). Effect of diet and smoking intervention on the incidence of coronary heart disease. *Lancet* ii, 1303–10.

Hypertension Detection and Follow-Up Program Co-operative Group (1979). Reduction in mortality of persons with high blood pressure, including mild hypertension. *J. Am. med. Ass.* 242, 2562.

Jachuck, S. J., Brierley, H., Jachuck, A., and Willcox, P. M. (1982). The effect of hypotensive drugs on the quality of life. *J. R. Coll. gen. Practrs* 32, 103–5.

Kannel, W. B. and Dawber, T. R. (1974). Hypertension as an ingredient of a cardiovascular risk profile. *Br. J. hosp. Med.* 2, 508–23.

—— —— (1981). Systolic blood pressure, arterial rigidity, and risk of stroke. *J. Am. med. Ass.* 245, 1225–9.

Klatsky, A. L., Friedman, G. O., Siegelaub, A. B., and Gérard, M. J. (1977). Alcohol consumption and blood pressure. *New Engl. J. Med.* 296, 1194.

Mann, A. H. (1977). The psychological effect of a screening programme and clinical trial for hypertension on the participants. *Psychol. Med.* 7, 431.

Medical Research Council Working Party on Mild to Moderate Hypertension (1977). Randomized controlled trial of treatment for mild hypertension: design and pilot trial. *Br. med. J.* i, 1437–40.

—— (1981). Adverse reactions to Bendrofluazide and Propranolol for the treatment of mild hypertension. *Lancet* **ii**, 540–2.

—— and Lovell, H. G. (1967). Relation between change of blood pressure and age. *Br. med. J.* **ii**, 660.

Miall, W. E. and Chinn, S. (1974). Screening for hypertension: some epidemiological observations. *Br. med. J.* **iii**, 595.

—— and Oldham, P. D. (1955). A study of arterial blood pressure and its inheritance in a sample of the general population. *Clin. Sci.* **14**, 459.

—— —— (1958). Factors influencing arterial pressure in the general population. *Clin. Sci.* **17**, 409.

Multiple Risk Factor Intervention Trial (1982). Risk factor changes and mortality results. *J. Am. med. Ass.* **248**, 1465–77.

NHLBI Working Group (1982). Management of patient compliance in the treatment of hypertension. *Hypertension* **4**, 415–23.

O'Brien, M. and Hodes, C. (1979). High blood pressure: public views and knowledge. *J. R. Coll. gen. Practrs* **29**, 234–9.

Oliver, M. F. (1982). Does control of risk factors prevent coronary artery disease? *Br. med. J.* **285**, 1065–6.

Ostfeld, A. M. and Shekelle, R. B. (1967). Psychological variables and blood pressure. In *The epidemiology of hypertension* (ed. J. Stamler). Grune & Stratton, New York.

Peart, W. S. (1978). Mild hypertension. *Adv. Med.* **14**, 87–92.

Pickering, G. W. (1968). High blood pressure. Churchill Livingstone, Edinburgh.

Puske, P., Tuomilehto, J., and Salonen, J. (1979). Changes in coronary risk factors during comprehensive five-year community programme to control cardiovascular diseases (North Karelia project). *Br. med. J.* **ii**, 1173–8.

Ritchie, L. D. and Currie, A. M. (1983). Blood pressure recording by general practitioners in north-east Scotland. *Br. med. J.* **286**, 107–9.

Robinson, J. O. (1969). Symptoms and the discovery of high blood pressure. *J. psychosomat. Res.* **13**, 157–61.

Roe, G. (1969). Symptoms of prevention: lessons from cardiovascular disease. *Br. med. J.* **282**, 1847–51.

Tuckett, D. (1982). *Final report on the patient project.* Health Education Council, London.

Veterans Administration Study Group on Antihypertensive Agents (1967). Effects of treatment on morbidity in hypertension: results in patients with diastolic blood pressures averaging 115 through 129 mmHg. *J. Am. med. Ass.* **202**, 116.

—— (1970). Effects of treatment on morbidity in hypertension II. Results in patients with diastolic blood pressure averaging 90 through 114 mmHg. *J. Am. med. Ass.* **213.** 1143.

WHO/ISH Mild Hypertension Liaison Committee (1982). Trials of the treatment of mild hypertension. *Lancet* **i**, 149–56.

—— (1983). Guidelines for the treatment of mild hypertension. *Lancet* **i**, 457–8.

Wilson, J. M. G. and Jungner, G. (1968). *Principals and practice of screening for disease.* WHO, Geneva.

10 Ischaemic heart disease and heart failure

Michael Kenworthy-Browne

INTRODUCTION

This chapter deals with the long-term illnesses which affect much of the circulatory system. Particular reference is made to ischaemic heart disease and heart failure which form the commonest group of chronic disease in the community. Aspects of peripheral and vascular disease are covered in other chapters.

DEFINITION

Ischaemic heart disease implies a lack of effective fusion to the heart muscle from any cause. In many patients there is likely to be widespread vascular damage as well. Systemic diseases and states which affect the heart, for example diabetes, tobacco addiction, and hyperlipidaemia will also affect peripheral blood vessels and cause widespread degenerative lesions.

It has been clearly shown that in the Western World the development of atheroma and degenerative diseases of the circulatory system start early in life and are widespread by the age of 30. Most causes of ischaemic heart disease under the age of 60 present with chest pain or frank infarction. Sudden death within two hours occurs in one-third of cases without medical intervention. Such a dramatic efent of a coronary or myocardial infarction (MI) is the end point of many years of degenerative pathology, but may be quite unheralded.

There is at present no adequate screening procedure for early diagnosis and reversal of this degenerative disease. Most of us will have patients who we rarely, if ever, see or who have consulted for the first time in an emergency. Such cases will stand out in most family doctor's memories, as will the patients we never actually reached because of sudden death.

The diseases which are dealt with in this chapter are:

Angina

Acute coronary insufficiency

Infarction

Interference with conducting systems:

(a) arrhythmias

(b) heart block

Heart failure

Valvular lesions

Therefore by definition anybody who has had a myocardial infarction has ischaemic heart disease (there are rare cases of coronary embolism which has no disability and where the rest of the cardiovascular tree is intact). In the same way for practical purposes the diagnosis of angina pectoris means ischaemia of the heart muscles.

INCIDENCE

In the average family practice a general practitioner can expect to see each year for every 1000 patients:

   (i) 5 patients with myocardial infarction;

  (ii) 7 patients with angina;

 (iii) 9 patients with heart failure.

These bland figures by themselves mean very little in an annual workload of 7000–12 000 consultations per year. The national statistics should help to put the picture in perspective.

Table 10.1 shows the commonest causes of death in this country for 1978. Even allowing for some errors in death certification these figures are alarming. While it is not unreasonable for death to occur over the age of 70 from degenerative disease, the proportion of cardiac deaths in the 40–70 age groups is considerable and is still increasing in the United Kingdom.

In the United States acute heart disease causes twice as many deaths as all forms of neoplasm, but in recent years the overall incidence of heart disease has shown a decline.

Table 10.1. *1978 United Kingdom—deaths*

From cancer	128 000
From hypertension	7000
From circulatory disease	296 000
Deaths from	
(a) Ischaemic heart disease	
Males	92 380
Females	68 078
(b) Acute infarction	
Males	65 412
Females	42 749

DIAGNOSIS AND APPROPRIATE INVESTIGATIONS

Ischaemic heart disease

The natural age range is 40–70, though younger patients may present with chest pain and be shown to have true angina. By the time the chest pain or a frank myocardial infarction occurs, the blood supply through the coronary arteries has already become critical.

Table 10.2. *Causes of cardiac ischaemia and angina*

Smoking	Aortic stenosis
Vascular disease	Hyperthyroidism
Anaemia	Myxoedema
Hypertension	Hypertrophic obstruction cardiomyopathy
Polycythaemia	Polyarteritis
Severe pulmonary hypertension	Syphilitic aortitis
Hyperlipidaemia	

Table 10.2 lists some conditions which are treatable, but which may cause or aggravate ischaemic heart disease and need to be excluded as part of the diagnosis. In particular, aortic stenosis, hyperlipidaemia and the rare cases of obstructive cardiomyopathy should be excluded in young people presenting with chest pain. It is never appropriate to dismiss anyone with central chest pain because he is thought to be too young: angina or ischaemic heart disease can occur at any age and myocardial infarction has even occurred in infancy.

Older patients, particularly over the age of 70, tend to have less typical chest pain or even none at all in acute infarction. A silent myocardial infarction may give rise only to severe confusion due to inadequate cerebral perfusion, and additional heart failure under these circumstances may be missed for several days. Table 10.3 lists some of the important common causes of chest pain which may be confused with angina and particularly confused with myocardial infarction.

Table 10.3. *Important causes of acute chest pain*

Acute pericarditis
Pulmonary embolus
Pneumothorax
Aortic aneurysm
Oesophageal spasm
Hiatus hernia
Gall-bladder colic
Acute pancreatitis
Intercostal neuralgia

Investigations

A number of investigations must be considered mandatory to confirm ischaemia, and additional tests may need to be used to exclude aggravating conditions (Table 10.4). A full blood count and film will exclude anaemia or polycythaemia and a high ESR may indicate polyarteritis or impaired plasma proteins – indicating the possible cause of a hypercoagulable state. A chest X-ray is advised, as an enlarged heart may not be detectable clinically and ventricular

Table 10.4. *Useful investigations in ischaemic heart disease*

Chest X-ray
ECG
Full blood count
ESR
Blood urea
Cholesterol
Triglycerides
Blood glucose

hypertrophy may give rise to heart failure if the angina is treated with a beta-blocker on its own: bronchogenic carcinoma can cause angina by local pressure effects.

A normal electrocardiogram does not exclude angina and therefore an exercise or treadmill tracing is advised with appropriate precautions. Hyperlipidaemic states may produce angina in those under 60 years of age, and the younger the patient the more important it is to estimate his cholesterol and triglycerides. It is still debatable whether any treatment will reverse lesions, but some treatment is available which is at least likely to prevent extension of the lesions.

Cardiac failure

Any heart disease may lead to cardiac failure and many reversible systemic diseases cause congestive failure (Table 10.5).

Table 10.5. *Causes of cardiac failure*

Ischaemic heart disease
Anaemia
Infections, especially pneumonia
Pulmonary embolism
Chronic lung disease
Hypertension
Drugs (e.g. Phenylbutazone)
Arrythmia
Cardiomyopathy (especially alchoholic)
Beriberi
Heart block
Hypothyroidism
Hyperthyroidism
Pericardial constriction

Heart failure is classically divided into three types, left failure, right failure, and congestive failure. They can also conveniently be thought of as due to three causes:

1. **Pressure over load** as with valvular stenosis or systemic hypertension.
2. **Volume overload** as in valvular incompetence.

3. **Pump failure** due to myocardial disease – ischaemic or other forms of cardiomyopathy.

Left ventricular failure

Left ventricular failure in its minor form is readily missed. For example, it may only cause insomnia due to an unaccountable nocturnal cough or restlessness. Orthopnoea, nocturnal dyspnoea, and frothy white sputum at night are more well-known signs but may need to be elicited by direct questioning. It is not possible to measure pulmonary venous pressure clinically, but fine crepitations at the lung bases indicate transudate fluid in the interstices as a result of increased pulmonary venous pressure. This clinical sign should be elicited after several deep breaths have been taken, as it is present in most people who breath shallowly especially if they have been lying down.

The cardiovascular causes of left ventricular failure include aortic stenosis and incompetence, hypertension, ischaemia, or left ventricular hypertrophy from any cause. In general diagnosis and treatment are simple clinical ones and if other diseases can be excluded, no particular investigations may be necessary.

Right ventricular failure

The classical signs are raised jugular venous pressure, an engorged tender liver, and dependent oedema. Sacral oedema accumulates when lying down.

Congestive cardiac failure

Congestive cardiac failure usually implies right ventricular failure in addition to left ventricular failure, the latter normally starting first and eventually producing right ventricular overload.

Particular emphasis should be laid on some of the pitfalls which may occur in diagnosis. Any infection, especially chest infections, may precipitate heart failure, particularly in the elderly. Myocardial infarction may give rise to severe confusion and the additional heart failure may be missed; or confusion may be the only presenting feature of heart failure or myocardial infarction.

Multiple pulmonary embolii in the absence of any identifiable clinical focus may only present as heart failure or sudden bouts of breathlessness. Resistance of heart failure to treatment should stimulate further investigation.

Heart block, atrial fibrillation, and other arrhythmias cause failure in elder people. The appropriate treatment for the condition often resolves the failure without specific failure therapy. The same may be true of hypertension – once blood pressure is controlled, failure therapy may be withdrawn or reduced to a minimum.

Investigations

The aim must be to exclude aggravating non-cardiac causes (see Table 10.5) as well as to define the extent of the cardiac disability: appropriate tests for the heart (Table 10.6) include a mandatory chest X-ray, preferably with a lateral

Table 10.6. *Useful investigations in heart failure*

Chest X-ray (with barium)
ECG
Full blood count
ESR
Blood urea
Electrolytes
Liver function tests

---

view, and if possible taken with a barium swallow, which helps to outline the atrial chambers. Calcification in valves, in the aorta, and the relative sizes of the heart chambers, together with an assessment of lung fields, can give more information very simply than any other single cheap investigation. An electrocardiogram, a full blood count, and biochemical analysis will give further information including liver function, in view of back pressure from congestive failure, and renal function, together with any electrolyte problems. The mechanisms of salt and fluid retention are intricate in heart failure and by the time detectable dependent oedema is present at least 5 litres of fluid are retained in the body. It therefore also becomes of great importance to ensure that relief of the failure and reduction of the retained fluids is not accompanied by electrolyte problems induced by inappropriate or excessive use of diuretics.

It cannot be over emphasized that thyroid disease, particularly over active thyroid states, can be extremely difficult to diagnose in the elderly and estimation of thyroid hormone status should always be considered.

Careful history taking may also reveal recurrent complaints of palpitation which the patient often finds difficult to define. A normal electrocardiogram may be severely misleading as cardiac arrythmias, particularly atrial fibrillation or flutter, may be very intermittent in their early stages. Many hospitals now have facilities for 24-hour recording of heart rhythm, which can be rapidly analysed, thus demonstrating the nature of the dysrhythmia.

MANAGEMENT

Ischaemic heart disease, without infarction

Cardiovascular disease is common enough for most people over the age of 35 to know of several people with acute heart problems and to have personal or family experience of sudden death. It is important for the family doctor to be able to define, and to have an overall plan of campaign for anyone who presents with angina. A similar plan can be used after recovery from the acute illness or myocardial infarction.

Aims of treatment are:

1. To relieve anginal pain and other symptoms.
2. To prevent myocardial infarction.
3. To improve survival.

Up to 1970 or so there was little help available even for the high-risk patients; but considerable advances are being made now which make it necessary for the family doctor to be able to identify and to refer the high-risk patients to a cardiological centre. The flow chart in Fig. 10.1 sets out a method of developing care. Some aspects of specialist care are included, because it is important for the family doctor to know what is likely to happen to his patients and to be able to explain it to the relatives.

It becomes of paramount importance to detect high-risk patients. People with the following six characteristics should be considered for further investigation, usually by a cardiologist. It remains important to consider the overall condition of the patient, the presence of other diseases and to consider the patient's own ability or desire to cope with prolonged investigations, operations, and treatment.

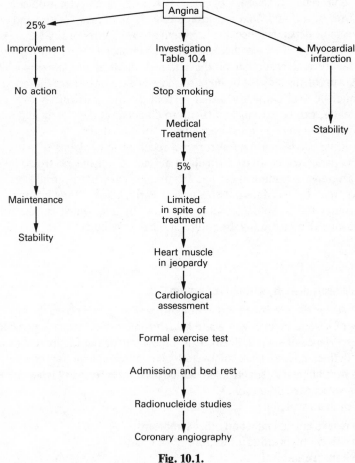

Fig. 10.1.

1. Unstable angina especially if the pain persists after bedrest.

2. Limiting angina persisting on medical treatment especially if it is of long duration.

3. The presence of dizziness with angina.

4. Continuing angina after an acute myocardial infarction.

5. A strongly positive exercise test, especially if the blood pressure falls with exercise.

6. Persisting positive exercise tests after an acute myocardial infarction.

For the vast majority of people, where surgery is not envisaged, there are three groups of appropriate drugs: nitrates, beta-blockers, and calcium blockers. Once treatable causes of angina (Table 10.2) have been excluded or treated, drugs from one or more of these groups will be appropriate. These are referred to in detail later in the chapter.

Care of acute myocardial infarction

It is not proposed to deal with acute myocardial infarction in great detail. In uncomplicated cases home care may be preferable to hospital. Most recently, however, there has been a return to the feeling that hospital facilities, with the ability to monitor anticoagulation, beta-blockade, and dysrhythmic drug administration may provide better overall results. Factors which need to be taken into account are:

(i) The state of the patient:

1. Is he shocked?

2. Is heart block or marked brachycardia present?

3. Is heart failure, especially left ventricular failure, developing?

4. Is he hypertensive?

5. Is arrhythmia present?

(ii) The home circumstances:

1. Can wife or relatives cope?

2. Are they calm enough not to worry the patient?

3. Are urgent communications easy both between the relatives and the patient, and between the doctor and the relatives?

(iii) The practice:

1. Is frequent follow-up feasible, initially even up to three times daily?

2. Can the receptionists and partners be alerted that coronary care at home is being undertaken?

3. Is medical care available rapidly round the clock?

It is generally agreed that bed rest, allayment of anxiety, and adequate pain relief, together with the control of heart failure, arrhythmias, and heart block are essential and the basis of active medical treatment. Early mobilization appears to have advantages after the initial acute episode of pain has resolved. Up to five days bed-rest, at least, is still advised, though with a minor infarction with obvious rapid clinical recovery, it is quite reasonable for the patient to sit out after two or three days. Calm confidence on the part of the doctor, wife, and relatives, together with a minimum of visiting from outside remains essential. Visiting even from close friends, can be extremely tiring if prolonged for more than five or ten minutes, and this is not often appreciated, except by those who have been through a major illness or operation.

Constipation is a factor which is frequently forgotten and may be extremely distressing to the patient.

Existing hypertension may settle completely or temporarily after myocardial infarction, so that treatment may be withdrawn. It is important, however, to monitor this for several months, as blood pressure often rises again with the return to active life.

Heart failure

The overriding principle in the management of heart failure is the treatment of any underlying cause (Table 10.5). Such causes are often difficult to identify, or the possibility of their existence may not occur to the general practitioner. But in any event, treatment of heart failure need not wait until the diagnosis is made, and must be treated in its own right.

Diuretics remain the mainstay of treatment, but are particularly effective in left-sided heart failure. The section on therapeutic notes gives a broad guide to the diuretics available. In general there is a great tendency in practice to use powerful short-acting loop diuretics in mild heart failure when a simple effective thiazide may well be just as effective, just as acceptable to the patient, and considerably cheaper.

It is also true that in many cases of heart failure, powerful diuretics are continued at unnecessarily high doses after the heart failure has resolved. As a result cardiac output is reduced unnecessarily, and increased fatigue is caused to the patient, together with a raised blood urea.

Potassium loss is also unpredictable. Potassium supplements are no longer added routinely in the absence of Digoxin but the following plan of campaign can be suggested:

1. Careful biochemical monitoring of potassium levels, especially in the early stages of treatment of acute heart failure requiring a considerable diuresis.

2. Six monthly or annual monitoring of potassium levels.

3. Avoid giving potassium in the same dose, and at the same time as the diuretic, as this merely causes rapid excretion of the absorbed potassium.

4. Potassium-sparing diuretics may considerably increase blood potassium levels, particularly when renal function is embarrassed, and the blood urea is rising.

Digoxin and other cardiac glycosides remain the second line of treatment for heart failure. Digoxin is essential in cases of atrial fibrillation, but in other situations the benefit may be relatively small, and the margin between therapeutic and toxic levels is rather narrow. Most patients in sinus rhythm and mild heart failure will not require Digoxin, but one or two may deteriorate if chronic Digoxin treatment is stopped, and these are probably the patients who remain on the borderline of heart failure. The section on Therapeutic Notes below covers further aspects of Digoxin treatment.

Vasodilators have fairly recently been recognized as important therapeutic agents in the treatment of heart failure. They may produce an improvement in cardiac performance, better than that achieved by cardiac glycosides. The nitrates act predominently by venous dilatation, Hydralazine and Nifedipine act by arteriolar dilatation, which reduces peripheral vascular resistence, and results in improved cardiac output, while Prazosine, Salbutamol, and Captopril act by both arterial and venous dilatation. Their use is likely to be effective when heart failure is severe, but their effect is somewhat unpredictable, and their use in general practice may be limited by the need to titrate and monitor the effects closely. Several of the drugs in this group are also well known as hypotensive drugs, but their use in heart failure is unlikely to produce troublesome hypotension.

General care and nursing measures are important in the early stages of treatment of heart failure, when mobility is impaired, and sore places may occur on the heels, as well as sacral or buttock areas. Acute heart failure in the elderly can be particularly rewarding to treat without admission to hospital, but again emphasis must be made on the need for close monitoring during the first few days of extensive diuresis.

IMPACT OF THE DISEASE – PATIENT, PRACTICE, AND SOCIETY

A label of 'heart illness' or 'heart disease' is one with considerable implications for the patient. The heart is central to life in most people's minds, and the statement 'it's his heart' may have as much overtone as the statement 'he's got cancer'.

'Heart failure' is a technical term which should never be used without adequate explanation. It is a label which sticks, and even with explanation is still taken to mean impending death. The terms 'heart attack' or 'coronary' are probably better understood, but time should still be taken to explain to the patient and to the relatives exactly what is meant.

Time is perhaps the one commodity which all doctors feel they are short of, but time is the one thing which will help more than any other – time spent in complete and simple explanation, time spent in finding out what the patients and relatives have really understood from these simple explanations time spent in going over, if necessary, again and again, the simple explanations, and ensuring patiently as much comprehension as possible. Time spent almost invariably saves a considerable amount of time later, but more importantly it creates an important bond of confidence.

Inevitably, considerable folk-lore surrounds conditions of heart disease and heart failure. When patients consider the future after a serious myocardial infarction, their recovery and will to recover will be affected by several factors, including, for example, the knowledge of friends or acquaintances who have had a similar problem, and may have died. Doctors may tend to consider a coronary as a temporary disability, but patients and their families correctly feel that it frequently involves major long-term adjustments, which disturb their existing assumptions of their future, the families' future, and their current patterns of living. While physical recovery from an infarction may be apparently objectively complete, the emotional recovery from an infarction is a process similar in its stages to adjustment to such forms of loss as blindness, or bereavement. As a profession we are probably at fault here, because we make great efforts to tell patients that they are now physically normal, and should be expected to get back to a totally normal life. At the same time we tell them that certain regular features of their normal lives are harmful, such as their diet, their alcohol intake, their smoking habits, their obesity and their lack of exercise. For some patients the change in life-style may be totally abhorrent: they would rather live dangerously and die suddenly. For others the knowledge of the factors involved in further prevention, may be just what is required by the patient and his family, and it would be wrong not to offer this advice.

PREVENTION: RISK FACTORS INVOLVED IN HEART DISEASE

For ischaemic heart disease the factors involved in prevention are those factors which may well contribute to an improved prognosis, even where quite severe ischaemia is established. Table 10.7 lists some of these risk factors, which are known well enough not to need very much comment. Unfortunately, not all of them are preventable or reversible; but smoking, cholesterol and abnormal blood fats, obesity and hypertension remain the most important factors in the whole group. If these factors are recognized and acted upon, then the prognosis is considerably improved.

Table 10.8 lists simple preventative aspects which must go hand in hand with consideration of the risk factors. Family practitioners should not feel they have to do everything themselves, and it is particularly in the aspects of prevention that they should call on the use of other professionals, and involve the patient in his own management.

Table 10.7. *Risk factors in ischaemic heart disease*

Smoking	
Raised cholesterol	
Hypertension	Main risk factors
Obesity	
Diabetes	
Type A personality	
Anxiety or psychosocial problems	
Physical inactivity	
Family history of ischaemic heart disease	

Table 10.8. *Preventative aspects of ischaemic heart disease*

Appropriate diet
Adequate exercise
Stopping smoking
Avoiding stress
Good diabetic control
Care of relatives of younger sufferers

However, to be realistic, preventative medicine has really not started in the field of ischaemic heart disease. The Health Service cannot finance the national screening procedures necessary to estimate cholesterol and blood fats, and there are many undiagnosed hypertensives and diabetics. Lip service only is still paid to the dangers of smoking, and also to the dangers of alcohol and obesity. The reduction of the prevalence of infections in the nineteenth and early twentieth century owes far more to preventative measures and hygiene than has ever occurred with the use of antibiotics. In an analogous way prevention of heart disease must involve changing the attitudes of the general population.

Prognosis and long-term care of heart failure depends much more on continuing active treatment than does prognosis in ischaemic heart disease. Explanations remain important, but much more important is the correct use in long-term monitoring of the drugs and their effects on the body. These aspects have been covered in the management section, and also in the pharmacological section of this chapter. In general, long-term heart failure occurs in older groups of patients, than in the more dramatic middle-age ischaemic heart disease cases. Consequently the management of heart failure tends to be bound up with the management of multiple pathology. This high-risk group of patients is increasing in size, and it is appropriate to consider the organization of the practice in terms of their overall care. This can be looked at in terms of, for example, the medical standards and mechanisms of audit within the practice, the use of the practice team and other associated professions, and ensuring that the organization of the practice itself, together with record systems and practice equipment are satisfactory.

MEDICAL AUDIT AND STANDARDS

Cardiovascular disease form a group of illnesses well suited to practice analysis and audit. The constituent diseases of cardiovascular illness are well circumscribed and defined, and the diagnosis may be considerably more certain than in many other clinical conditions.

Audit of a group of patients with a particular disease does not imply producing complicated research papers for general publication. The purpose of audit within a practice is to monitor the effectiveness of one's own medical care, to maintain standards, and to keep abreast of modern developments in therapy. It is possible to develop a broadly based practice protocol to provide consistency in the management of particular conditions.

Patients tend to follow guidelines more readily, as symptoms recur usually, if treatment is left off. If the symptoms do not recur, then the treatment may no longer be necessary. Patients are also more likely to attend for follow-ups, since they need prescriptions regularly. It may be entirely appropriate to arrange for a system of repeat prescriptions, but, as in other illnesses and conditions, there is obligation to ensure that the medical condition is unchanged, but organizing a regular, though not necessarily very frequent, system of follow-up.

More practices are developing a system of repeat prescriptions, described in Chapter 4, whereby the patient must be seen after a set number of repeat refills. Intervals depend on the doctor, the patient, and the condition being treated. For example, a stable treated congestive failure patient may be on a Thiazide diuretic, a potassium supplement, Digoxin, and salt-limited dietary advice. So long as his condition remains stable, it is entirely appropriate to see him once every three or four months, and estimate his blood urea and electrolytes once a year. The exact frequency of follow-up must be a matter of concern to the doctor, but it is not appropriate to repeat prescriptions indefinitely without attendance; and it is not appropriate to leave a patient on long-term powerful diuretics without occasional monitoring. It would also be reasonable from time to time to estimate a random blood sugar given the effect of Thiazide and other diuretics on glucose tolerance. Equally, it would be appropriate to estimate the serum uric acid occasionally as diuretics may precipitate clinical gout after a time.

To summarize:

1. Patients with ischaemic heart disease and heart failure are usually on long-term treatment.

2. All patients with these conditions should be followed up regularly, though not necessarily frequently.

3. A fool-proof system of repeat prescriptions with a recall system after a definite number of repeats should be organized within the practice.

4. The purpose of follow-up is to (i) review the necessity for treatment; (ii) to consider biochemical monitoring and other investigations.

THE USE OF OTHER PROFESSIONALS

It is clear that with increasing complexity of medical care the general practitioner neither has a monopoly of knowledge and skills or of time to be able to give complete advice in all fields to his patients, nor is it appropriate that he should do so.

District nursing sister

The district nursing sister is an essential member of the primary care team, and is particularly helpful in home care of the elderly patients with cardiac failure.

But she will also be of considerable use in assisting with a patient with an acute myocardial infarction when home treatment is planned.

Domiciliary physiotherapist

Domiciliary physiotherapy must also have its place, particularly in mobilizing the patient with heart failure after a period of inactivity; and also helping with chest expansion and breathing exercises, where there has been a significant chest infection as a complication of myocardial infarction or heart failure.

Most patients hope, and expect, to maintain their independance in their own homes, and a *domiciliary occupational therapist* is able to give advice and recommendations concerning all manner of appliances. These include stair rails, wall rails by baths and lavatories, and non-slip coverings for baths and showers. The experienced eye of the professional may well detect needs which escape a busy general practitioner.

In situations where a change of housing is likely to be necessary, referral to the Social Services Department is better done sooner rather than later. A change of home from an awkward and ageing council house to a sheltered flat or to a place in an old peoples home or Part III accommodation may well be foreseen near the start of an illness. The time taken to arrange such a transfer may coincide with the stabilization of the failure.

Dietician

A Dietician is particularly useful for obesity, diabetes, or hyperlipidaemic states.

PRACTICE ORGANIZATION, EQUIPMENT, AND RECORDS

It is the function of the practice to provide adequate service and constant professional availability for the patient. With ischaemic heart disease, it is clear that this is an area of medical practice where acute medical emergencies often occur. The organization of the practice needs to be geared to rapid communication and remedial action.

Communication systems

Communication systems are becoming more comprehensive even for remote country areas. A telephone system is taken for granted, and it is entirely appropriate to record telephone numbers on the records, or even the telephone number of a close neighbour. The use of the Post Office Paging System or an alternative Paging System is now becoming widespread, and it may not be too long before it is taken for granted that all doctors should have some form of paging system.

Equipment

Equipment specifically for monitoring chronic and acute heart disease is relatively expensive. An electrocardiograph, a portable defibrillator, and a cardiac monitor may all be considered useful adjuncts. However, it is only the electrocardiograph which is a common piece of equipment for general practice, and this is by no means universal yet. The real questions that have to be asked are:

1. Will the use of the equipment change the way the doctor can practice and increase the quality of care?
2. Does he have the expertise to use the equipment?
3. Will the equipment be used frequently enough to maintain his experience?

There are also the practical problems of ensuring that the doctor on call has the equipment readily available. With the increasing number of special care ambulance teams with defibrillators it may be difficult to justify the expense of a defibrillator in the practice which may be used less than once in every two years.

In general it may be said that most practices probably justify the use of an electrocardiogram, and there may be a few high-risk areas in the country where other equipment would be justified as well.

For investigations, it is always helpful ot have ready access to a haemoglobinometer and an ESR tube. A centrifuge is an important piece of equipment for spinning down heparinized blood samples so that no overnight increase in potassium leaking from the red blood cells produces a false electrolyte level.

Practice records

The practice records should provide some basic information on all patients who have long-standing heart trouble. An absolute minimum is a list of current treatment and drugs, because reactions with other drugs can so easily occur. All normal standards of record keeping should apply, with summary sheets, clear diagnoses, and readily accessible investigation results.

INDICATIONS FOR REFERRAL

The short- and long-term management of cardiovascular disease is well within the scope and competence of family practice. The ability to exclude associated causes and factors requires open access to laboratory and X-ray facilities, which are generally now available. Even if they are not, a personal phone call to the appropriate department should obtain approval.

There may remain a small proportion of patients in whom the doctor is unhappy about the diagnosis, or wishes to have a second opinion. Referral may, therefore, be necessary in some circumstances;

1. Unusual age or presentations of the disease.
2. Possibility of advanced medical or surgical help.
3. To have the support of the hospital department in long-term management.

4. Doubt about the diagnosis or its underlying causes.

5. Deterioration of the patient in spite of apparently adequate therapy.

Acute hospital admission may well be necessary, but the use of a domiciliary consultation may provide just the extra support and advice that the practitioner needs. The domiciliary consultation, when attended both by the specialist and the general practitioner, is still a most useful means of both rapport and education.

PHARMACOLOGICAL AND THERAPEUTIC NOTES

This section deals with many of the drugs which are in current use in various aspects of heart disease, other than hypertension, though many of them are also used in antihypertensive therapy. It is not a comprehensive list and individual doctors will still have their own choices and preferences.

Particular reference is made to some of the known side-effects and the precautions which may be necessary in their use.

The list is not a substitute for the normal sources of therapeutic information. Two important principles may be stressed:

1. It is essential for the doctor to get used to the actions of a small number of drugs in any one category.

2. One should not be afraid to try newer drugs.

Drugs used for angina

These are divided into vasodilators and beta-blockers. There are two forms of vasodilators: the nitrates and the calcium antagonists.

Nitrates

Glyceryl trinitrate is still one of the most effective drugs for providing symptomatic relief, and on occasions is useful in the absence of other facilities for making a diagnosis of angina. It is safe in long-term use, but is ineffective in infarction unless given parenterally. Side-effects with frequent use may limit therapy – flushing, headache, and postural hypotension.

Isosorbide dinitrate is also active sublingually and orally. Likewise it can be given parenterally and will reduce temporarily the cardiac load in acute infarction.

Many new formulations of nitrates are available including a multi-dose nitrate aerosol spray, which as the advantages of a reasonably long shelf-life. There is also a nitrate paste which is absorbed transcutaneously.

Calcium antagonists

Nifedipine reduces peripheral and coronary vascular resistance: useful in angina, hypertension, and heart failure. Parodoxically it can cause fluid retention, and ankle swelling is common. Palpitation and headache may occur. Use with beta-blockers precipitates cardiac failure.

Verapamil is effective both as a vasodilator and for depressing supraventricular arrythmias. But its use is limited in general practice without adequate diagnostic facilities. It is contra-indicated in patients with AV node or sinus node malfunction, digitalis toxicity, or in the presence of beta-blockers. Intravenous verapamil is especially contra-indicated in these circumstances.

Beta-blockers

Since the introduction of Propranolol in the early 1960s the beta-blockers have become one of the most widely used groups of drugs. At least ten beta-blocking drugs are currently available and they all have the same basic action: they block competitively the action of catacolamines at beta-adrenergic receptor sites. There are, however, many differences in the detailed properties which may influence the choice of drug. It is on these differences that the beta-blockers are currently promoted and sold. They include cardio-selectivity, differences in half-life, and in metabolism and elimination, and the property that some beta-blockers have in producing a weak stimulant effect on the receptors (partial agonist effect). Table 10.9 shows some of the properties of ten currently available beta-blockers.

Table 10.9. *Properties of beta-blockers*

	Half-life	Lipophilic	Hydrophilic	Elimination	Cardioselectivity	Partial agonist activity
Acebutolol	3	+	−	Liver	?	+
Alprenolol	2	+	−	Liver	?	+
Atenolol	8	−	+	Kidney	+	−
Metoprolol	3	+	−	Liver	+	−
Nadolol	20	−	+	Kidney	−	−
Oxprenolol	2	+	−	Liver	−	+
Pindolol	4	+	−	Liver	−	+ +
Propranolol	4	+	−	Liver	−	−
Sotalol	16	−	+	Kidney	−	−
Trinolol	4	+	−	Liver	−	−

The half-life varies considerably between them, but even those beta-blockers with a short half-life can be given twice daily if the dosage is large enough.

In general the liphilic beta-blockers are metabolized in the liver and the metabolites excreted through the kidneys, so their doses should be reduced both in liver disease and in severe renal disease. The hydrophilic beta-blockers should be reduced in severe renal disease, but are not affected by hepatic disease, and in general do not easily penetrate the blood–brain barrier.

If it is essential to use a beta-blocker in a patient with a tendency to bronchospasm, it is less likely to occur with a cardio-selective beta-blocker. But great care must always be taken to ensure that beta-blockers, if possible, are not used in patients who have a past history of asthma, as it may precipitate rapid and very resistent bronchospasm. Cardio-selective beta-blockers are also best used where cold extremities or Raynaud's phenomenon can be a problem, and those with partial agonist activity will also help in this situation.

Beta-blockers should not be given to patients who are in heart failure, or who require large doses of diuretics. Partial antagonist activity will not prevent heart failure.

A number of cases of sudden death have occurred in patients due to myocardial infarction and with unstable angina, where beta-blockers have been withdrawn suddenly. Beta-blockers should never be withdrawn in patients with angina, except slowly to a gradual reduction of dosage.

THE TREATMENT OF HEART FAILURE

Conventionally diuretics remain the mainstay of treatment, particularly in left-sided chronic congestive heart failure. The addition of Digoxin and vasodilating drugs has been mentioned previously and it is worthwhile taking a little space on the choice of diuretic.

Twenty-three diuretics were available in 1982 in the United Kindom. There is an enormous difference in price, and few advantages to be gained by prescribing expensive ones. Thiazide diuretics are by far the cheapest, are very well tolerated, and their properties are very similar to more expensive introductions such as Metolazone, Indapamide, and Xipamide. Incidentally Indapamide is marketed as an anti-hypertensive agent, but is, in fact, a diuretic, and combining it with a diuretic may produce very considerable electrolyte disturbances.

Loop diuretics such as Frusemide, Bumetanide, and Ethacrynic Acid produce a much shorter rapid diuresis lasting 4–6 hours. It is not generally known that repeating the dose in less than eight hours has no diuretic effect at all, and if a loop diuretic is given at eight-hourly intervals all diuresis is lost.

Loop diuretics should not normally be the first-choice treatment for mild heart failure, but should be reserved for patients with more severe heart failure and for those with nephrotic or hepatic oedema. They can safely be added to Thiazide diuretics. The use of intravenous Frusemide, together with intravenous morphia or heroin is life saving in acute left ventricular failure and acute pulmonary oedema.

Potassium sparing diuretics on their own are very mild, and are usually combined with a Thiazide in order to prevent dangerous potassium retention.

Potassium supplements

There is still considerable confusion about the use of potassium with diuretics, and it is very difficult to predict in the individual case where potassium supplements may be required. It is, therefore, totally appropriate to estimate serum electrolytes within a month of starting treatment, and regularly every six months, or annually in stable cases. Plasma potassium values lower than 3.0

mmol/l are uncommon. Loop diuretics at ordinary doses are less likely than Thiazide to cause important hypokalaemia, and patients with cardiac failure are less likely than those with hypertension to become hypokalaemic. The juice of an orange contains as much potassium as a tablet of slow-release potassium chloride and in general this quantity of potassium is too small to be of real value.

It is, therefore, important that patients should be identified in advance where it is necessary to avoid even mild hypokalaemia. These are:

1. Patients with arrhythmias, myocardial infarction, or severe ischaemic heart disease.

2. Patients with chronic liver disease or elderly patients on a poor diet.

3. Patients taking Digoxin and corticosteroids (which deplete potassium).

4. Patients taking drugs which interfere with ventricular repolarization such as Inothiazines and tricyclic antidepressants.

It is suggested that patients in these groups should be given potassium-sparing diuretics from the outset as potassium supplements can be so unreliable. Their plasma potassium should be kept at least above 3.5 mmol/l.

Cardiac glycosides

Digoxin can be of particular use in the control of heart failure, but once stability is reached it is worthwhile trying to withdraw it. It does, however, remain essential treatment where atrial fibrillation or atrial flutter exists, and if there is any doubt about dosage then Digoxin assay is now widely available and should be performed. (Normal therapeutic range 1.2–2.6 nmol/l.)

The plasma half-life of Digoxin is approximately 36 hours, but the myocardial half-life may be much longer, and therefore it is sensible to stop Digoxin for a week or more before concluding that it is no longer responsible for toxic effects. Digitoxin has a much longer plasma half-life and should no longer be used.

Vasodilators

As mentioned above, the use of vasodilators in heart failure has been shown to be valuable where conventional therapy alone has been ineffective. Nifedipine was discussed under Angina. It dilates arteries, but has a negative inotropic effect on the heart, which may make it undesirable for patients with heart failure.

Hydrallazine relaxes directly the arterioles, and is in common use for hypertension. In heart failure it causes a fall in peripheral resistance, and increases the cardiac output with an improvement in renal blood flow. Under these circumstances effects on blood pressure are small in heart failure, and therefore the use of Hydrallazine in normotensive patients is not contra-indicated. It should, however, be noted that dosages in excess of 200 mg daily are frequently associated with the appearance of a drug-induced lupus erythematosis.

Prazosin acts by both arteriolar dilation and in increasing the venous capacitance. It causes an increase in cardiac output and a fall in the venous filling pressure. As in hypertension, it is advisable to start with a very small dose at night, but again its use is not contra-indicated in normotensive patients.

The use of vasodilator drugs in the treatment of heart failure is relatively recent, but is appropriate in situations where the response to Digoxin and diuretics alone has been inadequate. If breathlessness is the major problem, then a nitrate is indicated and one of the long-acting nitrate preparations should be used. Where peripheral oedema is refractory, arteriolar vasodilators are best used. When both peripheral oedema and breathlessness co-exist then it is appropriate to use both a nitrate and a peripheral vasodilator.

SUMMARY

Ischaemic heart disease and heart failure, and generalized vascular diseases are areas where considerable advances are being made on two fronts. First, a great deal of publicity has been given, not only to the high level of mortality from vascular disease, but also to advances in therapeutic and surgical techniques, particularly heart transplants. It is totally unrealistic to expect that heart transplants and, to a lesser extent, coronary artery grafts, will ever be available to more than a very small minority of severe cardiac sufferers.

The second front of advances, therefore, must come with preventive medicine, and with the concern of the medical profession and family practice in particular with patients' lifestyles. The Western diet and the Western habits, including smoking and obesity, are proven major factors. While the exact relationships of the fatty fractions of the blood, high-density lipoproteins, low-density lipoproteins, and so on, have yet to be determined, and are constantly a matter of changing opinion, the overall message is clear. High-cholesterol and high-fat diets produce vascular degeneration and ischaemic heart disease. Prevention of disease, and health education, will need to start at a much earlier age. It is certainly becoming too late by the age of 30.

PERFORMANCE REVIEW CHECK LIST

General

1. Can the practice identify all patients with continuing angina or cardiac failure and those with a history of myocardial infarction?
2. Does the practice have a policy for the general management for these diseases?

Patients on treatment

1. How many of the following were recorded at initial assessment: smoking history, family history, presenting symptoms, social consequences?

2. How many of the following have been recorded at initial or subsequent assessment: blood pressure, weight, glucose, full blood count, urea and electrolytes, lipids, chest X-ray, ECG.
3. Is there any record of the patient's ideas or of the information given to the patient?
4. Are the current drugs and dosage clearly recorded?

Emergencies

Is there a practice policy for the management of acute myocardial infarction and acute LVF?

PATIENT ASSOCIATIONS AND SELF-HELP GROUPS

The Chest, Heart and Stroke Association,
Tavistock House,
North Tavistock Square,
London WC1N 9JE
For advizing and helping patients.

The British Heart Foundation,
57 Gloucester Place,
London W1H 4DH
Provides leaflets and sponsors research.

PATIENT BOOKS AND LEAFLETS

Produced by organizations above.

11 Physical disabling disease

John Toby

The concept of disability and its relation to impairment and handicap are discussed elsewhere in this book (Chapter 3). For the general practitioner it is the effect of an impairment on a patient's life-style which is most important and disability can be regarded as the difference between what he might reasonably want to do and what he is able to do.Limitation of consideration to specific activities such as housework or employment will grossly under-estimate patients' difficulties in coping with many chronic diseases. Conversely, if a patient is able to lead what he regards as a normal life, his view of his disability should be understood. A large subjective element in both the patient's and his advisers' assessments is unavoidable and must be recognized.

The most striking disabilities are usually motor but sensory impairments, especially those of the eyes and ears, may be equally disabling. Disability also results from other physical handicaps which are classified in Chapter 3 (p. 46) under the headings visceral, invisible, and aversive. In some of these cases it is society which determines the patient's disability but the effect on the patient may be the same as if he was himself physically disabled.

The commonest causes of physical disability are arthritis, multiple sclerosis, low back pain of various aetiologies, cerebrovascular diseases, ischaemic heart disease, and diseases of the chest. Many of the remainder are due to trauma, particularly at birth. Some of these problems are discussed in other chapters and consideration here is limited to diseases of the joints and nervous system. The impact of physical disability is felt most by the patient but his family are deeply involved and there are very important implications for the organization of medical care and society at large. The social and psychological aspects have been discussed in detail in Chapters 3 and 2 respectively. Some of these issues are briefly reviewed here from one general practitioner's point of view.

IMPACT ON THE PATIENT

Disability occurring in the course of an illness creates a burden which is added to the problems of the illness itself. The patient frequently suffers from pain, as in the case of arthritis, and possibly fear. The fear may arise from ignorance of the likely outcome of his disease or from a realistic expectation of severe handicap. In the acute stages of a disease the patient may be isolated by virtue of necessary rest and treatment and in the long term this isolation may continue as a result of its effects. In the case of children education may be difficult and for adults personal development may be severely curtailed. Normal relationships are difficult to maintain if the patient becomes physically dependent. Sexual activity may decline or cease leading to frustration of both partners and this may in part be due to difficulty caused by the physical problems. A vicious circle may be created with loss of self-esteem and status within the family leading to psychological dependence and withdrawal which confirms the patient's low standing with himself and others. Problems with employment will frequently aggravate the situation and the financial hardships which may be a consequence can serve to hasten the patient's general decline. His mental response to his misfortuenes may amount to a bereavement reaction. This is particularly the case where there is sudden deterioration and in progressive diseases the cycle may be reporduced on a number of occasions. Initial disbelief may interfere with treatment while resentment and aggression will almost certainly strain the relationships between the patient, his family and his advisers. If he becomes depressed to a significant degree the withdrawal that this induces will be added to any isolation resulting from his disease.

The full horror of the developments outlined are seldom realized although the elements are present to a greater degree than is often recognized. There is, however, much that the doctor and others working with him can do to alleviate the situation. Anticipation of the patient's reactions and discussion of these with him may reduce their severity and specific provisions may alleviate some of the isolation. The importance of the patient's self-esteem must be brought to the attention of those caring for him and the maintenance of a normal adult relationship between the doctor and patient is both an example to others and helpful in itself. The patient will usually benefit from adequate explanation of his situation and the potential for recovery, e.g. following a stroke or during an attack of multiple sclerosis, should be stressed. However, unreasonable expectations must not be encouraged because of the danger of consequential loss of credibility of the doctor and disappointment in the patient.

IMPACT ON THE FAMILY

The role of the family in the patient's support has already been mentioned. However, it has to be remembered that the family itself will often be suffering and that individual members will have needs of their own. An attempt should be made to understand something of the dynamics of the family and therefore the likely effects that this added stress will have on its members. These should be openly discussed in the reasonable expectation that such discussion will produce a more positive approach to caring. It may be necessary to provide specific support for individual members of the family and this may be more easily carried out by seeing the person concerned separately in the surgery. This, however, carries the risk that the patient will feeel that discussions about him are taking place behind his back and the reason for any such discussions should be made clear to him if possible. Any financial loss will usually be shared by members of the family and if this is severe all possible advice should be obtained as to how the situation can be rectified. Time will often be a problem for the principal person responsible for caring. Consideration should be given to getting relief in the form of a sitter-in to allow some freedom and time to do simple chores such as shopping without undue pressure. Short-term admission of the patient to hospital or other accommodation may be necessary to allow the members of the family to have a rest or holiday.

IMPACT ON SOCIETY

It is probable that 10 per cent or more of the population are disabled at any one time and the demands made on society are considerable. Perhaps the most important demand is that society should recognize the problem and not seek to confine the disabled to places out of sight such as their own homes or hospitals. Education in schools and through the media should aim to stress the 'normality' of the disabled. There are also needs in relation to the provision of financial support, transport, access to buildings, educational provisions, and employment. The financial support applies not only to the patient and his immediate family but to the services which are involved in caring. All doctors have a duty to bring these issues to the attention of those responsible for forming public opinion at every opportunity.

IMPACT ON THE PRACTICE

The first requirement for the doctor is time. The complex problems suffered by patients with physically disabling diseases are seldom capable of solution in very brief consultations, particularly when these occur at infrequent intervals. Where time is short the tendency to offer prescriptions of drugs and then repeat these without seeing the patient may be overwhelming. Planning is therefore necessary to avoid this and if the normal rate of consultation is rapid one solution is the provision of a certain number of longer consultations for particular patients. Alternatively, some form of 'mini clinic' may be organized which has the advantage of making it easier to involve other members of the practice team. The concentration of the efforts of general practitioners on acute medical problems and those presented urgently by patients has led to an organization which militates against proper care for complicated conditions and a conscious effort of thought is necessary to overcome this.

Disabled patients often have difficulty both in getting to the surgery and, once there, in getting to consulting rooms. Reception staff should be made familiar with these difficulties and devise techniques for overcoming them where possible. Appointments should be made available at times when patients can attend with reasonable convenience or be brought by relatives or friends. If it is possible to arrange a transport system, perhaps using volunteer services, this may add to the patient's convenience.

Consideration has to be given to the advisability of consultations in surgery or at home. One of the main aims of long-term management of chronic disability is to increase the patient's independence and enable him to regard himself as nearly normal as possible. It is therefore beneficial for him to come to surgery and this is also in the doctor's interest. On the other hand, assessment of the patient in his own environment is also important. If the doctor's policy is to bring the patients to the surgery whenever possible he should plan the occasional, or at least an initial, home visit to enable him to understand the patient's environment. Visits by other workers, however helpful in different contexts, do not give the doctor personal understanding of his patient's home conditions. When surgery buildings are planned the needs of the disabled should be borne in mind as should possible modifications to existing buildings to allow access by a wheelchair and the provision of appropriate toilet facilities.

ASSESSMENT OF DISABILITY

Apart from the physical arrangements and the allocation of time, the general practitioner must be sure that he has a system for assessment of patients suffering from disabling disease and be prepared to co-ordinate the work of specialists and other professionals who may be involved. The following points should be included in any assessment of such patients:

1. Disability as seen by the patient and doctor.
2. Diagnosis.
3. Symptoms of disease process.
4. Treatment, including drugs and side-effects.
5. Management of bowels and bladder.
6. Sexual function.
7. Self-care, including dressing and undressing, provision and preparation of food.
8. Care of feet.
9. Mobility.
10. Housing.
11. Occupation and employment.
12. Finances.
13. Family support.
14. Social contacts.
15. Specialist supervision.
16. Other professionals involved.
17. Information given to patient.

Such a list can be made the basis for a special record sheet which can then act as an *aide mèmoire* and as a prod to the doctor when dealing with the problems of disability. The preparation and completion of such a record also enables other members of the health care team to have access to essential information.

MANAGEMENT OF DISABILITY

It is not possible to discuss all the items listed above. In many cases the revelation of a problem will in any event suggest possible solutions. It is, however, very important to ensure that the patient is put in touch with all the agencies capable of helping him. Nurses, health visitors, occupational therapists, physiotherapists, and social workers may all have an important part to play. There is still a feeling that occupational therapy is mainly concerned with basket making and needlework but in reality it covers many aspects of living and therapists are the best source of information on aids. These range from simple gadgets like 'helping hands' and modified electric plugs to wheelchairs and complex electrical equipment. Social workers may be able to arrange family support, home helps, meals on wheels, and, depending on local arrangements, co-ordinate contributions from voluntary organizations. Domiciliary chiropody is often available but the extent of the service varies considerably from one area to another.

While advice about benefits will often come from social workers, the doctor should ensure that the patient has as much financial assistance as possible. This is discussed in Chapter 3. Special facilities are also available for getting patients to and from their place of employment if they do not themselves have transport. These are available through the disablement resettlement officer (DRO) who can be contacted at local Job Centres. The DRO can also advise both patients and their employers about modifications which can be carried out at the place of work to enable a disabled person to continue in employment. Financial assistance can be given to employers for necessary provisions but many are unaware of this. The DRO should be consulted as to whether or not a patient should be registered as disabled but this is not always of benefit and should also be discussed with his Trade Union.

ALTERNATIVE MEDICINE

Many patients feel the need for treatment other than that available from the conventional services. This may simply result from a desire to do something for themselves. It may be prompted by anecdotal accounts of successful regimens or reflect lack of confidence in their medical advisers. Self-help groups are important in the dissemination of information about such treatments. The offhand dismissal of the value of alternative medicine by doctors may be a potent source of discontent and there is always the possibility that such treatments may have some merit, as yet unproven. While the doctor should only promote treatments which are of proven value he should not discourage patients from those which are likely to be harmless and not prove too great a financial burden. Such treatments include acupuncture, osteopathy, many diets, homeopathy, and herbal remedies. With regard to diets, it is important to ensure that they provide adequate nutrition. Where rest or vigorous exercise are • a part of the treatment any possible harmful effects should be explained. The patient should also be encouraged to retain an open mind as to the outcome to avoid possible disappointment.

The contribution of self-help groups is discussed after the following sections as specific problems.

ARTHRITIS

Definition and terminology

This is difficult because the field is wide and encompasses both inflammatory and non-inflammatory diseases of varying duration. In the context of continuing care the general practitioner is concerned with chronic joint disease which largely excludes those of viral, bacterial, and traumatic aetiologies. The common arthritides which cause recurrent or persistent pain and usually swelling in one or more joints may be classified as follows:

Inflammatory
  (i) Rheumatoid arthritis (RA)
 (ii) Other connective tissue diseases such as sytemic lupus erythematosus (SLE)
(iii) Spondarthritides:
     including ankylosing spondylitis, psoriatic arthropathy, enteropathic arthropathy (such as those associated with ulcerative colitis and Crohn's disease)
     Reiter's syndrome
Degenerative
    Osteoarthritis (osteoarthrosis)
Miscellaneous
    Gout
    Pyrophosphate arthropathy (pseudo gout)

The term spondarthritis is a useful one in that it collects together those arthritides which usually involve the central joints, particularly the sacro-iliac joints. Controversy remains about the nomenclature in osteoarthritis. The familar term is retained although it is clear that in many patients inflammation is not a prominent feature and perhaps, for these, osteoarthrosis is a better description.

Arthritis in children is uncommon and is usually caused by juvenile rheumatoid arthritis (Still's disease). This is not discussed further nor is the management of gout which is that of the metabolic disturbance. It is, however, worth remembering that gout may present with a persistent arthritis in one or more joints rather than the more common intermittent inflammation. The problems associated with purely degenerative and traumatic lesions of the spine tend to present with recurrent acute episodes and therefore pose less difficulties in continuing care.

In the remainder of this discussion rheumatoid arthritis and osteoarthritis are assumed to be the most important conditions but many of the considerations apply to the other arthritides.

Incidence and prevalence

Accurate figures for the incidence of the various arthritic conditions are hard to obtain because of problems with definition and the fact that they are often included with other musculoskeletal disorders in large-scale studies. Approximately 20 per cent of all consultations are for musculoskeletal diseases and perhaps slightly more than half of these are due to soft-tissue lesions. This would suggest that just under 10 per cent of all consultations are for some form of chronic arthritis. RA and other inflammatory conditions account for between 2 and 4 per cent of new cases presenting to the general practitioner. RA itself has a prevalence of 3 per cent in the female population and 1 per cent in the male population. Estimates of the prevalence of ankylosing spondylitis vary but it, too, may have a prevalence of as much as 1 per cent. The prevalence of osteoarthritis is impossible to determine since virtually all patients will have some evidence of it from middle age onwards although many of these will not consult their doctors on this account and may not suffer significant symptoms.

Impact of the disease

The relatively high prevalence of rheumatoid arthritis and the increasing importance of osteoarthtitis in an ageing population make the management of these diseases a major demand on general practitioners and the hospital service. Many have felt that the education of doctors, particularly those who will become general practitioners, has been inadequate in this respect and it is noteworthy that patients with rheumatic diseases have a much higher referral rate to hospitals than those with all other chronic diseases. This is the more surprising because many of the problems are amenable to diagnosis and management in general practice.

Clinics with the services of a rheumatologist are not always available to general practitioners but this is becoming less common. The National Health Service has failed, and continues to fail, to provide necessary facilities for surgical treatment. The present waiting lists for operations on osteoarthritic hips is the most obvious example but the same applies to other surgical procedures. This is particularly unfortunate because new surgical procedures are being developed for the relief of arthritic conditions and the potential demand is considerably greater than the present waiting lists suggest. Although general practitioners are clearly unable to reduce the demands on surgical services they can ensure that the best use is made of the other hospital resources by the investigation and management of many rheumatic problems in general practice.

The effects of joint disease on individual patients vary considerably according to the severity of the disease and the circumstances of the patient. While most patients are not severely disabled some require much assistance and a small proportion will strain the combined resources of family, friends and the medical and social services. For society as a whole there is a specific problem in the treatment of rheumatic diseases, in addition to those posed by all causes of disability, and this relates to the costs of drugs. The total cost continues to rise and a significant proportion of this is for drugs used in the treatment of arthritis which tend to be expensive. It is the duty of all those dealing with such patients to bear in mind the cost of treatment when a wide variety of medications are available, some much cheaper than others.

Investigation and diagnosis

The presence of an arthropathy is usually clear from the history except in the elderly who may complain of weakness or unsteadiness on the feet. In this situation joint disease, especially of the knees and hips, may be unsuspected unless an appropriate examination is carried out. It should be remembered that pain from the hip is often felt lower down the leg, particularly just above the knee, and that pain in the region of the hip may be referred from the spine. The main problem, however, is usually to define the cause of the arthropathy.

A family history of rheumatoid arthritis, ankylosing spondylitis, osteoarthritis, psoriasis, and gout is helpful and should always be sought. It is often difficult to evaluate the report that an elderly relative had 'arthritis' but with rheumatoid disease and ankylosing spondylitis the history is often clear. The presence of extra-articulr associations of arthritis such as iritis, skin lesions, bowel disturbance, or genito-urinary abnormalities may tend to suggest a particular cause for the joint inflammation. These extra-articular manifestations may precede the development of arthritis and specific enquiry should be made. In osteoarthritis the occupation may be relevant.

The pattern of the disease is the most important part of the history and should be defined with as much accuracy as possible. Inflammatory arthritis tends to be worse in the morning and after sitting while osteoarthritis is worse with exercise and at night. An intermittent arthropathy suggests the possibility of gout or palindromic rheumatism. The latter is an uncommon but important presentation of RA in which one or more joints become acutely inflamed for 24–48 hours which is rather shorter than the inflammation of gout. The joints return to normal after an attack but the attacks recur with varying frequency. Involvement of the back, especially the sacro-iliac joints, suggests one of the sponarthritides. However, ankylosing spondylitis not uncommonly presents with large joint disease, particularly of the knees, before the spinal inflammation declares itself. In the fingers, involvement of the terminal interphalangeal joints helps to distinguish osteoarthritis from rheumatoid arthritis in which proximal inter-phalangeal joint involvement is much more common. Psoriatic arthropathy also tends selectively to involve the terminal inter-phalangeal joints.

Examination of the patient tends to act as an amplification of the history and to provide objective evidence of joint inflammation if this is present at the time. However, the absence of such inflammation should not necessarily be regarded as significant early in the disease unless there are reasons for believing that the patient's history is open to other interpretation. In addition to examining the joints, search should be made for extra-articular manifestations and, in particular, skin nodes or nodules. Rheumatoid nodules are commonly found on the extensor surfaces of the forearm whilst Heberden's nodes develop in relation to the terminal inter-phalangeal joints of the fingers in osteoarthritis. Where a monarthritis is present the possibility that it might be due to an infective lesion such as tuberculosis or brucellosis should be considered as these may last for a considerable period of time.

An error which occasionally occurs is to mistake non-articular problems for arthritis. In particular this applies to tennis elbow, nerve entrapments, such as carpal tunnel syndrome, polymyalgia rheumatica, and soft-tissue lesions around the shoulder. These may be chronic and if an obviously diseased joint cannot be found to explain the symptoms other diagnoses should be considered.

Investigation of joint disease is generally simple and well within the scope of the general practitioner. Unless the cause is clearly osteoarthritis the ESR should be done. This is usually raised in the presence of inflammatory joint disease. Very high levels, however, might suggest polymyalgia rheumatica or possibly myeloma if back pain is one of the symptoms. The haemoglobin should be checked as there will often be anaemia. This will usually be normocytic owing to the chronic inflammatory process but may be microcytic especially if there is any gastro-intestinal bleeding resulting from treatment with salicylates or possibly other drugs. If bleeding is suspected the stools should be examined for occult blood and in case of doubt a specialist opinion obtained.

Tests for rheumatoid factor are very useful providing that their limitations are understood. The most widely performed test is the Rose Waaler but some laboratories do a simple latex fixation test and others the differential agglutination (DAT). In case of doubt the laboratory should be contacted. A positive Rose Waaler at a titre of 1:64 is generally accepted as significant while a titre of 1:32 is borderline and should be interpreted with care. The Rose Waaler is positive in approximately 70 per cent of patients with rheumatoid arthritis and in about 25 per cent of patients with SLE. It follows that a negative Rose Waaler does not exclude RA. For a classification of RA and the relation to it of the various diagnostic investigations reference should be made to the criteria of the American Rheumatism Association. Unfortunately the Rose Waaler is also positive in 4 per cent of the apparently normal population and this, too, should be taken into account.

Where the presentation is atypical or there are any suggestive skin or other lesions SLE is a possibility and most laboratories will carry out a screening test for anti-nuclear factor (ANF). A positive ANF screening test should be confirmed by a test of the DNA-binding capacity which is virtually specific for SLE. This condition is probably underdiagnosed although it may only be mild cases which are missed. However, early treatment of SLE is important and the management varies significantly from that of other conditions associated with arthritis. In ankylosing spondylitis the HLA B27 antigen may be useful but it only increases the probability of the diagnosis. Ninety per cent of patients with ankylosing spondylitis have this antigen but so do a proportion of normal subjects. Other tests have been investigated as markers of joint disease or as measures of their activity and discussion with local rheumatologists and pathologists may be helpful in working out a policy for investigation in any particular locality or more generally in the future. Finally, investigation may include estimation of the level of serum urate with a view to a possible diagnosis of gout. This should be interpreted with care since the urate levels may be normal between exacerbations and as a result of treatment, especially with salicylates in low doses.

The other important component of investigation is radiology. This should include chest X-ray in cases where the patient is generally unwell. RA may itself produce lung lesions as may other related connective tissue disorders. Studies of the large bowel will be necessary where there is an associated disturbance suggesting the possibility of disease there. X-ray of the affected joints will often yield useful information although in early or mild arthritis there may be no bony changes or only some osteoporosis of the peri-articular bone. The classical erosions tend to occur later and in patients more severely affected. Unsuspected changes may be found in the small joints of the hands and feet even if these are not obviously involved and X-rays should include these parts. X-rays are also of value in assessing the progress of an arthritis but this is more usually the province of the rheumatologist. In suspected cases of ankylosing spondylitis the X-rays should include the sacro-iliac joints and possibly the remainder of the spine.

One further investigation which may be relevant is the examination of aspirates from joints with effusions. This will be carried out relatively infrequently in general practice but is particularly useful in cases of suspected pyrophosphate arthropathy in which it may be needed to confirm the diagnosis.

Management

The main elements of management are:

1. Reassurance and education of the patient.
2. Control of pain and stiffness.
3. Prevention of function.
4. Correction of associated problems.
5. Detection and treatment of extra-articular manifestations.
6. Referral to specialist units.
7. Referral to other professionals.

Reassurance and education of patient

This is the most fundamental aspect of management because until the patient's condition can be discussed with understanding on both sides it is not possible to make realistic plans for treatment. Most patients equate joint disease with severe disability and know of one or more people. possibly related to them, with severe arthritis. They need to understand that this is an uncommon outcome. Likewise there is a common belief that severe pain is unavoidable. Until the patient's beliefs have been explored and any fears have been allayed as far as possible it is difficult to make an assessment of the situation. Excessive anxiety prevents calm reporting of symptoms and disabilities and frequently leads to an apparent failure of treatment. Apart from reassurance, the patient also needs to feel that a firm diagnosis has been made so that the prognosis offered is credible and the management plan acceptable. On the other hand, it must be admitted openly that early arthritis may be unclassifiable and honesty about the doctor's uncertainty in these cases seems the only satisfactory basis for a useful relationship.

The patient must not have unreasonable expectations of any medication or referral because this will lead to disappointment. At the same time he should be encouraged to believe that important problems are capable of some solution because otherwise these will not be brought to the attention of the doctor. In connection with drugs, minor side-effects are very likely and should be anticipated. The extent to which more serious and less common unwanted effects should be discussed will depend on an individual judgement in any particular case. However, the patient must be told the reason for special precautions such as those required for corticosteroids and gold or penicillamine in order for him to play his part in any arrangements made. He should also be told of the possible need to try a number of different regimes, that this does not imply experimentation and is made necessary by individual variations in the response to drugs. This is of particular importance in the light of widespread anxiety about antirheumatic therapy. The patient should be given an opportunity to air any worries he has about therapy so that they can be discussed.

Control of pain and stiffness

This will usually be an early consideration in management and is necessary to demonstrate the ability of medical treatment to help. Doctors should develop a rational approach to drug therapy using a limited number of drugs ranging from those with the least side-effects to those that require special precautions. All effective anti-inflammatory drugs produce unwanted effects, particularly in the gastro-intestinal tract, and the greater the anti-inflammatory activity the more likely this is to happen. It is also important to avoid changing medication too frequently or in response to transient events. A period of at least two weeks should be allowed to elapse between changes in simple therapy and much longer in the case of longer acting drugs. An orderly progression of medication might be as follows:

1. Simple analgesics such as Paracetamol.
2. Non-steroidal anti-inflammatory drugs (NSAID).
3. Prednisolone 5 mg at night.
4. Gold or penicillamine (probably in conjunction with rheumatologist).

Any personal list of drugs will be open to criticism. Simple analgesics are particularly appropriate for patients with osteoarthritis and some with mild inflammatory disease. These will be intended for use from time to time as the patient's condition dictates. There are now a great number of NSAIDs and each doctor must consider his own policy. The longer established drugs such as Ibuprofen are amongst the cheapest and although they may have less anti-inflammatory activity than others they are generally well tolerated. Most rheumatologists would agree that aspirin has now been supplanted as the regular treatment of first choice. In the event of the first-line NSAID proving insufficient many doctors would prefer to use one of the propionic acid derivatives with greater activity such as Flurbiprofen before prescribing some of the newer preparations. There is no advantage in using more than one propionic acid derivative at a time. While newer drugs probably have a better safety record salicylates remain of value providing that they can be tolerated. As anti-inflammatory agents they should be given in dosages of 3.6 g per day if this is possible and more may be beneficial if the patient can tolerate it. Indomethacin should probably be used after a trial of other agents since it causes unwanted effects in many patients, some of them serious.

Morning stiffness is commonly a serious problem in patients with inflammatory arthritis and may not respond to general anti-inflammatory treatment. The use of Indomethacin 50 or 75 mg at night either in a long-acting oral preparation or suppository form may be beneficial. However, a small dose of corticosteroids at night such as Prednisolone 5 mg often has a dramatic effect. This should not be prescribed without due thought. Although this dosage is seldom associated with any problems it may cause adrenocortical suppression and the patient should carry a steroid card. There must also be some anxiety that the use of corticosteroids in this way may lead to the prescription of larger doses. This can be prevented by prior discussion with the patient and firmness on the part of the doctor. There is no place for the prescription of larger doses of corticosteroids by general practitioners without special advice although they are of considerable value in a small number of patients, particularly those with widespread extra-articular manifestations of the disease.

The use of a planned progression through a range of drugs such as this with an adequate trial of each preparation and attention to the other details shortly to be considered should results in reasonable control of symptoms in the majority of patients. However, a small proportion require further therapy. This will rarely be necessary during the first six months of the disease although occasionally an aggressive arthritis may have clearly failed to respond to any of the therapies outlined above within a shorter space of time. The main indications of the need for further treatment are persistently active joint inflammation and the development of continuing inflammation as is the development or extension of erosive change in X-rays of joints. In this situation a different range of drugs may be indicated and these are currently described as remission-induced drugs (RIDs). There is a common belief that these drugs actually slow joint damage or possible stop it altogether although this cannot be regarded as proven because of great difficulties in obtaining the necessary evidence. RIDs include gold, penicillamine, antimalarial drugs, cytotoxic drugs Dapsone, and Sulphasalazine but the use of these, apart possibly from the first two, will be a matter for the specialist rheumatologist. Regular blood tests are necessary with most of them and antimalarial drugs may cause retinal damage and require supervision by an ophthalmologist.

Attention should be given to the records of patients with rheumatic disease but opinions vary as to the advantages of using a special record card. Specific features such as the amount of pain, perhaps marked on a scale from 0 to $+++$, joint tenderness, swelling and range of movement, together with therapy and appropriate investigations, can be easily recorded in this way and act as a valuable guide to management. On the other hand, some find such aids difficult to use. Each general practitioner must consider these options and find the most satisfactory solution for himself.

One reason for the inappropriate use of drugs is the treatment of local problems in the same way as generalized active disease. Patients often have their main difficulty associated with one joint and, if so, consideration should be given to local treatment. It is not possible to list all the treatments available but the general practitioner should be aware of the value of joint aspiration if there is an effusion, local injection of corticosteroids, particularly into the knee, and splinting, especially of the wrists. Patients with RA are more likely to suffer from carpal tunnel syndrome and possibly other nerve entrapments which may respond to local steroid injection or splinting. There is no reason why aspiration and injection of corticosteroids cannot be carried out in surgeries and doctors unfamiliar with these techniques will usually find local rheumatologists only too happy to provide instruction and advice. Other local measures include support for joints in patients with osteoarthritis such as simple walking sticks and crutches.

Preservation of function

This is the other main aim of management and requires an understanding of the likely difficulties which may be encountered by patients. It is also necessary to understand the lifestyle of each individual patient and to ask them specifically what their disabilities are. Problems which may be insignificant to some patients are of major importance to others, e.g. the concert pianist with relatively minor arthropathy of the fingers. For many patients function is only limited by pain and stiffness but in others the problem may require more then simple relief of these. In RA the main problems occur with the shoulders, wrists, hands, knees, ankles, and feet and the doctor should make sure by questioning or by examination that function of these parts is adequate or at least being treated to the best of his ability. A particular problem occurs with the knees because when they are inflamed the position of comfort is in partial flexion. Prolonged rest in this position, particularly with a pillow under the knee, may result in flexion deformities. It is important that patients are advised of this danger and a regular check kept on the knees. If there is any sign of flexion deformity which cannot be rapidly corrected the patient should be referred to a rheumatologist with a view to splinting in the extended position. Serial splinting may be necessary to correct established deformities.

In the past much emphasis was placed on physiotherapy and, although this is now used less, it may have a valuable part to play. The physiotherapist can show patients how to ensure that the muscles around the affected joints, which tend to waste, can be kept in the best possible condition. This is of particular importance in the case of the knee and any patient who has inflammation there should be instructed in quadriceps exercises. Hydrotherapy can be a valuable aid to the mobilization of patients and where this is available the possibility should be borne in mind. An old-fashioned treatment which may still be of value is the use of wax baths for the hands and the requirements for this can be prescribed.

Particular problems occur with the back and chest of patients with ankylosing spondylitis. There is a tendency for movements to be progressively diminished and any doctor responsible for the long-term management of this condition should measure the degree of spinal movement, which is most easily assessed by the distance between the outstretched fingertips and the floor in full flexion, and chest expansion regularly. Patients with ankylosing spondylitis should have at least an initial instruction from a physiotherapist and ideally some continuing supervision. They should be very strongly advised not to smoke.

There has been much confusion about the relative merits of rest and exercise in rheumatic conditions and this should be discussed with all patients with significant arthritis. Some believe that they must rest as much as possible with the risk of joint deformity and disuse muscular atrophy while others are firmly convinced that they must indulge in vigorous exercise with the danger of increased inflammation and joint destruction. An acutely inflamed joint should be rested while satisfactory treatment is established. Patients with very generalized acute joint activity are probably best admitted to hospital where they may, in addition to other measures, receive a short course of ACTH. It is possible for such treatment to be carried out at home providing the necessary supervision and assistance can be given and the social circumstances are appropriate. While rest is the correct treatment in acute inflammation, moderate exercise should be encouraged with more prolonged problems. These considerations apply as much to osteoarthritis as to rheumatoid arthritis although the problem in the former is likely to be more localized and to present fewer difficulties.

Correction of associated problems

Mention has already been made of the anaemia which may accompany arthritis or its treatment. Where treatment is implicated this should be reviewed and if the anaemia is iron deficient it should be treated. However, the anaemia associated with inflammatory disease will only improve as a result of control of the disease process and iron will not be beneficial.

Patients suffering from arthritis often feel depressed. This may be due to uncontrolled pain and stiffness, limitation of activity, side-effects of drugs, endogenous depression or other life-events. If the depression is of sufficient severity it may prevent adequate assessment of the arthritis and lead to inappropriate treatment. It should therefore be sought whenever progress is unsatisfactory. Specific questioning may reveal typical disturbances but it must be remembered that sleep disorders may be due to the arthritis and poor appetite is often due to the side-effects of the drugs or to active RA. Depression must be relieved if that is at all possible but the extra burden caused by the side-effects of the drugs should be borne in mind.

Detection and treatment of extra-articular manifestations

These will tend to occur in patients who are already suffering from more severe forms of arthritis and who will therefore be attending rheumatology clinics. However, they may occur in patients who have relatively mild arthropathy and frequently present between clinic attendances. In the eye the most common lesions are iritis and scleritis and in such cases an urgent appointment should be made with an ophthalmologist. Significant disease of the lungs or pleura will lead to shortness of breath or pain and if this is suspected a chest X-ray should be performed. Many of the problems associated with rheumatoid arthritis are due to a vasculitis and this may cause small necrotic lesions in the skin, particularly of the nail folds. The presence of rheumatoid vasculitis is indicative of severe disease and an early consultation with a rheumatologist should be arranged. On the other hand, subcutaneous rheumatoid nodules are common and do not require any specific treatment. The other relatively common sites for extra-articular lesions are the nerves. A peripheral sensory neuropathy is not uncommon and others, including mononeuritis multiplex, occasionally occur. The possibility of nerve entrapment syndromes has already been mentioned. Those with neuropathies require early referral because more energetic treatment of the rheumatoid process may be indicated and attention may also be needed to the affected part such as a dropped foot.

Specialist referral

Patients suffering from inflammatory arthropathy will often be referred to a rheumatologist and the indications in general terms will be diagnosis, medical treatment, specific problems, consideration of surgery, and surveillance. The diagnosis of most patients with joint disease lies within the compass of general practice and there is no reason why hospital referral should be a routine procedure. However, it may be necessary with atypical presentations and where one of the less common arthropathies is suspected. Certainly patients with SLE and the more severe forms of spondarthritides should have the benefit of a consultant opinion. Treatment of uncomplicated and relatively mild arthritis should be regarded as part of general practice but those requiring potentially more dangerous treatment should be referred to hospital. There are two other specific instances where referral to hospital is required. The first is where there is a possibility of septic arthritis. Patients with advanced rheumatoid disease are most liable to suffer from this condition which is usually associated with a definite focus of infection elsewhere. The diagnosis should be suspected when there is a sudden exacerbation of inflammation in one or more joints associated with general malaise and shivering. It is important to realize that the condition may not be accompanied by very severe systemic disturbance and the the joints may not be very inflamed. The diagnosis can only be made or excluded by aspiration of affected joints. Admission to hospital is a matter of urgency in these cases. The other situation in which an urgent referral is necessary is that of destruction of the extensor tendons of the fingers which can be involved in synovial proliferation on the dorsum of the wrist. This results in dropping of the fingers which cannot then be extended at the metacarpophalangeal joints. Tendon repair is a matter of urgency. This condition should be anticipated in patients with marked synovial proliferation on the wrist and in these cases prophylactic clearance of the offending synovium should be considered.

The main matter for debate is the role of the rheumatologist in the surveillance of patients with moderate or severe RA. Most rheumatologists would like to see all such patients as well as those suffering from the less common arthropathies. The reasons for this are their greater expertise in assessment, familiarity with treatment, and their access to other professionals. The general practitioner, however, may be able to work with other professionals to a considerable extent. On the other hand, he cannot hope to achieve the same level of expertise in diagnosis and management. It seems reasonable, therefore, to suggest that patients with moderate or severe RA should be referred to a rheumatologist but attendances at his clinic need be infrequent if the general practitioner makes known his willingness to take an active part in follow-up. These issues should be discussed from time to time by general practitioners with their local rheumatologist and the threshold for referral can then be adjusted on the basis of expertise acquired and mutual trust.

General practitioners should continue to follow-up their patients even if they are attending a rheumatology clinic since the patient has a need for a doctor to whom he can bring urgent problems and the general practitioner will usually be prescribing medication and is therefore responsible for its supervision. A particular problem occurs with patients taking gold and penicillamine who require frequent, usually monthly, checks of blood and urine. This is best done by the general practitioner who can provide the necessary continuity and can avoid the dangers of divided care. The passage of information between general practitioner and rheumatologist may be improved by the use of a 'Co-Operation Card' which contains details of therapy and the results of regular investigations. This card can then be held by the patient for use both in surgery and hospital clinic.

The other main point of referral of patients suffering from arthritis is the orthopaedic surgical department. The problems which such departments are experiencing have already been mentioned. However, most patients with osteoarthritis should be referred directly to the surgeon as the interpolation of a rheumatologist in these cases is unlikely to be helpful. The same may be true of isolated surgical problems occurring in otherwise mild rheumatoid disease but where the problem occurs in the context of more severe generalized RA or where there is doubt about the appropriateness of surgical treatment the opinion of a rheumatologist should be sought before referral to the surgeon.

Referral to other professional services

The wide range of other professional services available has already been described but particular mention should be made of daily living units which are available in most district general hospitals and which compromise a simulated home environment where the patient's performance can be assessed and various aids tried. These are usually supervized by occupational therapists and are often inaccessible to general practitioners. It is access to facilities such as this which form part of the argument for referral to a specialist clinic.

Prognosis

Apart from the relief of immediate symptoms the question uppermost in the minds of most patients with joint disease will be the outlook for the future. It is therefore a matter of great concern that we are unable to answer this question which may not be made explicit. It is, however, possible to make general statements which are likely to be of some reassurance to the majority of patients who fear progressive and severe disability. It is fair to say that most patients will do well, particularly those who have suffered for some time from mild seronegative arthropathy. The Rose Waaler test does have some predictive value in that patients with a strongly positive reaction are more likely to suffer from severe disease. However, even some of these patients suffer little disability and an optimistic attitude is therefore entirely justified. The possibility of deterioration cannot be denied but the extent to which frankness is advisable must depend in part on an assessment of the patient's psychological make-up and his need for practical information in the making of important decisions. In this context female patients should be told that pregnancy is often associated with remission of the disease but that there may be an exacerbation after delivery. If it is appropriate the problems of raising a family with a handicapped parent should be discussed.

In osteoarthritis the prognosis is also very variable. However, patients can often be assured that acute exacerbations may be due to short-lived inflammation and that these do not necessarily predict continued deterioration. Surgery is now frequently of great benefit to patients with osteoarthritis of the hips and, to a lesser extent, the knees, together with the metatarsophalangeal joints of the great toes and the carpometacarpal joints of the thumbs.

The prognosis of most of the other arthritides is also difficult to determine and a matter which should be raised in any referral letter. Ankylosing spondylitis has received a bad press but the majority of patients suffer from relatively mild forms of the disease. Those with severe spondylitis may have some reduction in their life expectancy but the majority are able to lead a fairly full life and probably have a normal life expectancy.

CHRONIC DISEASES OF THE NERVOUS SYSTEM

These may be static or progressive. Examples of the former are brain injury at birth and other trauma, neural-tube defects, poliomyelitis, and surgery, e.g. for cerebral tumour or spinal-cord lesions. In these cases the management is that of the resulting disability. Progressive lesions include multiple sclerosis, motor neurone disease, Parkinson's disease, and some forms of peripheral neuropathy. In other cases it may be difficult to say whether or not neurological damage will be progressive or static. This is the case in cerebrovascular disease either localized or diffuse, spondylitis and some cases of multiple sclerosis and peripheral neuropathy. The same considerations also apply to the much rarer diseases of muscles which are not discussed here.

In many patients the diagnosis is obvious but in others a high degree of suspicion is necessary to avoid labelling symptoms as being 'functional'. Where this diagnosis is considered close attention must be paid to the psychological circumstances and in the absence of a clear psychiatric disturbance repeated search should be made for abnormal neurological signs. The diagnosis of difficult neurological problems will usually be a matter for hospital specialists but it is important that a definite decision is reached as early as possible to retain the confidence of the patient. It is also important that the diagnosis should be as complete as possible. Motor abnormalities tend to be more obvious than those affecting the sensory system but the presence of the latter may be of more significance in the management of the patient. Thus in cases of stroke successful rehabilitation may depend on recognition of a hemianopia or impairment of spacial awareness and in the absence of this recognition attempts at mobilization will frequently be doomed to failure.

Further consideration here is limited to multiple sclerosis and Parkinson's disease which, apart from stroke, will be most commonly met with in general practice.

Multiple sclerosis

Multiple sclerosis (MS) is due to plaques of demyelination which may occur at any site in the central nervous system interfering with a wide variety of functions. Characteristically there is evidence of damage at several sites in different parts of the nervous system or a history that these have occurred together with an evolving pattern of relapse and remission. The prevalence in most parts of the United Kingdom ranges between 0.05 and 0.1 per cent although in parts of Scotland it is much higher. It is more common in women than men in a ratio of 3:2 and usually presents in young adult life, although not uncommonly in the older patient.

It is perhaps the most feared of the chronic diseases. Various factors contribute to this fear. The cause remains unknown despite intensive research. The mechanism is difficult for patients to understand and there are no visible changes other than its effects. It usually affects healthy young people and its course is generally unpredictable. The publicity given to it has been of great value in producing money for research and in helping patients' problems to be appreciated, but as a result an unjustifiable anxiety exists in many members of the community.

It is important that MS be differentiated from other diffuse disorders such as neurosyphilis, connective-tissue disorders, and sarcoidosis. Where the presentation is that of a hemiplegia it must be distinguished from vascular disease and cerebral tumour. In the case of lesions limited to the spinal cord the possibility of a remediable cause of cord compression or subacute combined degeneration must be borne in mind.

In the vast majority of cases the diagnosis should be confirmed by a specialist opinion. This will usually be required by the general practitioner but even when there is little doubt the implications are such that most patients will benefit from a second opinion. Apart from the greater experience of neurologists there are some investigations which may be useful although there is no diagnostic test.

The management of MS is, in general, that of chronic neurological disability but function must be preserved in parts affected by relapses so that if and when recovery occurs permanent disability is minimized. The physiotherapist has a valuable part to play in this process although there is little evidence that regular attendance at physiotherapy departments has a beneficial effect on the course of the disease.

Many patients with established MS have some difficulties with their bladder and bowels. These aspects should be regularly reviewed and in some cases appliances may be necessary. Occasionally drugs such as Emepromium bromide may be of assistance to patients with urinary incontinence but more often patients learn to cope with their difficulties by the regulated passage of urine and the restriction of fluid intake when necessary.

Drugs may be of limited value in some other problems associated with MS. Muscular spasms of the legs are common and painful. When these occur they may respond to treatment with Baclofen and analgesics. Patients may also be subject to trigeminal neuralgia which will frequently be helped by Carbamazepine. There is no evidence that long-term corticosteroids have any beneficial effect on the course of the disease. There is, however, little doubt that the use of ACTH in relapses results in earlier remission. This is normally given in courses of between two and four weeks starting with 80 units daily and tailing off after an initial one or two weeks on the full dose. It may be that oral steroids would have the same effect but this has not been investigated and there is a greater likelihood of their long-term use. In recent years there has been considerable interest in treatment with polyunsaturated fatty acids such as linoleic acid. The rationale of this is far from clear and the benefits have not been established. On the other hand, the use of vegetable oil and soft margarine rather than butter causes little disruption to the patient or his family and should not be discouraged. This, however, is not the case with gluten-free diets which have also enjoyed a vogue and are without any benefit.

The prognosis for patients suffering from MS or a probable demyelinating episode is very uncertain. A small number of patients will follow a rapidly downhill course, dying within a matter of months or a few years. At the other extreme, a rather larger number of patients will suffer little or no permanent disability over several decades. The majority of patients, however, will suffer relapses at a rate of perhaps one every year or two for a number of years before suffering increasing disability. Onset at a young age and presentation with optic neuritis with complete remission are favourable indications. There seems little doubt that where a diagnosis of MS is established the patient should be told and the implications explored with them. However, one episode of probable demyelination such as an attack of optic neuritis may never by followed by another and may possibly have some different expanation and unless there are very strong reasons to the contrary it is not justifiable to tell the patient of the suspicion.

Parkinson's disease

Parkinsonism is a syndrome characterized by tremor, rigidity, and akinesia due to disease of the basal ganglia of the brain. There are no specific tests and the diagnosis rests on recognition of the pattern of clinical signs. It is predominantly a disease of older people and about 0.5 per cent of the population are affected at 60 years of age. Many of these, however, are not severely disabled.

The idiopathic form of the syndrome is the most common and usually presents in the fifth or sixth decade. It is to this that the name Parkinson's disease or paralysis agitans is attached. Many of the remainder are suffering from Parkinsonism secondary to the effects of drugs of which the most commonly implicated are Phenothiazines and Butyrophenones such as Haloperidol. Rarely other drugs may be involved and this possibility should also be considered.

There has been some debate concerning the role of atherosclerosis in Parkinsonism. Some authorities recognize this while others do not. The typical signs are frequently observed in patients who have other evidence of cerebrovascular disease and this becomes increasingly common with age. The prevalence of

Parkinsonism is therefore much commoner than that given above when the entire elderly population is considered.

The main difficulties with the diagnosis of Parkinsonism occur in its early stages. Patients may suffer from a variety of symptoms including shakiness, cramps, and transient sensory disturbances before there are any marked physical signs. It is very easy for these to be regarded as neurotic in origin. Depression is a common association of Parkinson's disease, perhaps due to an organic disturbance in the brain or possibly to the consequences of the disease. Where the presenting feature is mainly akinesia it can easily be confused with the retardation of depression. Unilateral Parkinson's disease can be mistaken for hemiplegia and this may be suggested by the failure of an arm to swing properly when walking. On the other hand a diagnosis of Parkinson's disease may be made in the case of tremors of other origins, in particular because tremors become increasingly common in the elderly or previously existing essential tremors may become worse then. The tremor of Parkinsonism has a lower frequency than that of essential tremor and is usually of 'pill-rolling' type. It tends to increase with anxiety and to disappear at rest.

Patients with Parkinson's disease may show dementia and this was described infrequently in the past but seems likely to be a common feature. This must not be confused with the mental states resulting from treatment of the disease or from the use of drugs which may themselves have caused the Parkinsonism. The withdrawal, if at all possible, of such drugs, preferably before instituting anti-Parkinsonian therapy, is an important part of management and may also be necessary for diagnosis. Where the disease may be drug induced it can be necessary to wait for up to two years after its withdrawal to establish whether or not it was the cause of the problem. Before considering the use of anti-Parkonsonian drugs the presence or absence of depression must be established as far as possible since treatment of depression with such drugs as tricyclic anti depressants may reduce or eliminate the need for other measures.

There are two main lines of drug treatment open to the general practitioner: anticholinergics and laevodopa. The long-established use of anticholinergics remains valuable for tremor and rigidity in less severe cases. The preparations commonly used include Orphenadrine, Benzhexol, Benztropine, and Procyclidine. These all produce dryness of the mouth and some degree of constipation. The latter may be severe in the elderly who may also suffer from confusion, hallucinations, and urinary retention. Attacks of glaucoma may be precipitated in patients with shallow anterior chambers.

It may be asked why anticholinergic drugs should be used now that laevodopa is available. There can be no doubt that the use of the latter has had a very significant effect on the medical management of Parkinson's disease. Unfortunately, however dramatic its effects may be in individual patients they are not permanent and it is probably wise to restrict the use of laevodopa to those who are suffering from moderate to severe disability. If laevodopa is to be used it should usually be given in combination with Carbidopa which reduces the degradation of dopa outside the brain allowing smaller doses to achieve the same levels of dopamine within the brain. The smaller dose reduces unwanted effects but these remain problematical for many patients. The most common effects are nausea and vomiting but it may also cause arhythmias, postural hypotension, exacerbation of glaucoma, and the precipitation of urinary retention. Postural hypotension is a major problem because patients with Parkinson's disease already have a tendency to fall. This is probably due to a combination of the flexed body posture together with inability of the musculoskeletal system, and in particular the muscles around the ankles, to make rapid adjustments when the body's balance is unstable. These side-effects occur early and later the patient may suffer from hallucinations, confusion and dyskinetic movements which can be very distressing for both the patient and his relatives. In order to minimize the early side-effects the dose should be built up gradually starting with drugs such as Sinemet '110' daily or Madopar 62.5 mg daily. The latter contains laevodopa together with Benserazide which is another decarboxylase inhibitor. The dosage of these drugs should not be pushed to the maximum tolerated because when failure of response occurs later there may be some improvement if the dose can be increased. It is suggested that the aim should be a dose consistent with reasonable activity.

The problem of late failure of treatment is the major disadvantage for those patients who are able to tolerate laevodopa in the first place. After a number of years the response diminishes and although there may be some benefit from increasing the dose to tolerance this is also usually short-lived. The failure of treatment may occur in a number of ways and some specific patterns have been observed. There may be an increase in the side-effects, there may be a 'wearing-off' effect or an 'on–off' effect. The 'wearing-off' effect describes a shortening period of benefit from each dose which may be partly offset by more frequent taking of tablets. The 'on–off' effect is characterized by rapid swings from near normality to almost complete rigidity.

There have been a number of attempts to assist patients to benefit from the smallest possible dose of laevodopa. Amantadine has a slight adjuvant effect in doses of 100–300 mg daily but this drug is expensive and the benefits from it are relatively limited. More recently much work has been done on the use of Bromocriptine which acts as a dopamine agonist. Unfortunately this drug also has severe side-effects in some patients and at present its use should probably be restricted to centres with experience. Even more recently Selegiline Hydrochloride has been introduced. This is an inhibitor of the enzyme monoamine-oxidase-B which destroys laevodopa in the brain. Once again it has been shown to have serious side-effects and its place in treatment has yet to be established.

The emphasis here on the use of drugs is not to suggest that the other aids to management which have been stressed throughout the chapter should be neglected. It is, however, an area of chronic neurological disease in which the correct use of drugs may assist the patient a great deal and may have a significant effect on longevity. Until more accurate figures for the incidence of the disease and the outcome of treatment are available it will be difficult to advise patients with any precision. However, prior to the introduction of laevo-dopa about two-thirds of patients were either dead or severely disabled within seven years of the diagnosis. This is no longer the case and some studies have suggested that patients on laevodopa may have a normal life expectancy. This, however, conflicts with clinical experience of this treatment already referred to suggesting that its effects. although beneficial, are not permanent.

It is thus possible to be relatively optimistic with patients suffering from Parkinson's disease and to stress that many suffer from fairly mild disability, that treatment has a great deal to offer and that advances are still being made which should have a beneficial effect on the management of most patients whose disease is now being diagnosed.

WRITTEN INFORMATION FOR PATIENTS

This is a valuable adjunct to explanations that the doctor may give to the patient in the course of consultations. Nearly all patients with disabling diseases have a need to understand what is happening to them to the limit of their intellectual abilities which are often under-rated. The possibilities range from simple lists of instructions such as exercises, to books written by specialists which contain information previously regarded as the province of medical practitioners. General practitioners should have a list of publications making use of advice from specialists and patients' associations. The provision of such information is widely appreciated by patients and there is no record of any harm having resulted from them. Practices may find it useful to have copies of those publications dealing with the more commonly encountered diseases which can be loaned to patients.

In the list at the end of the chapter there are a number of organizations which relate to specific conditions and almost all these produce leaflets and reading lists. With respect to the diseases specifically discussed within this chapter the Arthritis and Rheumatism Council have produced pamphlets for patients suffering from the common arthritides and the Multiple Sclerosis Society have amongst their publications a very useful leaflet intended for newly diagnosed patients entitled 'So you have MS?' There are two books relating to MS which many patients find very helpful: *Living with multiple sclerosis* by Elizabeth Forsythe published by Faber & Faber and *Multiple sclerosis: the facts* by W. B. Matthews published by Oxford University Press.

PERFORMANCE REVIEW

There have been few attempts in the past to measure the quality and provision of care for patients suffering from disabling diseases. Problems of definition and the establishment of appropriate standards perhaps provide some explana-tion for the relative paucity. However, the use of a list of facts which should be known and recorded about disabled patients would provide a satisfactory basis for examination of general practitioners' knowledge and records of their patients' disabilities. The relatively limited scope of investigations required in rheumatological disease and the rates of referral to hospital are other areas which might usefully be considered as could the efficiency or otherwise of the supervision of patients on specific medications such as gold or penicillamine. The frequency of consultations and the use of repeat prescriptions for patients with arthritis is another area which would raise issues of significance.

A more challenging study might be that of the patients' perceptions of the care of chronic disease. These studies would call for the establishment of a disease register and for many practitioners the construction of a register for all patients with significant handicap is likely to be a major task. However, a reasonable expectation might be the production of a list of patients with major handicaps and those with progressive disease which would be used in the study to follow-up and the involvement of other professionals.

PERFORMANCE REVIEW CHECK LIST

1. General

    (a) How accessible are the practice premises for disabled patients?

    (b) Can the practice identify their patients who have major handicaps?

2. Assessment and management of patients

From the records of handicapped patients, can the following items of care be identified?

(a) Diagnosis – history and symptoms, examination, appropriate investigations.

(b) Assessment of disability – including

    Self-care

    Mobility

    Bowel and bladder function

    Sexual function

    Family support

    Finance

    Housing

    Occupation and employment

    Social contacts

(c) Patient resources and education

(d) Management and follow-up

    Degree of control of pain and stiffness

    Preservation of function

    Drugs: side-effects and monitoring

    Detection and correction of associated problems

(e) Appropriate referral to other professionals and agencies

(f) Appropriate referral to specialists

SELF-HELP GROUPS AND OTHER BODIES

A large number of groups have been attempting to help patients with the chronic physically disabling diseases. Most of these have been set up by sufferers from the disease or other interested people with two main aims. These are to assist individual sufferers and to foster research into prevention and treatment. The enthusiasm and activities of local branches varies and local specialists with a particular interest in the disease or diseases concerned are likely to know the local situation. There are also groups and organizations which seek to help all disabled people with particular aspects of their life such as mobility.

The decision to recommend that a patient considers joining such a group should not be taken lightly. On the one hand patients can expect support and understanding from fellow sufferers together with advice, education, organized activities, and possibly material assistance. However, they are also exposed to patients with serious forms of the diseases and some of those who join such groups may be patients of a rather dependent nature. Contacts of this sort may affect some people adversely. It is necessary, therefore, to weigh the advantages and disadvantages of joining a group and to discuss these with each individual patient. The following organizations and their addresses, while not comprehensive, may be found useful. Many of the organizations have local branches whose addresses can be obtained form the Head Offices.

General

Age Concern England,
National Old People's Welfare Council,
Bernard Sunley House,
60 Pitcairn Road,
Mitcham,
Surrey CR4 3LL   Tel. 01–640–5431

Age Concern N. Ireland,
N. Ireland Old People's Welfare Council,
2 Annadale Avenue,
Belfast,
N. Ireland BT7 3JR   Tel. 0232–693117/8

Age Concern Scotland,
Scottish Old People's Welfare Council,
33 Castle Street,
Edinburgh,
Scotland EH2 3DW   Tel. 031–275–5000/1

Age Concern Wales,
1 Park Green,
Cardiff CF1 3BJ   Tel. 0222–371821/371566

Disabled Living Foundation,
346 Kensington High Street,
London W14 3NS   Tel. 01–602–2491

Disability Alliance,
4 Nederhall Gardens,
London W3 53G

PHAB (Physically Handicapped and Able Bodied),
42 Devonshire Street,
London W1N 1LN   Tel. 01–637–7475

Royal Association for Disability and Rehabilitation,
23–25 Mortimer Street,
London W1N 8AB   Tel. 01–637–5400

SPOD (Sexual and Personal Relationships of the Disabled),
The Diorama,
14 Peto Place,
London NW1 4DT   Tel. 01–486–9823

Motoring

Disabled Drivers' Association,
Ashwellthorpe Hall,
Ashwellthorpe,
Norwich NR16 1EX   Tel. 050–841–449

Motability,
Boundary House,
91/93 Charterhouse Street,
London EC1M 6BT   Tel. 01–253 1211

Arthritis

Arthritis & Rheumatism Council for Research in GB & The Commonwealth,
41 Eagle Street,
London WC1R 4AR   Tel. 01–405–9572

British Rheumatism & Arthritis Care,
6 Grosvenor Crescent,
London SW1X 7ER   Tel. 01–235–0902

Back Pain Association,
31–33 Park Road,
Teddington,
Middlesex TW11 0AB   Tel. 01–977–5474/5

National Ankylosing Spondylitis Society,

c/o The Royal National Hospital for Rheumatic Diseases,
Upper Borough Walls,
Bath,
Avon BA1 1RL   Tel. 0225–65941

Muscular diseases

Muscular Dystrophy Group of GB,

Nattrase House,
35 Macauley Road,
Clapham,
London SW4 0QP   Tel. 01–720–8055

Neurological disease

Association for Spina Bifida & Hydrocephalus,

Tavistock House North,
Tavistock Square,
London WC1H 9HJ   Tel. 01–388–1382

Friedrich's Ataxia Group,

12c Worplesdon Road,
Guildford,
Surrey GU2 6RW   Tel. 0483–503133

Motor Neurone Disease Association,

245 Popes Lane,
London W5   Tel. 01–567–5521 (evenings)

Multiple Sclerosis Society of GB & N. Ireland,

286 Munster Road,
Fulham,
London SW6 6AP   Tel. 01–381–4022/01 385–4146/8

Parkinson's Disease Society of the UK,

81 Queen's Road,
London SW19 8NR   Tel. 01–946–2500

Spinal Injuries Association (Paraplegics and Tetraplegics),

5 Crowndale Road,
London NW1 1TU   Tel. 1–388–6840

Skin diseases

Eczema Society,

5/7 Tavistock Place,
London WC1H 9SR   Tel. 01–388–4097

Psoriasis Association,

7 Milton Street,
Northampton NN2 7JG   Tel. 0604–711129

Visual handicap and deafness

British Association of the Hard of Hearing,

6 St. James Street,
London WC1 3DA   Tel. 01–405–5182

Guide Dogs for the Blind Association,

Alexandra House,
9–11 Park Street,
Windsor,
Berkshire SL4 1JR   Tel. 075–35–55711

National Library for the Blind,

Cromwell Road,
Bradbury,
Stockport,
Cheshire SK6 2SG   Tel. 061–494–0217/9

National Listening Library (Talking Books for the Handicapped),

49 Gt. Cumberland Place,
London W1H 7LH   Tel. 01–723–5008

Royal National Institute for the Blind,

224 Gt. Portland Street,
London W1N 6AA   Tel. 01–388–1266

Royal National Institute for the Deaf,
105 Gower Street,
London WC1E 6AH   Tel. 01–387–8053

Acknowledgements

I am very grateful to Dr E.D. Sever for helpful comments in the production of this chapter. He is, however, in no way responsible for its shortcomings.

12 Psychological problems

Gordon Lennox

THE SIZE OF THE PROBLEM

That mythical beast, the average general practitioner, with a list of 2500 persons, finds mental diseases the condition of highest incidence, at 460 persons per annum, second only to 'colds' and their complications (Fry 1979). Should he seek out, among those attending surgery, the hidden psychoneurosis, he will find that he has failed to diagnose a large number. Johnstone and Goldberg (1976) found that of those who attended, some 32 per cent were found to have a conspicuous psychiatric disorder and a further 11 per cent a hidden psychiatric disorder, that had been missed by the general practitioner. Surveying the general population Brown and Harris (1978) found in married women, some 15 per cent suffering from undiagnosed depression, while others have found point-prevalence figures for psychiatric disturbance, at 10–20 per cent of the population. In the face of a problem this size, and a largely chronic problem at that, it is obvious that care – not cure – will be the predominant therapeutic activity. Many doctors find this a difficult concept and continually attempt to intervene with the aim of ending the problem. It would appear to be more helpful to utilize the continuous relationship which the general practitioner makes with his patient, and to provide long-term care in repeated small doses. For an overview, see Goldberg and Huxley (1980).

Happily, the general practitioner no longer works alone, but as a member of the primary health care team, along with district nurses, health visitors, and midwife. The receptionists form a critical link between the professional members and their practice: their capacity to recognize problems at the desk and their ability to manage them is a crucial part of the team's care. The team can be extended to include the social worker (Graham and Sher 1976; Gilchrist *et al.* 1978; Williams and Clare 1979), counsellor (Waydenfeld and Waydenfeld 1980; Anderson and Hasler 1979), community psychiatric nurse (Touch *et al.* 1980), and clinical psychologist (Johnstone and Goldberg 1976; Bhacat *et al.* 1979; Earll and Kincey 1982). Each brings a particular orientation to the team and provides an educational as well as a service function. In extended teams, the poverty of the medical model becomes rapidly apparent: the so-called soft areas of sociology demands a place (see Table 12.1).

Part of the difficulty in general practice is that the false distinction between medicine and psychiatry is almost always blurred. The specific question, 'Is this

Table 12.1. *Models of illness*

Medical model	Social model
Affects individual alone, e.g. gene	Affects the family relationships, e.g. marriage
Defined pathological process, e.g. biochemical change	Disturbed functioning in the group, e.g. delinquency
One diagnosis	Multiple factors
Aetiology usually single	Causes usually many
Single treatment, drug	Multiple therapies usually together

condition organic or functional?' becomes meaningless, as almost always there is a dual diagnosis, e.g. migraine in a trait anxiety, sexual dysfunction following a myocardial infarction. The law of parsimony was never intended to apply to this area. A further difficulty is that:

1. Organic disease may present as psychological, e.g. anxiety in thyrotoxicosis.

2. Psychiatric disease may present as organic, e.g. weight loss in depression.

3. Organic illness with a psychological overlay, e.g. angina associated with cardiac neurosis.

Nothing less than the diagnosis of the whole person can encompass the problems: on each occasion, the whole diagnosis must be examined (Schulman 1977). This is usually performed in general practice by history taking (a lot), examining (some), and investigating (a little, specifically). However, once the diagnosis has been made, it must always remain to some extent provisional: beware the new symptom developing in chronic psychiatric disease, as it may well be new organic illness. The first mental illness in middle age has a high chance of being organic: carcinoma of the pancreas is well known for its ability to mimic depression, and alcoholism seems to mimic each and every psychiatric disease. The general practitioner must always feel that he has to wear two hats, that he is never either a physician or a psychiatrist; he is always both.

A further danger lies in the seductiveness of the psycho-dynamic constructs – so much can be explained by them: the wise doctor regards all diagnoses as provisional, except the last. In the field of psychiatry, patients are frequently unfaithful to their well-established diagnosis, the schizophrenic develops an anxiety state, the depressive becomes agoraphobic: our diagnostic/problem list must allow for this without surprise. The most splendid traps await those who diagnose hysteria, more especially in the presence of organic type signs: it is worth remembering that the mortality of 'hysteria' is high, and that neurotics get ill with increasing frequency and die of it. Few will have practised psychiatry for any length of time without gathering a series of horror stories of the classic presentation of psychiatric syndromes that turn into organic disease as time progresses. Once the doctor has accepted that the interface between psychiatry and medicine is slightly more than semi-permeable, his patients can relax (Simms and Prior 1978).

Perhaps the most difficult area in medicine is the psychiatric care of the physically ill: while remaining in contact with the realities of say, secondary carcinoma, and seeking out the unusual calcium disturbances, the general practitioner must also enter the intricacies of the patient's internal life, his hopes of survival and his fear of death. To treat the whole man demands a whole physician, and often the doctor's personal resources are unequal to the task: in this area, as in all types of psychotherapy, the doctor requires support from colleagues to be able to cope, and it is here that the team approach has the most to offer.

The GP, with his long-term relationship with the patient, has a good opportunity to develop skills in recognizing and noting the personality of the patient, the obsessional who will continue to take the tablets long after the dyspepsia would have stopped lesser breeds; the anxious, whose major complaint melts with reassurance, only to return a week later; the dependent, who so long, and only so long as his dependency needs are met, displays the behaviour of the perfect patient, but who bites the hand that feeds him the moment it is suggested that he grow up. These stereotypes of human behaviour are well known and easily recognized. Of more importance is the apparent change in personality that occurs in illness indicating the severity of the life threat experienced by the patient, the normally stoic who becomes acutely anxious can be a marker of the perceived organic disorder. Late-onset 'neurosis' is always suspect: it is usually organic in aetiology and often cerebral.

Illness behaviour, what the patient does when ill, is very variable. Mechanic (1966) illustrates three types:

1. The culturally learnt response, e.g. the Italian response, and its florid symptomatology, which to British eyes is often thought to be neurotic even in the presence of organic illness.

2. The intense anxiety, that is always reactivated by life threats.

3. The urge to exploit illness, and attempt to obtain more from illness than is usually allowed. The adoption of the sick role leads to the exaggeration of the complaint and a ready excuse for failure, claiming attention and seeking solace.

Medical men as a whole are intolerant of any illness response that is not logical, honest, and scientific. Their wives have been noticed to raise rather cynical eyebrows when the subject is discussed.

The GP's role in relation to this considerable problem of psychiatric is highly complex: with his open access and the therapeutic alliance hopefully established, he is in an ideal situation to handle most of the disorder. He is situated ideally to consider the family aspect of illness, and to help over a long period. He requires a broad eclecticism, using each and any tool to obtain the ends he and the patient have chosen: he will find the need to refer to specialists uncommon. The immense amount of the problem he will handle himself, but when further aid is required, he will need rapid deployment of resources under his specialist colleagues' control. His major tool will never be pharmacological; this hope is rapidly passing and it is likely that he will depend more on his skills as a psychological manipulator, listening and advising, analysing and responding. It seems in the next few years that a rapid move forward into increased psychotherapeutic skill is likely: but the hope of specific drugs, happily without significant side-effects, capable of making marked alteration, has almost gone.

ANXIETY

The commonest presentation in general practice, anxiety is a considerable problem. The first aim is to establish what the patient is anxious about, although this is far from easy. The presentation may be organic: headache or migraine is frequent. Certain syndromes are classic, the left inframammary pain syndrome and the hyperventilation syndrome being examples. Often the anxiety has produced physical dysfunction, varying from dyspepsia to failure of sexual function and a complete history is required to sort out the cause from the effect. A somatic facade is often presented with the patient demanding relief for his headache, while the doctor demands knowledge of the patient's social life. Clearly the chance of misunderstanding is high, and the doctor will do well to begin by stating that the problem is complex and a full history will be required: education of the patient in the psychosomatic relationship is needed before this history can be taken, for unless the doctor and the patient share something of the same health belief system, communication will be very limited.

Traditionally, the anxieties have been divided into the trait type and the state type, but this is unhelpful. Most anxiety patients have a family trait to anxiety, which is both learnt and genetic: the recognition of this is often helpful, as it enables the patient to realize that others he knows have shared his lot. The doctor's knowledge of the family may well enable him to recognize the problem, but he must be aware of easy dismissal of the patient's problem inherent in this diagnosis. If the problem is a trait of personality, it is unlikely that drugs will help, and much psychological work will be required to effect change. The anxiety states occur both in those with trait anxiety and in more stable people. It is described as being reactive to stress or life events, and is often quite short lived. Tennant *et al.* (1981) have described a study of neurotic disorders, mainly anxiety states; they found rapid remission was the rule, half being recovered within one month, the recovery being independent of psychotropic agents. They suggested that such conditions might best be regarded as normal distress responses. As the risk of addiction and dependency on tranquillizers and hypnotics is now apparent, care should be taken to restrict their use in self-limiting disorders.

The chronic 'acute anxiety state' is hardly a name likely to commend itself to those who invent psychiatric glossaries, but the patient is well known to all family doctors; usually female, she suffers a series of anxiety related syndromes, never being completely free from problems and often becoming dependent and demanding in relation to drug treatment. These patients make poor relationships, both within the therapy situation and in real life, finding self-absorption in the illness more rewarding than life itself. They are hard to inveigle into therapy and do badly if forced: in the one to one, dependency on the doctor is rapidly induced, but the transference is hard to use therapeutically, while within a group therapy, less neurotic members are critical of the life style adopted. Chemotherapy is of little or no value and the pain for both the doctor and the patient is considerable. Happily some improve over time, and some seek other doctors and other therapies (Groves 1978).

Two problems in diagnosis have to be recognized: first, that depressive illness can often present as an anxiety state, turning later into an agitated depression, with a marked suicidal risk. Careful assessment of mood and suicidal ideation is mandatory in all psychiatric illness. Secondly, all the effects of an acute anxiety state are mimicked by thyrotoxicosis and other endocrine disorders. An organic basis should always be considered, and alcohol intake carefully reviewed.

Where the first two syndromes of anxiety, the trait and the state anxiety are generally non-specific in the source of an anxiety, by contrast, phobic anxiety is directly induced in one or more specific situations. Agoraphobia, usually presenting as anxiety experienced when away from home, for example, out shopping, has a markedly limiting effect on not merely the patient but on the whole family life.

Management of anxiety

Anxiety is a symptom, not a disorder, and before treatment plans are made, it is essential not to begin symptomatic treatment. Once serious illness, physical and psychiatric, is eliminated there is time to consider possibilities. The urgent pressure to treat, now, fully, with the nostrum of the previous doctor, should be resisted despite the inevitable pressure. A plan or programme agreed with the patient, minimizing or ignoring drug therapy is undoubtedly the best. If drugs must be used, care should be taken to ensure that the patient understands that they are short-term props only, and that long-term use has more problems than help. Should careful history taking have led the doctor to believe, as is often the case, that anxiety is a product of unresolved conflict, conscious or unconscious, then to exhibit drugs is both to block the patient's ears to any interpretation, and also to minimize his capacity to help himself by problem solving and decision making.

The first stage of management is to explain and convince that the symptoms are a reasonable reaction given the circumstances: that the patient is not going mad and that shortly the complaint will pass. It is essential to convey to the patient that the doctor is interested: it takes a modicum of medical insight to realize that drugs are used to get rid of patients when the doctor is bored or lacks the essential repertoire of responses.

Secondly, a management plan, appropriate to the problem must be organized. Critical to this is a decision as to which mode of therapy is required and what resources are available. It may be that the doctor feels able to offer therapy himself, in the form of one-to-one psychotherapy: should this be the case, in general practice, he would be well advised to inform the patient at the onset of the limited nature of the contract, say, 4–5 half-hour discussions; it must be made quite clear that the therapy will be time limited and goal orientated. Much can be done in this short time, and at weekly intervals, the transference effect is easily controlled: longer, more frequent and sustained psychotherapy demands training, as badly managed transference reactions are damaging. Should the doctor feel that such a treatment is required, he must refer the patient to an appropriate professional: it is not likely that the local psychiatric service will have much to offer, except perhaps a young doctor in supervised training, and if the need is serious, the best resource is the lay psychotherapist consulted privately. If the problem springs from the family, and is either marital or sexual, then a focal therapy arranged by the Marriage Guidance Council or the Family Planning Association may be appropriate. Surprisingly good results can be obtained, even if in patients with marked problems by focal therapy limited to one area of their lives, and to short or moderate duration. Family therapy may well be available through the social work department. If a place can be found in a group psychotherapy, this type of patient does well: the sharing of problems with others, the discovery that the problem is not unique and the weekly experience of others improving has a marked effect, expecially in the area of commitment and work in therapy.

Clearly the major problem in anxiety is tension, and as relaxation is obviously the opposite, it has much to offer: it is, however, simply a symptomatic relief unless the patient chooses to use it as a life-controlling exercise. Autohypnotic relaxation by imaginal conditioning has the benefit that it enables the patient to use his imagination to take charge of his internal situation and to some extent, to dictate his feelings. The technique is rapidly learnt and is taught by the British Medical and Dental Hypnosis Society whose weekend courses are advertised in the medical press. A full description can be found in Kroger and Fezler (1976) with a series of useful scenarios for specific treatment situations. In use in general practice, the training of the patient requires three half hours, after which improvement is usually obvious or the patient is not interested in trying.

Access to a clinical psychologist is limited, but should help be available, behavioural techniques in anxiety reduction, including biofeedback, are of proven value. Perhaps the greatest value is to be found in the treatment of phobias, where behaviour therapy is clearly the most effective treatment.

Although drugs are often used as the treatment of first resort, they have been left to last in this review because their efficacy is so low. This is strange in view of the vast quantities consumed, but for the past three years the literature has been bombarded with reports of the failure of drugs to consume anxiety, of the dangers inherent in their use, their propensity to be increased and to be used in overdose situations and the constant problem of addiction. General practitioners are becoming much more cautious in their use (Murray *et al.* 1981). Prior to the benzodiazapines, barbiturates were in common use, especially phenobarbitone for the reduction of tension. Only moderately effective, some became addicted, and in overdoses, they proved potent respiratory depressants. Barbiturates are now virtually abandoned, with only occasional use in institutions under close supervision. Their replacement by benzodiazapines was hailed as a great advance: they are safe. This statement is true of their effect in overdose, as they are much safer than barbiturates, but risk of dependence remains. There is little to choose between the benzodiazapines except the duration of half-life. This is a vexed issue, as a commonly used hypnotic, nitrazepam has a half-life of 43 hours, and so becomes an excellent next day sedative, not exactly its intended use. Equally, the ultra short life hypnotic, triazolam, with a half-life of four hours, has the effect of increasing anxiety next day by a withdrawal effect (Morgan and Oswald 1982). This withdrawal reaction is an interesting effect of a small group of related drugs, alcohol, barbiturates, and benzodiazapines. In each case, withdrawal leads to anxiety and insomnia, and clearly it is worth asking if the exhibition is worthwhile to the patient: clearly, there is a price to be paid. If the patient is not warned of the withdrawal effect, he will certainly experience it as a recrudescence of the symptoms he began taking the drug to be rid of: however, the well-prepared patient manages withdrawal relatively easily.

The neuroleptics, composed of the phenothiazines, the thioxanthenes and the buterophenones, have a very small part to play: although free of dependency effects, they are much more toxic for other than very short-term use as the risk of tardive dyskensia is present even in small dosage.

Careful choice among the antidepressives can produce a useful sedative effect and if depressive features are present, this is a useful side-effect. Amitriptyline has a good night sedative quality and this avoids at least the worst of the anticholinergic side-effects. Mianserin is markedly sedative in the first few days, which is often when the effect is required, and a moderate dose again at night is helpful for sleeping. The monoamine oxidase inhibitors have a marked anti-anxiety effect and have been considered almost specific for phobic anxiety. While this use of them is perfectly justified, the usual care must be exercised with diet, and the drug is only possible with selected patients with high compliance.

Current interest is focused on the β-blocker drugs which exercise their effects not centrally but on the peripheral symptoms, such as palpitations. Their particular benefit is that they reduce specific symptoms without general sedation, but they remain toxic substances and the usual contra-indications apply, asthma, diabetes, and heart failure.

It remains important not to consider drugs as the answer to anxiety: they all have side-effects of varying severity. They are not problem solvers and in the last analysis they play much the same role in our culture as alcohol in stress: few physicians take pleasure in the image of themselves as either barmaid or pusher. Certainly to turn to drugs first in the treatment of anxiety is the resort of the therapeutically destitute.

AFFECTIVE DISORDERS

Changes of mood in both an upward and a downward direction are the common lot of mankind, rarely causing major problems unless the swing is rapid or severe, or unless the swing is in one direction only and is sustained. The difficulty in general practice is in deciding when the change is significant and to do this requires an adequate taxonomy and an accurate assessment.

To the surprise of the profession, recent community surveys, particularly Brown and Harris in (1978) in Camberwell and the Outer Hebrides, have produced results showing the frequency of depression of types normally thought to be serious and requiring therapy to be the order of 15 per cent. Most of these cases are unknown to the family doctor and are, in our terms, untreated: clearly most of them recover spontaneously. A second subset of the first group do attend the doctor, and of these, the majority are treated by the GP without referral to a specialist service. Some few, probably not only the most sick, are referred to specialist psychiatric care by Outpatient Department, Domiciliary Visit, or admission to the mental hospital.

Within this categorization, there may be variants from the transient alteration in mood within the norm, through to the psychomotor retardation of the severe endogenous depression. All carry with them the problem of suicide. The importance of recognizing depression as a potentially fatal disease must always be acknowledged and remain in the forefront of the practitioner's mind in continuing care. Should the serious depression be missed, the results can be catastrophic.

Perhaps the simplest classification of depression is to categorize on the severity of mood change. Most patients who claim depression mean that they are fed up, miserable, bored, unhappy, feeling lost. Usually the mood change is transient and responds to an invitation to a party or better than expected exam results. This group is largely young and mainly female. The second group, the reactive depressives show a more marked lowering of mood and this lowering is sustained. The patient attributes the change to an event in his life, e.g. a bereavement, or loss of a job. There may be reactive features in an upswing sense in that for a while a patient can cheer up in relation to company but soon relapses when left alone. It is in this area that most attempted suicides occur. Although the endogenous depression merges into the severe reactive, there is usually little doubt when true endogenous depression is encountered. The quality of mood is markedly low and quite unresponsive: usually the illness is not reactive and does not react to any stimulus. Physical elements tend to dominate the picture: the patient is obviously ill and often deeply suicidal. It is in this group that suicide, in the completed successful sense, is so common.

Mania, the upward swing, is relatively uncommon and usually requires admission and expert help.

Suicide

The epidemiology of attempted or para-suicide and suicide, is extraordinarily difficult.

1. All attempts do not go to hospital and so are not known to the hospital: many are probably unknown to anyone at all – they simply recover and go on with life.

2. All suicides are not recorded as suicides: a considerable number are labelled 'accidental death' either by reason of the nature of the 'accident' or by the decision of the Coroner.

However, more than 4000 patients per annum do take their lives against a background of perhaps 600000 per annum para-suicides. The distinction between a 'successful' suicide and a 'failed' para-suicide is difficult: there are some deaths that seem to fall into the profile of low-risk attempters, perhaps those who have got the dose wrong or have chosen the wrong drug. However, most (93 per cent) of suicides are psychiatrically ill; 70 per cent depressed, 15 per cent alcoholic (Barraclough *et al.* 1974). Some survivors clearly intended death and go on to be successful later. The differentiation in the clinical situation is particularly difficult as the life-risking activity appears to have a considerable affect on mood: the majority of para-suicides are not depressed or at least only transiently.

Most para-suicides believe themselves to be safe in the overdose; this has led to the view that the attempt is to manipulate the psychosocial environment and the relationships around them. This somewhat superficial philosophy tends to omit that group of largely young women who clearly meant to die and finally succeed in doing so (Office of Health Economics 1981) (Table 12.2).

Figure 12.1 illustrates the way the medical viewpoint has altered over the past 20 years: we began by considering that some attempters were successful and implied that all attempters were serious attempts to die. The view was then put forth that para-suicide was a different disease on epidemiological grounds and so it proved to be. Later a large overlap group was reported. Long-term follow up tends to suggest that the para-suicide overdose continues to have a poor long-term progress: 10–20 per cent of them finally succeed. This makes them an important group for preventive medicine: a well-established therapeutic relationship may be drawn on in time of trouble.

The profile of attempted and completed suicides can be drawn up to appear to be quite different groups, as indeed the stereotypes are (Fig. 12.2 and Table 12.3). In practice the overlap area is quite large (see *British Medical Journal* 1975).

Table 12.2. *Statistics of deliberate self-harm*

In a practice of 2500 patients
each year there will be 400 patients with depression of which 100 will consult their doctor
3–4 attempted suicides
and *one* successful suicide every *3–4 years*.

Nationally (England and Wales)
there are 4000 suicides per annum
(probably 6000 if 'undetermined' deaths are included)
that is 0.7 per cent of mortality but one-third of all student deaths and in young men second only to road traffic accidents.
(These figures are probably low because of Coroners' open verdicts.)

93 per cent of these suicides are mentally ill and two-thirds visit their GP or psychiatrist in the month before dying, 24 per cent in the week before; 80 per cent are on psychotropic agents.

One-third of all suicides have made previous attempts.

'Overdoses' currently run at more than 100 000 cases per annum (not including the cases dealt with by GP alone or those known only to the patient!).

Of young women aged 15–30 one in a hundred attempt in any one year – 90 per cent by self poisoning.
16–25 per cent of attempters will repeat within the year;
15 per cent of all depressives, and
10 per cent of all alcoholics,
eventually commit suicide.

Table 12.3. *Profile of attempted and completed suicides*

	Para-suicide attempted	Suicide completed
Sex	Female	Male
Age	Young, one-third under 35	Older: rate increasing with age
Social status	Various	Divorced, separated or bereaved, living alone
	Not socially isolated	Social isolation
Class	Higher in social class IV and V	All but upper > lower > middle
Associated illness	Mild personality disorder, 80 per cent not ill	Depression, alcoholism, physical illness, 90 per cent ill
Aim of act	Relief of tension: manipulation of social and intra-personal situation. Impulsive	Most intend to die
Act	Thought to be 'safe' chance of rescue high, rarely violent	Planned Little likelihood of failure, e.g. firearms. Often violent

Management of depressive illness

It is useful to identify certain principles or rules first. First, as in the rest of medicine, nothing is so important as an accurate diagnosis, based on a careful history and examination. The value lies in identifying which patient will benefit from treatment and which needs hospital care, particularly which has suicidal

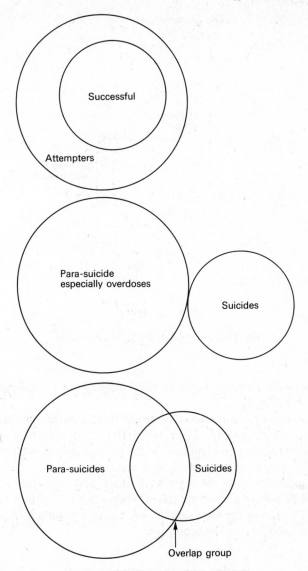

Fig. 12.1. Model of changing views of para-suicide and suicide.

risk. Without correct diagnosis, the exhibition of antidepressants becomes an unrewarding task, often leading to overdoses.

The second rule is always to assess the suicidal risk: in each and every patient who complains of depression, and on each occasion on which they are seen, unless obviously well. Failure to remember this leads to the patient feeling that he is not being taken seriously, and the doctor prescribing potentially lethal doses of tricyclics and failing to administer relevant care. It may be helpful to

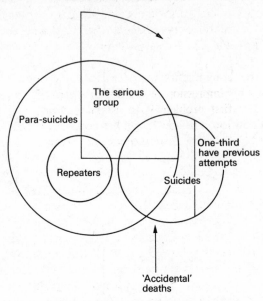

Fig. 12.2. A model of the factors in suicide.

tag the notes with a sticker which by implication warns of suicidal risk: one such is shown as Fig. 12.3.

Third, the doctor must always be ready to change his diagnosis as the situation alters. What appears at first sight to be a minor complaint may well be the onset of a more serious condition. Many patients present with anxiety and insomnia, who prove subsequently to have depression.

Psychological categories are not always stable, and frequently overlap: the doctor must be prepared to accept mixed diagnoses but to always manage the patient on the basis of the most serious one, e.g. in a woman with phobia and depression, he should treat the depression.

HISTORY OF	
OD	ALC
AS	PPH
DEPN	LOSS

Fig. 12.3. Sticker indicating suicidal risks.

Finally, if there are endogenous features, e.g. early morning waking, loss of weight, delusions of poverty or sickness, and the choice is made to treat with antidepressive medication, he should ensure that the dose is adequate e.g. 150 mg/day of tricyclic and of reasonable duration, rarely less than six months minimal.

The key must be set by the first interview, for it is from this encounter that the patient forms his impression of his doctor's capacity to understand and bear his pain. The first problem is to establish clearly and accurately the patient's mood, how low it is, how long it has been present and its reactivity. If a cause is offered it should be examined but not necessarily accepted as causal of the whole disturbance. The current state of hope in the patient should be examined hand in hand with the suicidal risk: has suicide crossed your mind? Would you like to end it all? Have you made plans, collected pills? Left a note? Physical disturbances should be asked for: alteration of eating habit and therefore loss of weight, bowel function, menses, sexual performance, sleep rhythm and quality. Particular attention should be paid to the early morning waking and the feelings experienced by the patient in the early hours of the morning. The patient should be questioned on drug taking as a cause of depression and of alcohol intake. Current relationships, marital and occupational, are worth examining in detail. Holidays planned should be noted: beware the holiday that will be the solution to all the problems.

The previous history, psychiatric and medical, is of great value; endogenous illness of the manic depressive psychotic type is notoriously recurrent. Previous overdoses warn of the liklihood of this behaviour being repeated. Before ending the first interview, make an appointment to see the spouse or relatives that day or the next. Decisions as to the treatment can often wait 24 hours, unless admission is required at once, as the viewpoint of the observer and a second look at the patient often proves helpful in making an accurate diagnosis. Should the second interview not be kept the GP has the difficult problem of following up the patient: difficult as it may be, it should not be neglected.

The second interview with the spouse or relative enables the evaluation to proceed. What has been noticed? How long has it been going on? How well can the problem be coped with at home? It is at this point that decision can be provisionally reached to treat at home, or to seek further advice, from out-patient department, from domiciliary visit or to admit to hospital. The criteria for admission are those of severity and safety (Table 12.4). Should the patient remain at home, the plans of management should now be made: follow up, at least weekly at onset, will be laid out, what to do if appointments cannot be kept explained, the possibility of time off work discussed, both in terms of capability for work and the problem of being left alone at home all day. If problems in the patient's life appear to be dominant, problem solving or crisis intervention technique can be applied. It is apparent that the psychotherapy of the depression has already begun and the patient is surrounded by concern and

Table 12.4. *Criteria for admission to hospital*

1. Suicidal risk, moderate or high
2. Severity of illness
3. Domestic circumstances are limited and emotional supports are low, e.g. family and friends absent or exhausted by duration of illness
4. Poor compliance with the drug regime or failure to respond to adequate dose of tricyclic (150 mg/day) over an adequate period (at least four weeks)

help: whether this approach should become more formal must be decided on the basis of the type of illness. Reactive depression can well be managed on psychotherapy lines alone, while endogenous depression demands by its physical characteristics a chemical or physical approach. Nevertheless, each patient needs much more than a quick prescription, and support is of the essence.

Psychotherapy can be carried out by the doctor alone, or in co-operation with a lay therapist, either a counsellor or psychotherapist. The doctor has a duty to continue his supervision in these circumstances until he is certain improvement is taking place, and the therapist has an equivalent duty to return the patient to medical care if the situation deteriorates. GPs can well learn psychotherapeutic skills by sharing the patient in joint sessions with the therapist. Most GPs develop styles of supportive therapy that they find useful for them. Therapy is a very individual affair and represents more of the therapist's personality than he may well care to admit. The psychologists have recently developed a new treatment named cognitive therapy as a form of behaviour modification. It is well described by Goddard (1982) and Mackay (1982), and can be considered for mild and moderate depressions: it can be well combined with physical methods. Its efficacy has been recently reported as being equally effective as chemotherapy, and the combination as more effective than each alone (Blackburn *et al.* 1981).

Depth or explorative psychotherapy is not usually considered suitable for depression: the major need is for support until the risks of the illness are over. It may well be that once the patient has recovered, there is therapeutic work to be done, both to consolidate the insights gained by the illness and prophylactically to prevent recurrence. The GP's major need is to develop skills in supportive psychotherapy, well described by Bloch (1979).

The use of drugs in affective disorder

So enthusiastic has been the prescribing of drugs over the past 20 years, that to the lay mind, depression and drug therapy are now linked: regrettably, some doctors share this simplistic view, although the evidence does not bear them out. It seems likely that the routine use of chemotherapy has been ill-advised, and that while their exhibition in serious cases makes marked differences, their overuse in minor cases is unrewarding, side-effects leading to low compliance, and a ready supply for ammunition for an eager overdoser.

Sedatives and hypnotics

Most depressives have anxiety elements in their history and it is tempting to treat them: equally, all depressives complain of sleep disturbance, the absence of this complaint would cast doubt on the diagnosis. Regrettably, sedatives and hypnotics are not of great value, and their routine use is to be depricated. Barbiturates have nothing to commend them and their danger in overdose makes an absolute contra-indication in depression except under the most closely supervised hospital conditions. The benzodiazapines, although safe in overdose, have problems – the long-acting, e.g. nitrazepam, make for sedation the next day which may be unwelcome; while the short-acting, e.g. triazopam, produce anxiety next day. If a problem-solving approach is used, or psycho-therapy attempted, it might be well to avoid their use. If sedation is required, the antidepressant can be chosen to have this most useful side-effect – e.g. day sedation with amitriptyline; night sedation with mianserin.

Antidepressants

The antidepressant drugs fall into three groups, the tricyclics, the newer anti-depressives, and the monoamine oxidase inhibitors. There are many examples of each type and the doctor is well advised to use only one of each, in order to get used to the side-effects of, and confident in the full dosage of each example. Among the tricyclics, amitriptyline is undoubtedly the standard against which others are measured: there is certainly no evidence that any other is better, although side-effects may be reduced. In the standard tricyclics, the proven useful dosage used in all the trials is 150 mg/day: the evidence that less is useful, except in children or the elderly, is hard to find. It seems a pity to use so powerful a substance with such unpleasant side-effects in dosages less than that likely to be useful. Full dose at the onset of treatment is, however, rarely tolerated, and must be worked up to over the first week. As the drug takes 10–14 days to produce measurable response, except for the side-effects, which begin at once, it could well be three weeks before the patient notices change: this must be discussed with the family and the need to tolerate the side-effects to reap the benefits made clear. Equally it is helpful from the onset, to state the necessity of long-term treatment to prevent relapse, for recurrence is extremely common in depression. Evidence is accumulating that the efficacy of tricyclics, in preventing relapse, is still present some eight months after the apparent end of the illness (Coppen *et al.* 1978). But it should be noted that this effect is gained on full dosage. Compliance, the patients co-operation in taking therapy, is gained by education and in this way by ensuring that the patient and doctor are on the same side. Bottles of tricyclics should be brought on each occasion in an attempt to avoid hoarding for suicidal purposes: prescribing such a drug by post or a repeat system seems inappropriate, for if the patient does not require more personal care, he may not require the drug. Tricyclics are contra-indicated in cardiac cases, especially recent infarction and arrythmias.

The newer antidepressives are legion: it is essential not to attempt to know them all, especially as there is no evidence that any one is superior to any other. Two useful members of the group, both of which are rapid acting, are mianserin and nomifensine. Mianserin shows marked reduction in complaints within four days but is, initially, markedly sedative: it is best to give the dose at night, starting with some 30 mg and increasing after four days to 60 mg a night. The patients should be warned not to work, or drive, or take alcohol in the four days after starting or increasing the dose. The sedative action rapidly reduces and the patient feels more alert than previously. Nomifensine has the opposite effect in that it is initially alerting and should be taken early in the day to avoid disturbance of sleep: 50 mg twice daily increasing to 75 mg twice daily appears optimal. In both these examples, much larger doses can be used if required: should an initial good response fade off after some weeks, a small increase in dose is often effective in producing a rapid response.

The role of the monoamine oxidase inhibitors is less clear: initially they obtained a poor reputation by reason of the so called tyramine/cheese reaction. If tyramine is taken, almost always in one of the prohibited foods, a severe headache is induced with marked hypertension, sometimes leading to sub-arachnoid haemorrhage. However, in careful hands, well instructed, with a dietary warning card, the problem is uncommon. While they are undoubtedly effective on occasions, they are thought to be less reliably so than the other two groups, seeming to work best when anxiety is predominant part of the depressive illness. Phenelzine is probably the safest of the group, used in a dose of 30–45 mg/day. Combination therapy, using monoamine oxidase inhibitors plus tricyclics is best left in the hands of those enthusiasts practised in its use. MAOIs work relatively rapidly, usually in a few days. However, most patients in view of the dietary restrictions, want to end treatment as soon as possible.

Hamilton (1982) has shown that in ordinary clinical practice, in severe depressive illness phenelzine and imipramine were equally potent.

Subsequent follow-up visits, which need initially to be of weekly frequency, can in due course become monthly. On each occasion several tasks require attention; the current mental state and suicidal risk must be assessed, continuance of treatment, evaluation of side-effects, and fresh prescription if indicated: care taken to ensure the correct dose is being taken and that the patient has not failed in compliance as soon as he feels better.

It may well be that at the onset of the depressive illness the psychodynamic elements of the illness are submerged by the physical: the patient may be so psychomotor retarded as to be unable to remember what made him unhappy. Further enquiry at a later stage may enable the physician to discover factors in the patient's life that require help, an unresolved bereavement being particularly common, a poor marital or sexual relationship being frequent. When the patient is particularly well and cheerful, it is important to exclude a swing to hypermania, either as a spontaneous shift, or as an effect of a tricyclic anti-depressant. Should this occur on tricyclic therapy, the drug should be stopped and haloperidol substituted pending a second opinion.

Care should be taken to avoid 'silly' doses of tricyclics taken as 'tonics' or as a talisman: dependence of this type is particularly easy to create and its avoidance depends on explaining clearly at the onset, and frequently during the course of the illness, the doctor's pharmacological intentions.

The problem of recurrent affective disorders

Reactive depression, with its usual personality element, not uncommonly recurs and although it is unlikely to respond to drugs, they are often used. Dependence in this situation is common, the patient presenting to the doctor, not to tell his story, but to obtain a prescription, and treated this way the situation seems to be quite incurable: the alternative strategy of problem recognition and, it is to be hoped, solving, requiring as it does an increase of interest and time invested, this seems to be more effective in the long run and at face value is better medicine. In contra distinction, recurring endogenous depression with its high mortality from suicide, demands the consideration of chemotherapy in the prevention of its recurrence. Two approaches have been tried: lithium therapy and long-term tricyclic administration. If tricyclics are used, it must be in adequate dosage, as the evidence that prophylactic tricyclic works is good only in the area of 150 mg/day (Coppen 1978; Coppen *et al.* 1978) with the usual proviso of the elderly and the very small. It is difficult to assess how good compliance is in this group and it seems easier, despite the side-effects, to use lithium and monitor the blood levels. Perhaps the doctor is more confident with the biochemistry report in his hand.

BEREAVEMENT

Bereavement provides a classic example of relatively short-term continuing care of a psychotherapeutic mode. A significant loss has occurred and support is needed as time provides its adjustment. As the GP has often been involved in the illness that initiated the loss, he is in an ideal position to offer help. Often help will not be required as the grieving process will be supported within the family network, no dysfunctional symptoms being reported either by the patient or relatives. Rarely, the swing from bereavement to depression is acute and dangerous, particularly in elderly men, who carry the highest suicide rate and here a chemotherapeutic or even a hospital regime will be indicated. There is an intermediate situation containing normal bereavement process that is unsupported, in which the GP plays a brief but significant role in allowing the mourning and encouraging the grief work. Also, and more relevantly, there is a class of morbid grief, that, though less than full-blown depression, remains more severe for a longer duration than normal. This latter group does poorly on chemotherapy and psychological methods are currently being developed which show promise. Forced grieving, or positive mourning, are names for the techniques of creating active grief work in the patient who has blocked. Grief work has always to be done and to be felt to be done: the techniques enable this process, which is diminished by reliance on drug therapy. It is often found in blocked mourning that passive listening and empathy, so relevant to normal grieving process, is without value: the pain has been blocked off often by denial mechanisms of an hysterical nature. Deep interpretations of ambivalence are wasted in this situation and cognitive restructuring is required to allow access to the more usual therapy. Of the many techniques available, some are obviously only suitable to group settings, for example, with a therapeutic community, where the pyschodrama of 'having the funeral again', re-enacting the funeral and commitment can loose floods of emotions and break up the blocked affect. More suitable for a one to one setting is a therapy designed round the repeated exposure to the facts of death, repeatedly re-examining both the events around the death and the feelings about them until they are passed. A visit to the grave, 'really to say goodbye' can be arranged, possibly with support: a precious possession, say, a photograph, may be found to be a block and it may be lent to the therapist, or even in a carefully planned and thought out way may be thrown away as a symbolic leaving behind and moving on: a letter may be written to the deceased, listing the pros and cons of the shared life to enable a balance to be struck and hate may have to be expressed. In all such therapy, care must be taken to ensure that sufficient support is available and that too great a pressure is not applied. The suicidal risk in bereavement is high and must be accepted: not to intervene is more dangerous than therapy, but at all times the doctor will be aware of the risk of depressive illness engulfing bereavement. Cognitive therapy will suggest that the patient's maladaptive thought pattern is at root cause and such thoughts as 'It's the end' must change into 'It's a new beginning', 'I've nothing to live for' to 'There's everything to live for'. Reality testing is particularly simple in this area and rational emotive therapy with its clear structure is easily appreciated (Beech *et al.* 1982).

THE USES OF LITHIUM

The place of lithium in treatment of acute mania, is limited to a small role in the hospital management, as originally described by Cade (1949). In the treatment of depression, the evidence of efficacy is limited: it is no longer used in the treatment of the acute attack but largely as a prophylactic agent. In this respect lithium is now an established treatment and is probably the only drug to continue to protect the patient against relapse after some six months. It is this effect that has caused lithium to be called the 'mood normalizer'.

The best evidence for the use of lithium comes from trials in which the affective disorder tends to be at the endogenous or severe end of the spectrum: bipolar is a particularly strong indicator. Recurrence is the prime criteria and more than two bouts per year or three bouts in two years provides a starting line. It should be noted by both physician and patient that relapse is not uncommon in the first 12 months of therapy but that continuing the treatment has its benefits and that apparent early failure of proplylaxis should not dishearten either.

There is no compelling evidence to enable a decision to be made as to when to stop prophylaxis. Maggs (1979) promotes the suggestion that after twelve symptom-free months treatment might cease: Baastrup *et al.* (1970) found nearly all their patients relapsed within one year of ceasing the drug. Experience in general practice suggests patients are not clamouring to stop and appreciate the benefits of stable mood and psychological health: but thyroid and renal function bear careful watching.

Withdrawal reaction has not been noted, so gradual withdrawal would seem unnecessary.

Preparations

In the United Kingdom lithium is marketed in two forms: lithium carbonate (plain and sustained release tablets) and recently as lithium citrate in sustained release form. There is no evidence that one is better than another but it is best to get to know one form.

Recent reports of renal toxicity attribute the damage to peak plasma levels: in view of this it is advised that the daily dose be divided. Amdisen (1980) believes the single-dose regime should never be used.

For effective prophylaxis it has long been thought that any plasma level between 0.5 mmol/l and 1.5 mmol/l was effective. With toxic effects common at a level of 2.0 mmol/l most physicians aimed at 1.0 mmol/l but this practice was based on little or no evidence. Studies now show that relapse rates did not rise significantly until plasma levels were below 0.4 mmol/l. It is now recommended that the desirable plasma level is 0.4–0.8 mmol/l.

Success in using lithium is dependent on complete compliance: if this is unlikely to be obtained it may be safest to avoid lithium. Compliance is best obtained by consideration of the patient's health belief model and in this situation the patient needs to understand:

1. Manic depressive illness is a recurrent illness and has been so in him. He can expect further hospital admissions unless he takes the drug.

2. The drug is dangerous only if used badly: with careful co-operation and regular blood tests all will be well: he can expect far fewer attacks while on lithium.

3. Side-effects are common at first but usually settle. Serious effects can occur and the patient must know them.

Starting therapy

It is worthwhile contacting the laboratory before commencing, as the staff may well perform the routine tests on only one day per week.

1. **Before treatment**
   ensure physical fitness
   examine urine for albumen and blood
   check blood urea and creatinine levels
   exclude hypothyroidism

2. **Day 0** – commence treatment with two tablets at night
3. **Day 7** – blood test – 12 hours after last intake:
   adjust blood level by adjusting dose *pro rata*
   i.e. if two tablets give 0.3 mmol/l; four tablets will give 0.6 mmol/l
4. **Day 14. 21. 28.** – repeat test and adjust
5. Thereafter monthly and later three monthly – blood test and adjustment of dose if required.

A patient instruction sheet for lithium is set out below.

A PATIENT INSTRUCTION SHEET

Manic depressive disorder

Your illness is one of swings of mood from normality to excitement or to depression: in your case these attacks are recurrent but it is well known that using lithium will reduce the frequency of attacks to about one-tenth. Lithium is not a once and for all cure but regular careful usage will prevent most of your expected attacks: the treatment may need to be continued indefinitely. You should not stop treatment without consulting your doctor, or take other treatment, again without consulting him.

The treatment is based on two factors.

1. The right doses taken at the same time each day – 8 a.m. and 8 p.m.
2. Regular blood checks to test the serum level taken some 12 hours after the last dose: omit morning dose on blood test day.

Side-effects The table below shows three groups of side effects. The slight metallic taste is reduced by taking the tablets with or after food.

1. MINOR　　　slight metallic taste
　　　　　　　slight loss of appetite
　　　　　　　slight thirst
　　　　　　　slight muscle tremor
　　　　　　　slight nausea and looseness of stool
　　　　　　　extra volume of urine

these are common at onset but tend to wear off.

2. MODERATE　weight gain
　　　　　　　swelling of ankles
　　　　　　　marked nausea
　　　　　　　marked tremor

these effects should be reported to the doctor and the dose reduced if the blood level is high.

3. SEVERE　　　vomiting
　　　　　　　diarrhoea
　　　　　　　coarse tremor
　　　　　　　sleepiness
　　　　　　　dizziness
　　　　　　　difficulty with speech
　　　　　　　– coma

these effects are dangerous. Stop taking the drug and report at once to the doctor.

Routine monitoring

At each interview the mental stage should be appraised: a routine health diary is useful, lest the interview simply tests the mood of the day.

A simple record placing mood on a scale

$$0 = \text{depression} \qquad 5 = \text{normal} \qquad 10 = \text{manic}$$

is sufficient to show swing and tendency of mood. Blood levels must be 12 hours after the last tablet so a morning test is preferable.

Blood tests should include blood urea and creatinine each six months with thyroid function at yearly intervals.

Overdose, by suicidal intent, concurrent illness or failing renal function, leads to toxic levels and requires urgent treatment. The symptoms develop gradually with vomiting, diarrhoea, sleepiness leading to coma, and vertigo. The tremor is coarse, with hypertonic deep reflexes and attacks of hyperextension and epilepsy may occur.

Side effects not mentioned on the patient instruction sheet

1. Blood changes: leucocytosis and granulocytosis are common as are changes in the ECG and the EEG. They are not dangerous and persist during the duration of therapy, disappearing when medication is withdrawn.

2. Muscle tremor can be sufficient to make the patient stop treatment. Beta-blockers, e.g. propranolol, 10 mg three times per day is helpful.

3. Hypothyroidism is usually found in the low thyroxine levels well before clinical myxoedema. Low levels may be tranisent but if TSH is raised, thyroxine is indicated 50 mg once or twice per day.

4. Persistent polydipsia and polyuria requires lower blood levels, especially if the polyuria is over 3.5 l/day.

5. Chronic renal toxicity is probably dose related: if not cleared by reducing the plasma level discontinutation is indicated. For a good review of the current situation see Srinivasan and Hullin (1980).

ALCOHOLISM

Few professionals have difficulty with the word 'alcoholism' or find difficulty in deciding that any individual is 'alcoholic'. If the person is damaging himself physically, mentally, socially, maritally, or occupationally – then he or she is alcoholic. It is, however, a word to keep to ourselves, as the use of it as a label in the presence of the patient almost always starts an unproductive row. Too many patients have protested 'I may have an alcohol problem, but I'm not an alcoholic': it is better to accept this and try to help with the alcohol problem: the term 'alcoholic' is usually used as a term of abuse. The alcohol problem is always a chronic one, it has usually been present for years before it comes to notice and will certainly be a problem for years to come. Unless it is recognized as a chronic relapsing condition, much harm will be done both to the patient and the doctor–patient relationship. Like diabetes, the problem remains, like rheumatoid it attacks every system, like trait anxiety it is never really over, like multiple sclerosis it tends to run from bout to bout: but it is equally right to go on treating, helping, and supporting the diabetic, the multiple-sclerotic, and the alcoholic, despite the considerable risk of relapse, even if apparently currently well controlled. It is this expectation of relapse, associated with a desire to help, that delineates the doctor's capacity to be of use. Further, like so many other conditions, it is a family affair and the doctor must remain aware of the dangers to, and the difficulties of, all the members of the alcoholic family. Unhappily, too often the best intentioned fall into despair and therapeutic indifference: too many alcoholics tell stories of medical neglect, and while some may be pleas for recognition, it is unlikely that all are historically incorrect. It may be that with our standardised mortality ratio of 311 for alcoholic cirrhosis, doctors could well bear a little sympathy for the plight of this chronic disease that lasts a lifetime (Office of Population Census and Surveys 1972) (Table 12.5).

Table 12.5. *Occupations in relation to alcohol. (After OPCS 1972.) Liver cirrhosis mortality (England and Wales 1970–72). Standardized mortality ratio*

Average occupation	100
Publicans and innkeepers	1576
Ships officers	781
Barmen, barmaids	633
Ships men	628
Fishermen	595
Hotel proprietors/managers	506
Restauranteurs	385
Medical practitioners	311

Detection

The absolute incidence of alcoholism, is, by the secretive nature of the disease, unknowable, but it is generally accepted that each GP has some 25 on his list, most of whom are undetected. They will be diagnosed only if a high index of suspicion is exercised and this must be based on concepts of correct sterotypes. The gutter alcoholic, always drunk, imbibing meths in a homeless men's hostel is so far from typical as to be almost useless. It is necessary to begin from an entirely different basis: remembering the teenager with the motorcycle accident, the bank manager with the cheerful style in the afternoons, the phobic housebound housewife, the successful salesman who wants to stop smoking, the elderly confused who has developed pneumonia, the husband of the wife with another manfriend, the consultant who isn't getting it right, and the partner who is losing his grip. All sorts and conditions of men and women become alcoholics: the disguise is infinite.

Special suspicion must be directed to certain areas:

Physical illness

GPs need to have an *aide mèmoir* to the physical findings in, and complications of, alcoholism: no-one can remember them all, but alcohol is a toxic substance and must be considered in every organ system. The diagram in Fig. 12.4, or the list in Table 12.6, may help: each must create his own from experience and reading. Gastrointestinal illness is particularly significant.

Table 12.6. *List of some complications of alcoholism*

System	
Hepatic	fatty liver
	alcoholic hepatitis
	cirrhosis
	primary neoplasm
Pancreatic	acute, chronic or relapsing pancreatitis
Haematological	elevated MCV without anaemia
	anaemia, micro- or macrocytic
	haemolytic anaemia
	thrombocytopenia (toxic)
Endocrine	hypogonadism
	gynaecomastia in male
	feminization with impotence and infertility
	pseudo Cushing's syndrome
Nutritional	vitamin deficiency, especially B group
Metabolic	raised lipids
	raised uric acid
	altered blood sugar

Psychological illness

Alcohol can play a part in any other psychiatric illness but is typically associated with the list given in Table 12.7, which may act as a reminder.

Some behavioural and sociological characteristics

Certain patterns of behaviour are well recognized as typical: the excess usage of medical services by alcoholics is renowned, e.g. the Monday morning certificate, the repeated minor illness attendance, possible neurotic, the repeated but unsupported D and V. Recurrent accidents, both major and minor, both at work and on the roads, particularly occurring after 10.00 p.m. and at weekends, are characteristic. Marital problems, rows and abuse, battering of wives and children, sexual failure are all highly suggestive and deserve investigation. Difficulties at work are common, the manager or foreman often recognizing the alcoholic long before the doctor. Legal difficulties, loss of driving licence and debts, particularly in relation to maintenance of a previous marriage are common. Typical in a general practice setting are those who repeatedly attend smelling of alcohol at the time of consultation, always worth a note in the

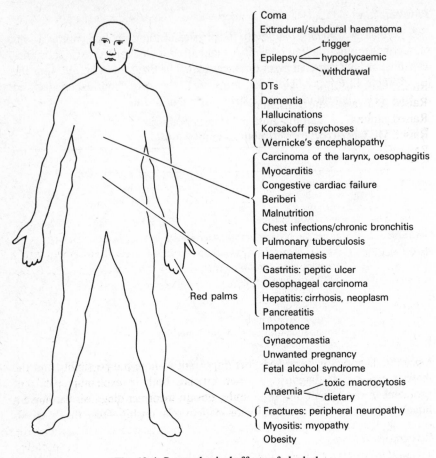

Fig. 12.4. Some physical effects of alcohol.

Table 12.7. *Some psychological illnesses*

Blackouts
Memory loss; dysmnesic syndrome
Reduced self-esteem, self-neglect
Withdrawal syndromes
  Shakes
  DTs
  Epilepsy
Psychosexual syndromes, especially impotency
Depression
Attempted and completed suicide
Aggressive, antisocial behaviour and violence { Battered baby syndrome
Psychosis – hallucinosis   Battered wives syndrome
Fuge
Morbid jealousy
Dementia

margin '?C_2H_5?'. A collection of such entries makes a diagnosis quite likely, and a random blood alcohol will often confirm the diagnosis.

Biochemical and haematological screening tests

Raised blood alcohol
Raised AST (aspartate transaminase)
Raised gamma GT (gamma-glutamyl transpeptidase)
Raised MCV (macrocytosis without anaemia)
Reduced folate
Raised PTT (prothrombin time)
Raised fasting triglyceridés
Raised uric acid

While there is no single unequivocal test for alcoholism, the finding of a disturbance of the above biological values should lead to a detailed history of alcohol intake. The use of random blood alcohol tests in association with other investigations has a particular value in that it frequently reveals the denial that is so characteristic. It should be noted that even the most sensitive tests may be normal at times, and further, that other liver and marrow bone toxins can give similar abnormalities, e.g. barbiturates and anticonvulsants.

Identification

Once the diagnosis is suspected, it is important to note the possibility and the reasons for it: the diagnosis is often crucial, both in explaining recurrent problems in the patient and the family, but an incorrect diagnosis can have a hugely deleterious effect on the doctor–patient relationship. Once the diagnosis is established, continuing care demands awareness at each consultation of the complications of the disease. A sticker on the notes, or an entry in the problem list is well worth while: it identifies the subsequent risks not merely of cirrhosis but of depression and suicide. Clark (1981) gives a good review.

Taking the history of acohol consumption in a suspected alcoholic

Of all approaches, the direct frontal, and of all questions, 'How much do you drink?' seem to be the least rewarding. The topic is best approached obliquely by a doctor with a non-judgemental approach: if by implication the question is suggesting an inferior status for the respondent, it is obviously doomed. Perhaps, 'When last did you have a drink?', 'What do you normally drink?', 'What would be a good night out for you?', 'How often a day do you have a drink?'; until gradually a daily and weekly drinking history is established. Withdrawal symptoms should be sought: 'How do you feel the next day?', 'How much does it affect you?' 'Do you ever need another drink?'.

The critical question is 'Has your drinking ever caused you problems?' but this requires a well-established relationship: when the time is ripe, the CAGE screening questions are most effective (Mayfield *et al.* 1974).

CAGE SCREEN

Have you ever felt you ought to **cut** down on your drinking?

Have people ever **annoyed** you by criticizing your drinking?

Have you ever felt **guilty** about your drinking?

Have you ever needed a drink as an **eye-opener**, to get rid of a hangover?

A simple formal questionnaire, well tried and proven, is the brief MAST shown in Table 12.8. Both these questionnaires are shown on one page of the *British Medical Journal* (28 November 1981, p. 1459) and a photostat copy on the

Table 12.8. *Brief MAST. (After Pokorny et al. (1972))*

	Circle correct answer	
Do you feel you are a normal drinker?	YES	NO (2 pts)
Do friends or relatives think you are a normal drinker?	YES	NO (2 pts)
Have you ever attended a meeting of Alcoholics Anonymous?	YES (5 pts)	NO
Have you ever lost friends or girlfriends or boyfriends because of drinking?	YES (2 pts)	NO
Have you ever got into trouble at work because of drinking?	YES (2 pts)	NO
Have you ever neglected your obligations, your family, or your work for two or more days in a row because you were drinking?	YES (2 pts)	NO
Have you ever had delirium tremens (DTs), severe shaking, heard voices or seen things that were not there after heavy drinking?	YES (5 pts)	NO
Have you ever gone to anyone for help about your drinking?	YES (5 pts)	NO
Have you ever been in hospital because of drinking?	YES (5 pts)	NO
Have you ever been arrested for drunken driving or driving after drinking?	YES (2 pts)	NO
Total score		

desk is a great help. A score of five points or more on a brief MAST is taken as diagnostic of alcoholism.

The function of denial in the alcoholic's defence

Denial is one of the most successful of the defence mechanisms, and is perhaps the commonest of the techniques the ego uses in conflicts which may lead to neurosis. In the general practitioner's ordinary day, he will make use of this mechanism simply to stay sane: the capacity to blot out anxiety and worry is an essential component of the healthy mind. However, when the risks involved in any behaviour becomes excessive, and denial becomes impossible, anxiety ensues. It is in this delicate balance that so many problems of management of the alcoholic flounder. The alcoholic will deny(i) the amount he drinks (ii) that he's been advised in the past to stop drinking (iii) that alcohol has damaged him in the past and is doing so currently (iv) he may even deny the evidence of blood alcohol levels, claiming he lost his driving licence over a police error.

To some degree, the stance can be understood, even admired, for to inform the physician exactly how much he drinks and that he was advised to abstain and has damaged himself is to lose his defence and to become neurotic. The alcoholic is usually aware at one level that his stance is foolish and precarious, but he fears to fall from it. Hence, many consultations can be wasted in lies and deceits, leading to an ever angrier doctor and an increasingly alienated patient. The end play of this particular game is to send the patient to the psychiatrist labelled 'mad' or 'bad' and as a punishment, presumably for having been so stupid as to attempt to delude the doctor.

If it is the case that denial is a normal defence mechanism, it might be asked why we attempt to breach it: some doctors do not attempt to, having found by bitter experience that one is unlikely to succeed by frontal attack and preferring to await a time of easier penetration. Strong (1980), in a study of doctors' attitudes to the problem, offers a series of insights into why the GP leans back from confrontation, particularly illustrating the feelings of helplessness so often experienced. He points out that alcoholics in no way satisfy the basic assumption of doctors about the doctor–patient relationship. It is, for example, commonly assumed that the patient has an illness, or at least a problem for which he wants help: yet the alcoholic is often a help-rejecting complainer. Thus the assumption of medical expertise and control over the situation is lost: doctor's orders are almost always broken by the alcoholic.

It is for these reasons, that denial is the commonest defence and that the doctor is commonly decommissioned in the encounter, that leads the enlightened physician into different patterns of management. The way lies in avoiding the frontal attack, instead using the patient's power to better ends. While this may be possible in early and middle cases of alcoholism, it is clearly not possible in the 'terminal' case. Much more effort is needed to screen out the cases in which a relatively high level of success can be expected. Pollak's (1978) study showed 64.9 per cent improved or better, sober over two years, a remarkable result. Edwards *et al.* (1977), in a controlled trial of treatment and advice found one-third of male alcoholics became free from the problem after one session of firm, honest advice offered in the presence of their spouse. It can no longer be held that alcoholism is untreatable.

Management

As in so many other areas of psychological medicine, the relationship is crucial; without a good basis the doctor is impotent. This relationship must never be assumed, no matter how good it has been before: in Western culture, the diagnosis is inevitably experienced as a slur on the character of the patient and always the relationship is under strain. It is tempting to draw on the investment of previous experience and be brutally frank about your opinion to the patient and his family: while this can on occasion prove fruitful, it is usually counter-productive, and it is better to plan to approach the diagnosis over several sessions – time is rarely of the essence in general practice.

1. Once the possibility is considered, establish the drinking habit from the patient.

2. Examine and investigate, biochemically.

3. Family members should be brought into the psychological and drinking history taking process.

4. The diagnosis should be debated in terms of the World Health Organiza-tion definition of damage to health, physical or psychological to relationship, occupation, etc. with the intention of delineating the problem or problems: avoid voicing the label 'alcoholic'.

In view of the high incidence of physical and psychological illness, a careful psychiatric history is mandatory and a full physical examination with simple blood tests (haemoglobin series and biochemical profile) is required. This is often much better put off for 24 hours to allow an appointment of say 15 minutes: it wastes time to hurry at the onset of treatment. It seems to be critical in the handling of the alcoholic's problems, to plan ahead on a relatively long-term basis, much like the care of a long-term depression in which one might arrange weekly appointments for a month and fortnightly for the next three months. The patient receives much security from this approach, knowing that the doctor has understood the long time scale of his condition.

Never make abstinence a prerequisite of further contact, as to do so seems always to stop further contact. As it is those who are sick who have need of the physician, and as alcoholism is a chronic relapsing disease, they should be warned like the depressives they so often are, to make contact when in relapse. Note, however, and tell them, that contact while drunk is of no value, and the surgery is the stage on which the interaction will take place.

Goals in relation to drink should be set early and be realistic: while the evidence that controlled drinking can be followed by the more severely addicted is hard to come by, many minor alcoholics can manage to reduce their intake to reasonable levels and with support, remain sober. The AA approach, effective as it may be, seems to effective in only some 10 per cent of contacts. It is easy for the general practitioner to find a member of AA with whom to relate: as this member becomes trusted, he or she can be used to introduce the new patient to the group, but medical expectations should not be high. Often the family will ask for help to force the patient into the grasp of AA: this is unlikely to be a useful ploy as the AA process is essentially one of conversion of a religious kind and has to be one of personal conviction.

Controlled drinking is the usual aim and to achieve this objective, the patient needs to bring his drinking into conscious critical perspective. It is important to look at the gains that drinking bring him in a behavioural analysis: a depth analysis of previous life experience and looking for a causal factor appears quite worthless. Most success will be found in the group of alcoholics, by far the majority, who still have a semi-stable home background and a semi-willing spouse. If she can be involved in the behavioural treatment, the chances of successful control of drinking are higher.

Behavioural analysis is the process of examining the precipitants, especially interactional, of drinking behaviour and the subsequent responses. Often the drinking bout is initiated by an unexamined breakdown in marital relationship or an excess of pressure at work without a response of extra support at home. If the therapist, and there is no indication that this need be a doctor, allows the family to discover the power of their interaction and if there is a will to a good and sober marriage, then relatively few sessions will enable the spouse to alter reactions in such a way as to make sobriety pay off. A full-blooded behaviourist approach can be attempted with a day-to-day diary of events and interactions analysed to provide a base line: rules can be written out and a contract signed. Such a contract will provide for mutual support and talk times, sexual relationships, and will delineate the pay offs. Breach of the contract usually results in withdrawal of the benefits of the contract but is not rewarded with negative feedback: a breach is a failure but dealt with in a neutral way. Some find value in contingency contracting, in which at the simplest, the drinker agrees with his spouse to 'pay' for his drinking behaviour (Miller 1972).

Drug treatment, except in response to withdrawal syndromes, is largely unrewarding. If the patient has a primary depressive illness, then the treatment of this by standard methods is obligatory and rewarding. However, often, the drinking pattern is not greatly altered. Should anxiety predominate, the anxiolytics, almost invariably the benzodiazapines can be given, but outside the withdrawal syndromes are relatively ineffective. The hope that the dangerous sedative, alcohol can be exchanged for the safer benzodiazapines is rarely fulfilled, the patient taking both in a random manner and often together. If one chemical is abused, the odds are that others will be too. Recently, attempts have been made to reduce anxiety with beta-blockers, especially propranolol, but this has largely been reported as ineffective. The use of lithium in alcoholics with associated depression, was successful, and it is suggested that lithium be used in depression with the same indications of repeated endogenous/psychotic bouts as usual.

Three substances that produce adverse effects in the drinker by the formation of toxic substances have been investigated: disulferam (Antabuse), citrated calcium carbimide (Abstem), and metronidazole (Flagyl) prove in practice to be disappointing and only the first is in common use. Careful analysis of the results show that no matter how interesting the aldehyde reaction is to a biochemically trained doctor, it has little effect on outcome and it could well be that the major effects are caused by compliance, that is to say, the patient is convinced of the seriousness of the doctor in carrying out this life-threatening procedure. The drug works best in the setting of twice weekly attendance at the clinic, suggesting that the contact is as important as the feared metabolic effect. Implants of disulphiram are equally effective, and this in the absence of assayable blood levels!

In the treatment of withdrawal states, chloromethiazole (heminevarin) is usually regarded as the optimal treatment, with benzodiazapines as a second string.

Alcohol withdrawal states

In the management of the alcoholic, withdrawal states are encountered from time to time. The minor episodes can be managed in practice, the major episodes of, for example, alcoholic hallucinosis, require a psychiatric admission, while full-blown delirium tremens deserves the facilities of the acute medical unit as it is so often accompanied by serious illness.

If the case is to be treated at home, the full co-operation of the family must be obtained and the following pattern established:

1. Alcohol is forbidden: while alcohol can be used in the prevention of delirium tremens, it is never an optimal treatment.

2. The use of sedatives, either benzodiazapines in heavy dosage, e.g. 10–20 mg six hourly reducing over five days, or chlormethiazole, 10–15 mg six hourly, reducing over five days, undoubtedly makes for a pleasanter withdrawal period but it carries the danger of further addiction. All concerned must realize that the next few months will be likely to be tense and restless, that resource to further drugs carries further dangers and that change of life-style comes from change of mind, not change of tablets.

The role of vitamins is uncertain but most practitioners give a mixture of vitamins B and C by intramuscular injection of Parentrovite HP. Careful watch

---

Table 12.9. *Table of withdrawal symptoms. (After Edwards and Grant (1977))*

1. Affective disturbance: fear, panics, stutter reaction
2. Tremor, going on to 'the shakes', coarse, generalized reaction to stress
3. Nausea, vomiting, and repeated retching, classically early morning 'Toothbrush' vomiting
4. Night sweats
5. Hallucinatory states – 'the horrors', disturbed sleep with vivid nightmares, hallucinations, visual and auditory
6. Epilepsy ('rum fits')
7. Delirium tremens, restlessness, overactivity, tachycardia, sweating, pyrexia, disorientated illusions, delirium and hallucinations, reduced attention span, confabulation

---

should be kept during domiciliary withdrawal, both of the general state of the patient (pneumonia at this stage is a common complicating illness), or some specific indication for hospital admission, e.g. dehydration, fever or fit. Withdrawal symptoms are listed in Table 12.9.

FAMILY THERAPY

The major problem of continuing care, as distinct from the episodic treatment of isolated major illness, is that so often the presenting patient does not contain the whole problem. The identified 'patient', the sick person, or the one complaining, is often representative either of the family or some social background, for example, the work set-up. Two situations are common, where the patient as the weakest member of the social setting breaks. First, as for example in marital distress, one partner presents, and second, where one person within the family presents, who is, albeit unconsciously, recognized by the family as the sick member and scapegoated. Loaded with family guilts, pressures, and failures, the identified member lives under the expectation of illness and social failure, and in due course, achieves this expectation. It is obvious that in presentations such as these, there is often difficulty in making sense of the consultation until the occult features are made clear and this can only be done by a full appreciation of the whole family. Happily, the general practitioner in his guise as family doctor has a relatively easy access to the whole family: it is interesting to observe that when great difficulty is found in seeing other members of the family, that the doctor's suspicion that there is something wrong in the relationship is usually correct. This easy access to the whole family is in marked contrast to consultant practice where it proves much more difficult to obtain the wider view, leaving it up to the family doctor to exploit his opportunities to the benefit of the whole family.

Experience with trainee GPs has shown that the major block to using the whole family as the unit of therapy lies in not knowing what to do with it, how to handle it, and particularly how much time family therapy will take. Happily, family therapy is short in duration and infrequent, of the order of once a month. The process begins by calling the family together, certainly the husband and wife, and usually all the children, noting at once that they are usually quite comfortable in being together and that the problem seems to lie in the doctor. The history of the presenting complaint should be taken, ensuring that each member has a say. At this point, the doctor's interest in each person's view-point begins the change within the family: for example, toilet training is traditionally regarded as mother's task but father's view on the child's eneuresis may be most relevant: it is only when one discovers that father was eneuretic until aged 10 that one sees the difficulty for the child of being dry by five! The double message to the child, by parents with opposing viewpoints, can never be resolved unless one viewpoint changes or the child become the adult. Again, the encopretic child, who carefully laid his offering in his mother's underwear drawer, was saying something his father could not understand: nor could the doctor until father's cross-dressing in love play became apparent in family therapy.

Adolescence is a crisis for the family, not merely for the young person: when, to the rigidities of middle age is added the problems of youth, the mixture can be explosive. Often in this situation the resulting outburst is violent or anti-social behaviour of a type almost designed to hurt the parents: unless the family as a whole sort out their internal tensions, there is little hope for the youngster's probation taking and driving away mother's occult depression and father's hidden drinking. Family therapy, putting all three in the same room at the same time, will alone achieve something worthwhile, as so many dysfunctional families operate by the myth 'divide and rule'. When this occurs within the family setting, it invariably means that children own loyalty to a split authority.

Family life tends to be begun for sexual and childbearing reasons and these two areas are fertile grounds for problems. Most women who present for family planning advice, have little or no difficulty, but some have constant problems from irregular bleeding on the pill, through pain with the coil to recurrent requests for termination of pregnancy. In all cases of difficulty in contraception, much can be gained by at least interviewing the couple, as only when both partners' attitudes to the method used and the ensuing failure is discovered, will the reasons become apparent. Should termination of pregnancy be requested, it would appear almost mandatory to discuss with both parties, if available: such interviews can be painful to all concerned, but form the foundation of continuing care and subsequent contraceptive practice. If, as happily, is usually the case, the continuing care period is trouble free, the doctor can claim success: if the follow up is stormy, at least the basic background is understood, and the doctor can be identified as a helpful and caring figure.

In a society with divorce rates at the current level, few days can pass without the doctor becoming aware of marital distress as a cause of the presenting anxiety or depression. Here again, a ready capacity to see the couple as a unit for a short series of interviews can prove therapeutic. It is not suggested that straight marriage guidance is by necessity every GP's forte, but few will be able to identify all the tension headaches as without cause. Psychosexual problems, so common as the precipitator of poor marital relationships, are a common place event in the psychiatrically orientated practice and many family doctors develop skills in dealing with these by such techniques as the Masters and Johnson exercises: unhappily, the distinction between sexual in the physical sense and marital in the relationship sense is often hard to make, and the behaviour therapy approach merges into the psychodynamic family therapy.

When the need for family therapy is apparent and the doctor decides it should be offered, the next choice is to decide who shall offer the therapy. The GP may do it himself, or in duo therapy with another person, often of the opposite sex, as this reduces the scapegoating that can occur where one gender gangs up on another. Co-therapists can be recruited from health visitors, social workers, community psychiatric nurses, marriage guidance counsellors, or lay therapists. If time is so arranged as to have 10 minute discussion at the end of therapy, each co-therapist will find in the other, both a tutor and a support. It is important to realize how much can be done in repeated small doses of time:

general practice need not be paralysed by the hour of the analyst, or the long interview of Balint. It is more important to obtain a spread of interviews across the weeks, than to pour all the effort into the first few hours. In all family therapy the key to change lies in time, and sometimes the most major and gratifying changes occur between interviews and for reasons that are far from clear: accurate information of contractual nature needs to be offered the client at onset. 'We'll meet for half an hour each fortnight for the next three months, and then assess where we are' makes an excellent starting offer. Initial treatment plans, that 'we will attempt to achieve this or that' are often failures; openess to what the family brings and a willingness to work at areas they consider important, refining, redefining, and clarifying the problems, listing the possibilities for change and above all, tolerating the tensions poured out seems the most productive approach. There are many styles of family therapy, so many that each therapist can be content with his own eclectic style: descriptions can be found in Minuchin (1974), Dicks (1967), but for a general text of low volume, Glich and Kessler (1974) is recommended. A general review of the family therapy literature is provided by Bentovim (1982): quite the most stimulating figure on the scene over the past 20 years has been Haley, all of whose writings are worth study (see Bentovim 1982).

Of all the areas of family therapy, the easiest for the GP beginner is sex therapy, for in this area there are clearly defined goals and very clearly defined techniques. Most medical students receive instruction in what has become known as the M and J techniques, a behaviour therapy introduced by Masters and Johnson (1970), best described by Kaplan (1974). A recent review by Hawton (1982*a*) gives a report of current therapy and an outline of treatment methods: a further review (Hawton 1982*b*) describes the common problems and treatments, giving an adequate review of the current literature.

SCHIZOPHRENIA

The continuing care of schizophrenia in the community is currently shared between the GP and the community psychiatric nurse: while the general practitioner continues to provide normal medical care, the community psychiatric nurse tends to maintain the psychiatric therapy particularly the depot phenothiazines. Unhappily, side-effects, trivial and serious, abound and the family doctor needs constant awareness of the problem. The common side-effects are dry mouth, blurred vision, constipation, and urinary retention. Postural hypotension can occur but these effects are usually found at the onset of therapy and offer few problems in maintenance therapy. Extrapyramidal symptoms vary with the drug used, its dose and frequency of administration: some tend to wear off over time, but others develop over quite long periods. Parkinsonism, with muscular tremor and weakness, rigidity and stooped posture is common, and tends to pass off: it has become traditional to treat with anti-Parkinson drugs, but not entirely effectively. The drugs used, such as benzhexol and benztropine can usually be withdrawn after a few months. More serious effects occur and can be more permanent: akathisia, known as 'happy feet', a motor restlessness; marked involuntary movements called dyskinesias can occur. Akinesia is a common side-effect giving a postural equivalent to the psycho-motor retardation of endogenous depression. Frightening to both patient and doctor are the spastic disorders of head and neck, acute dystonias and the occulogyric crises; these last reponse to intravenous procyclidine. Perhaps the worst effects because of their unpredictability and permanence, are the tardive dyskinesias, often presenting as abnormal facial and chewing movements. Clarification of these movement disorders has been brought about the the description of Marsden *et al.* (1975).

Two seasonal effects should be noted, the photosensitivity reaction often proceeding to blistering, and the hypothermia occuring in cold weather. However, at all seasons the phenothiazines interact, often alarmingly, with other therapeutic agents and care should be taken to mark the notes in such a way as to avoid adverse effects.

The long-term care of the schizophrenic does not consist, however, solely in drug manipulations: not merely do schizophrenics have the usual run of illnesses, they have marked tendency to anxiety and often depression. Even on depot phenothiazenes some 30 per cent relapse, a rate equivalent to oral usage. Hence, the GP must constantly be aware of the tendency to further psychiatric breakdown and the need for readmission. History taking recalls that life-events are common precipitants of breakdown (Brown and Brierly 1968; Leff and Vaughan 1980). A good relationship with the schizophrenic can ensure that early recourse to increased medication is available, and happily this may reduce the chance of needing readmission.

Recent research on breakdown in established schizophrenics has shown relatives expressed emotion, and the time spent face to face are two critical features. Much basic work has been done by Leff, and his review (1981) is well worth study. The difficulties in the long-term handling of the problem can be illustrated by the title of Freeman's (1980) review, 'Coping with a schizo-phrenic'. Cure is well outside current horizons: only a multifactorial approach in which chemotherapy plays but a small part can be considered adequate.

PERFORMANCE REVIEW CHECK LIST

General

1. Can the practice identify all patients who have a past history of overdose, alcoholism, and depression?
2. Can the practice identify all its patients on regular psychotropic medication?
3. Does the practice have a policy for the prescribing of hypnotics, minor tran-quillizers and antidepressants?
4. Has the practice considered employing a trained counsellor?

Patients on treatment

1. Are the reasons for starting and maintaining psychotropic drugs or other therapy clearly recorded?
2. Is there any record of the patient's (or relatives') ideas or the information given to the patient?
3. Are the current drugs and dosage clearly recorded?
4. Are the reasons for any referrals to psychiatrists or other agencies clearly recorded?

Emergencies

1. Does the practice have a policy for the management of overdoses?
2. What proportion are followed up?
3. Does every doctor understand the working of the Mental Health Act 1983?

PATIENT ASSOCIATIONS AND SELF-HELP GROUPS

Alcoholics Anonymous,
PO Box 514,
11 Redcliffe Gardens,
London SW10 9BQ

Compassionate Friends,
50 Woodways,
Watford,
Herts WD1 4NW
(An international organization of bereaved parents.)

Cruse, National Organization for the Widowed and their Children,
Cruse House,
126 Sheen Road,
Richmond,
Surrey.
(Counselling service.)

Gingerbread,
Minerva Chambers,
35 Wellington Street,
London WC2E 7BN
(One-parent families.)

National Schizophrenia Fellowship,
79 Victoria Road,
Surbiton,
Surrey KT6 4NS
(For the welfare of sufferers and their relatives.)

Phobic Society,
4 Cheltenham Road,
Chorlton-cum-hardy,
Manchester.

Release,
1 Elgin Avenue,
London W9

(Counselling on drug addition and other problems.)

Richmond Fellowship,
8 Addison Road,
London W14 8DL

(Halfway houses for the mentally ill and those with emotional, drug, or alcoholism problems.)

The Samaritans,
17 Uxbridge Road,
Slough SL1 1SN

PATIENT BOOKS AND LEAFLETS

Mitchell, R. (1975). *Depression.* Penguin, Harmondsworth.
Palmer (1980). *Anorexia nervosa.* Penguin, Harmondsworth.
Winokur, G. (1982). *Depression: the facts.* Oxford University Press.
Goodwin, D. (1982). *Alcoholism: the facts.* Oxford University Press.

REFERENCES

Amdisen, A. (1980). In *Handbook of lithium therapy* (ed. F. N. Johnson). Medical and Teaching Publishing Company, Lancaster.

Anderson, S. and Hasler, J. C. (1979). Counselling in general practice. *J. R. Coll. gen. Practrs* **203**, 352–6.

Baastrup, P. C. *et al.* (1980). Prophylactic lithium double-blind discontinuation in manic-depressive and recurrent depressive disorders. *Lancet* **ii**, 326.

Barraclough, B., Bunch, J., Nelson, B., and Sainsbury, P. (1974). A hundred cases of suicide: clinical aspects. *Br. J. Psychiat.* **125**, 355–73.

Beech, H. R., Burns, L. E., and Sheffield, B. F. (1982). *A behavioural approach to the management of stress. A practical guide to techniques.* Wiley, Chichester.

Bentovim, A. (1982). Reading about family therapy. *Br. J. Psychiat.* **140**, 425–8.

Bhagat, M., Lewis, A. P., and Shilitof, R. (1979). Clinical psychologist and the primary health care team. *Update* **18**, 479–88.

Blackburn, I. M., Bishop, S., Glen, A. I. M., Whalley, L. J., and Christie, J. E. (1981). The efficacy of cognitive therapy in depression: in treatment trial using cognitive therapy and pharmacotherapy, each, alone and in combination. *Br. J. Psychiat.* **139**, 181–9.

Bloch, S. (1979). *An introduction to the psychotherapies.* Oxford University Press.

British Medical Journal (1975). The suicidal profile. (Editorial.) *Br. med. J.* **i**, 525–6.

Brown, G. W. and Birley, J. C. T. (1968). Crisis and life changes and the onset of schizophrenia. *J. Hlth social Behav.* **9**, 203–14.

—— and Harris, T. (1978). *Social origins of depression.* Tavistock, London.

Cade, J. F. J. (1949). Lithium salts in the treatment of manic excitement. *Med. J. Aust.* **36**, 349–52.

Clark, W. D. (1981). Alcoholism: blocks to diagnosis and treatment. *Am. J. Med.* **71**, 275–85.

Coppen, A. (1978). Mianserin, lithium and the prophylactics for depression. *Br. J. Psychiat.* **133**, 206.

—— Ghose, K., Montgomery, S., Ramarae, V. A., Bailey, J., and Jorgensen, A. (1978). Continuation therapy with amitriptyline in depression. *Br. J. Psychiat.* **133**, 28–33.

Dicks, H. V. (1967). *Marital tensions.* Routledge and Kegan Paul, London.

Earll, L. and Kincey, J. (1982). Clinical psychology in general practice: a controlled trial evaluation. *Jl R. Coll. Gen. Practrs* **32**, 32–7.

Edwards, G. and Grant, M. (eds.) (1977). *Alcoholism. New knowledge and new responses.*

—— Orford, J., Egert, S., Guthrie, S., Hawker, A., Hensman, C., Mitcheson, M., Openheimer, E., and Taylor, C. (1977). Alcoholism: a controlled trial of treatment and advice. *J. Stud. Alc.* **38**, 1004–31.

Freeman, H. C. (1980). Coping with schizophrenia. *Br. J. hosp. Med.* **23**, 54–8.

Fry, J. (1979). *Common diseases.* Redwood Burn, Trowbridge.

Gilchrist, I. C., Gough, J. B., Horsfall-Turner, Y. R., Ineson, E. M., Keele, G., Marks, B., and Scott, H. J. (1978). Social work in general practice. *Jl R. Coll. gen. Practrs* **28**, 675–86.

Glick, I. D. and Kessler, D. R. (1974). *Marital and family therapy.* Grune and Stratton, New York.

Goddard, A. (1982). Cognitive behaviour therapy and depression. *Br. J. hosp. Med.* **27**, 248–53.

Goldberg, D. and Huxley, P. (1980). *Mental illness in the community: the pathway to psychiatric care.* Tavistock, London.

Goldfield, M. R. and Davison, G. C. (1976). *Clinical behaviour therapy.* Holt, Rinehart and Winson, New York.

Graham, H. and Sher, M. (1976). Social work and general practice. *Jl R. Coll. gen. Practrs* **26**, 95–105.

Groves, J. E. (1978). Taking care of the hateful patient. *New Engl. J. Med.* **298**, 883–7.

Hamilton, M. (1982). The effect of treatment on the melancholies (depression). *Br. J. Psychiat.* **140**, 223–31.

Hawton, K. (1982a). Behavioural treatment of sexual dysfunction. *Br. J. Psychiat.* **140**, 94–101.

—— (1982b). Sexual problems. *Br. J. hosp. Med.* **27**, 129–35.

Johnstone, A. and Goldberg, D. (1976). Psychiatric screening in general practice. *Lancet* i, 605–8.

Kaplan, H. S. (1974). The new sex therapy: active treatment of sexual dysfunction. Aailliere, London.

Korger, W. S. and Fezler, W. D. (1976). *Hypnosis and behaviour modification: imagery and conditioning.* Lippencott, Philadelphia.

Leff, J. (1981). Schizophrenia. *Practitioner* **225**, 37–42.

—— and Vaughan, G. (1980). The interaction of life events and relatives' expressed emotion in schizophrenia and depressive neurosis. *Br. J. Psychiat.* **136**, 146–54.

Mackay, D. (1982). Cognitive behaviour therapy. *Br. J. hosp. Med.* **27**, 242–7.

Maggs, R. (1979). Stopping lithium prophylaxis. *Br. med. J.* i, 623.

Marsden, C. D., Tarsy, D., and Baldessarini, R. J. (1975). Spontaneous and drug induced mental disorders in psychiatric patients. In *Psychiatric aspects of neurological diagnosis* (ed. D. F. Benson and D. Blumer). Grune and Stratton, New York.

Matsers, W. H. and Johnson, V. E. (1970). *Human sexual inadequacy.* Churchill, London.

Mayfield, D., McLeod, G., and Hall, P. (1974). The CAGE Questionnaire: validation of a new alcoholism screening instrument. *Am. J. Psychiat.* **131**, 112–13.

Mechanic, D. (1966). Response factors in illness: the study of illness behaviour. *Social Psychiol.* **1**, 11.

Miller, P. M. (1972). Use of behavioural contracting in the treatment of alcoholism: a case study. *Behav. Ther.* **3**, 593–6.

Minuchin, S. (1974). *Families and family therapy.* Harvard University Press, Cambridge, Mass.

Morgan, K. and Oswald, I. (1982). Anxiety caused by a short life hypnotic. *Br. med. J.* **284**, 942.

Murray, R., Ghose, H., Harris, C., Williams, D., and Williams, P. (1981). *The misuse of psychotropic drugs.* Roy. Coll. Psychiat. Gaskell, London.

Office of Health Economics (1981). *Suicide and deliberate self harm.* London.

Office of Population Census and Surveys (1972). *Occupational mortality.* HMSO, London.

Pokomy, A. D., Miller, B. A., and Kaplan, H. S. (1972). The brief MAST (Massachusetts Alcohol Screening Test). *Am. J. Psychol.* **129**, 342–5.

Pollak, B. (1978). A two year study of alcoholics in general practice. *Br. J. Alcoh.* **13**, 24–35.

Schulman, R. (1977). Psychogenic with physical manifestations and the other side of the coin. *Lancet* **i**, 524–6.

Simms, A. and Prior, P. (1978). Patterns of mortality in severe neurotics. *Br. J. Psychiat.* **133**, 299–305.

Srinivasan, D. P. and Hullin, R. P. (1980). Current concepts of lithium therapy. *Br. J. hosp. Med.* **24/5**, 466–75.

Strong, P. M. (1980). Doctors and dirty work: the case of alcoholism. *Soc. Hlth Illness* **2**, 24–47.

Tennant, G., Bebbington, P., and Hurry, J. (1981). The short-term outcome of neurotic disorders in the community: the relation of remission to clinical factors and to 'neutralizing' life events. *Br. J. Psychiat.* **139**, 213–21.

Tough, H., Kingerlea, P., and Elliott, P. (1980). Surgery attached psychogeriatric nurses: an evaluation of psychiatric nurses in the primary health care team. *J. R. Coll. gen. Practrs* **211**, 85–9.

Williams, P. and Clare, A. (1979). Social workers in primary care. *Jl R. Coll. gen Practrs* **29**, 554–8.

Waydenfeld, D. and Waydenfeld, S. W. (1980). Counselling in general practice. *Jl R. Coll. gen. Practrs* **30**, 671–7.

13 Skin disease

Martyn Agass

Diseases of the skin are common, not least perhaps because of the immediate and obvious manifestation of any pathology and its consequent recognition by the patient. A community survey in Lambeth (Rea *et al.* 1976) established that 22 per cent of the population sampled were suffering from a skin disorder of one kind or another, eczema was the commonest problem affecting 6 per cent of individuals followed by acne with a prevalence of 3.5 per cent. These findings are reflected in the work of the general practitioner, and the Second National Morbidity Study (Office of Population Censuses and Surveys 1974) recorded that 19.4 per cent of all consultations were for disorders of the skin and subcutaneous tissues. Ironically for both general practitioners and their patients, teaching of dermatology is relegated to a very lowly status in the undergraduate medical curriculum.

The high numbers of patients with dermatological problems consulting their doctors and the increasing numbers being referred for specialist advice has occurred despite the introduction of many new powerful therapeutic agents such as corticosteroids and antibiotics. Why is this? Patients, of course, are living longer and developing the associated dermatological problems of the elderly; and the vast array of pharmacological preparations now at our disposal has seen a rise in the frequency of drug-related rashes. However, the prime reason is probably a social one. We live in an age which is dominated by the media and an unblemished skin and faultless complexion represent the pinnacle of physical perfection to which we are all exalted to strive. The corollary of this is that for many patients diseases of the skin have sinister implications and carry great stigmata. Associations with infectious and venereal diseases or general uncleanliness abound.

Diseases of the skin impinge on every aspect of life – diet, dress and relationships with family, friends, and members of the opposite sex will be affected. Hobbies will be carefully selected and great determination and presence of mind will be needed to follow certain pastimes (e.g. swimming). Academic achievements, performance at interviews, and choice of career are similarly influenced. The development in later life of an occupational skin disease will necessitate the search for a new job.

Naturally the effects on other members of the family are profound. The reaction of parents to the development of skin disease in one of their offspring may initially be one of sadness followed by guilt. The family's past medical history may be examined in detail in order to detect the source of the affliction. With the passage of time these emotions can easily be transformed into over-indulgence and spoiling with the development of jealousy and resentment among siblings. Brothers and sisters have the additional problem of coping with the social stigmata of an abnormal sibling and may dread introducing their friends to the family circle.

School is often the first significant hurdle for the young patient with skin disease. His pathology adds an extra burden to the problem of making friends and settling down in a large establishment. Games and PE lessons acquire a special fear with the revelation of an unsightly rash to curious peers and often the exposure of clothes stained with strange ointments. It is necessary for the teaching staff to be educated about the nature of the condition and its manage-ment – perhaps to the extent of helping with the application of medicaments at intervals throughout the day.

The first task of the doctor who is managing a patient with a skin disorder is to encourage that patient to express all the fears and anxieties he may have and to reassure him appropriately. The most trivial lesions – from a medical view point – may hold untold significance for the patient. The progress of the disease and its response to treatment will be clearly demonstrable to the patient and so it is essential to explain the cause of the condition (if known) and the rationale of treatment. If the diverse social aspects of the illness are not recognized and their implications discussed, then much therapeutic endeavour will be to no avail. The doctor will envisage a long relationship with his patient over the course of many years and might anticipate that at times much of the patients or his family's wrath will be directed towards him. The doctor too must come to terms with the frustration of managing someone with an incurable ailment; his objective will be to encourage his patient – with the assistance of family, friends, and appropriate supporting agency – to accept his disability and lead a fulfilled life.

DIAGNOSIS

In dermatology, as in other branches of medicine, an accurate diagnosis is an ideal prerequisite to treatment. However, the unique circumstances of general practice, where disease is seen at an early stage in its evolution, frequently justifies the initiation of therapy on empirical grounds before a firm diagnosis has been made. Diagnosis is usually dependent on the nature and distribution of the rash supplemented by details from the history. The latter will include the site of origin of the rash, its subsequent spread, and the presence of any similar affliction in the family or colleagues at work.

Many common skin disorders, such as eczema, have an hereditary element. Knowledge of this, whilst of some diagnostic use, is of more value in the management of the patient enabling him to relate to other similarly afflicted relatives and so eventually come to terms with his disability more effectively. Environmental factors can precipitate or influence the presentation of symptoms; a hot environment will intensify pruritus and exacerbate those disorders aggravated by sweating and sebum formation – such as seborrhoeic dermatitis and acne. Exposure to light has its own distinctive influence – in the short term precipitating photosensitive dermatoses, herpes simplex, and disseminated lupus erythematosis and in the longer term, the actinic keratoses of the elderly.

A careful drug history must be taken encompassing both prescribed and proprietary medicaments, and including all topical preparations. Infective organisms transferred from animals can be implicated as causative agents and certainly papular urticaria secondary to insect bites presents a common problem in general practice.

An important but rather more nebulous factor is that of stress. The link between stress and many skin diseases is well recognized but little understood. Exploration in this direction is a necessary and important part of management if the patient is to derive the maximum benefit of subsequent therapy.

Examination of the skin is usually the most relevant factor in establishing the diagnosis. Individual lesions are best studied with a ($\times 8$) magnification hand lens, in good light, but the key to the diagnosis is most often to be found in the morphological distribution of the rash. A widespread rash is often synonymous with a systemic disease, such as psoriasis which has a predeliction for the extensor surfaces and scalp; eczema – affecting the flexures, and herpes zoster – the dermatome supplied by the affected dorsal root ganglia. On occasions skin diseases are a manifestation of more generalized pathology and an appropriate examination will be necessary. Sometimes examination of a patient's clothing will be indicated – when parasitic infestation or occupational exposure to certain chemicals is suspected.

DIAGNOSTIC PROCEDURES

In the vast majority of cases diagnosis of a skin disorder will be established without recourse to the following investigative techniques. Nevertheless they are, with the exception of patch testing, simple procedures and can clarify the diagnosis and expedite appropriate management.

Examination for fungus

Most general practitioners possess or have access to a microscope and hence have the facility to examine skin scrapings for fungal hyphae. Superficial layers of epidermis are scraped away with a scalpel blade – concentrating particularly on the advancing edge of the lesion. The scales are placed on a microscope slide and suspended in one or two drops of 10 per cent potassium hydroxide solution and then a coverslip placed over them. The slide is gently heated in the flame of a bunsen burner and then examined under the microscope using low power.

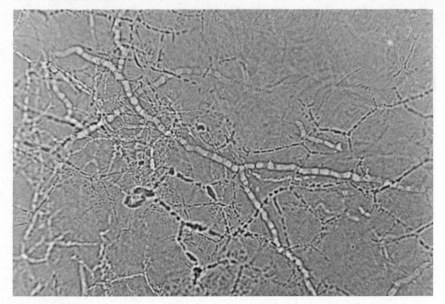

Fig. 13.1. Fungal hyphae in 10 per cent potassium hydroxide solution.

Any fungal hyphae present will be demonstrated (Fig. 13.1). If a more precise diagnosis is desired, or if the doctor does not have a microscope available, then skin scrapings can be sent to the local microbiology laboratory for mycological examination and culture. The collection of scrapings on dark paper facilitates their identification by the microbiology laboratory. Nail clippings can be sent to the laboratory for mycological studies in the same way as skin scrapings.

Another simple technique, usually confined to Departments of Dermatology, is the use of Wood's light. This produces ultraviolet light through a nickel-cobalt filter and will evoke a distinctive fluorescence in certain clinical situations, e.g. with ringworm of the scalp (*Microsporum audouinii*). The rash of erythrasma produces a characteristic pale coral pink fluorescence.

Examination for bacteria

Bacteriological culture has only a limited role in the management of skin disease. Although it could in theory be used to confirm the diagnosis and ascertain antibiotic sensitivities in certain conditions, such as acne vulgaris and impetigo, it is of little practical value. The clinical diagnosis is seldom in doubt and the response to appropriate therapy is usually rapid and uncomplicated.

It is helpful, on occasions, to define the flora of bacteria from a leg ulcer. This information is of value if the patient develops a subsequent cellulitis so that the nature and sensitivity of the causative organism will be known. Systemic antibiotic therapy has no role in the treatment of uncomplicated leg ulcers.

Chronic paronychia are often caused by *Candida albicans* and bacteriological examination will differentiate them from staphylococcal infections.

Patch testing

This is a technique for elucidating which, of a number of substances, may be responsible for a contact dermatitis. It is particularly appropriate in practice for those patients who endure repeated episodes of dermatitis and the group of patients with chronic venous ulcers of the legs who develop a sensitivity to one of the medicaments used to dress them. In the latter case administration of a reagent to which the patient has been sensitized causes great morbidity and delays healing.

The patient for whom patch testing has been recommended is referred to a dermatologist and a range of suspected allergens are applied to the skin of the back or upper arm in appropriate concentration. The application sites are inspected at 48 and 72 hours and the degree of reaction assessed. The interpretation of the reaction requires some skill as false-positive and false-negative results are common. When a substance has been identified as an allergen, the patient should be informed and given a list of all the preparations containing that allergen. A record of the findings and list of the prohibited preparations must be displayed prominently in the patient's notes so that their future use can be avoided. The nursing staff, both on the district and in the practice, are responsible for the greater part of the care of these patients and it is vital that they be informed of these findings and their significance.

It is essential that the skin is quiescent prior to patch testing and so before referral, any dermatitis must be appropriately treated.

Biopsy

Although biopsy of a lesion, and subsequent histological examination is a simple way of making a definitive diagnosis, it is primarily a tool of the dermatologist. The general practitioner is likely to send only those specimens removed after minor surgery for histological confirmation of diagnosis. In the case of a large lesion, the specimen sent to the laboratory should be representative of the lesion as a whole and should include some normal skin. Prior to transport, the specimen should be immersed in 10 per cent formol saline.

MANAGEMENT: GENERAL PRINCIPLES

Management of the patient with skin disease begins at the first consultation. The history and examination proceed in the way described earlier and it is reassuring for the patient if the doctor touches the rash during his enquiry, so indirectly dispelling any notions of uncleanliness on the part of the patient.

In most instances the therapy offered is topical although sometimes these agents will be supplemented by systemic treatment in the form of antibiotics, antihistamines, or steroids. Topically applied medicaments have two components – a vehicle or base and an active constituent.

The vehicle

The vehicle has a profound influence on the active constituent which it supports and selection of an appropriate vehicle is a most important part of therapy. There are three types of vehicle – powders (e.g. Calamine, zinc oxide), liquids (e.g. water, alcohol), and greases or ointments (e.g. lanolin).

Powders are used to impart substantiality to an otherwise bland preparation or to reduce friction and they are best employed on normal skins. Liquids, by their evaporation, exert a cooling influence and are principally indicated in the treatment of acutely inflamed skin. The application of liquids to a weeping skin encourages them to dry – exemplified by the use of potassium permanganate solution in the treatment of acute eczema. Ointments do not contain any water and when applied to the skin, make it feel greasy. They form a protective layer preventing loss of moisture and promoting the penetration of any accompanying constituents. These emollient properties make them useful when the skin is dry – as in atopic eczema or icthyosis. Ointments rarely need the addition of preservatives. They can be diluted with soft paraffin when they form an ideal vehicle for tar or salicylic acid or they can be diluted with emulsifying ointment to form a water miscible compound.

Powders, liquids, and greases form the basis for all compounds used in dermatology. Creams are emulsions and comprise a suspension of two immiscible liquids. Oily cream BP (water in oil emulsion) exerts a cooling effect but leaves a greasy residue and had useful emollient properties. By contrast aqueous cream BP (oil in water emulsion) has a drying influence and is more suitable for use on wet or occluded skin. The water content of creams enables them to support the growth of bacterial and fungi and to avert this, compounds such as parabens or chlorocresol are added. However, these are 'sensitizers' and in susceptible individuals can lead to the development of contact eczema.

Powders and liquids can be mixed to form 'drying pastes' whilst powder and grease together form a thicker protective paste such as zinc and castor oil BNF.

The inter-relationship of these compounds and the indications for their use were summarized by the Dutch physician Polano (Fig. 13.2). In therapy the spectrum of wet–dry skin should be treated by the corresponding spectrum of bases, namely liquids–powders–grease. Skin conditions are not, of course, static and their evolution from one form to another is an indication for an analgous change of base.

The active constituents

The advent of steroids and antibiotics has heralded a therapeutic revolution in dermatology, as in so many other branches of medicine. After the introduction of hydrocortisone there followed the next generation of steroids with a halogenated nucleus. These compounds were more potent and thus efficacious

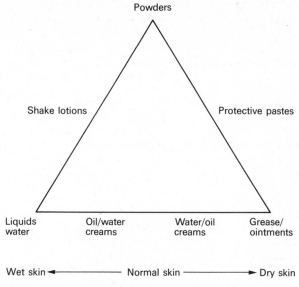

Fig. 13.2. Polano's triangle.

than their predecessors and of course had a correspondingly greater propensity to cause side-effects.

Steroids exert their beneficial effect in dermatology by suppressing inflammation, and reducing the rate of DNA synthesis and cell division. There is now a daunting array of steroid preparations but the choice of base is still vitally important. Dry eczematous skins respond much better to the application of ointment, but creams have a far higher degree of patient acceptability. In addition preparations combining a steroid with antibiotics, antifungal agents, or antiseptics are available and although these have their uses, it must be remembered that the presence of a steroid does not preclude the development of hypersensitivity to an additive – nor the antibiotic prevent a steroid-precipitated infection.

The dangers of steroid preparations are well known, with continued use causing thinning of the skin and atrophy, striae, purpura, and telangectasia. The face is particularly subject to the perils of continued steroid application with the development of these side-effects together with a peri-oral dermatitis. The thinner skin of infants and children is also more susceptible to iatrogenic damage. Potent steroid creams can induce adrenal suppression and any adult using more than 50 g of fluorinated steroid cream per week for longer than two months, can be regarded as being at risk.

The enormous range of preparations is bewildering but they can be conveniently classified according to their potency (Fig. 13.3). Most practitioners solve the problem by selecting one or two agents from each category and becoming

1. Strongest	*Active ingredient*
Dermovate	Clobetasol propionate 0.05%
Halciderm	Halcinonide 0.1%
Nerisone forte	Diflucortolone valerate 0.3%
Propaderm forte	Beclomethasone dipropionate 0.5%
Synalar forte	Fluocinolone acetonide 0.2%
2. Strong	
Adcortyl	Triamcinolone acetonide 0.1%
Betnovate	Betamethasone (as valerate) 0.1%
Locoid	Hydrocortisone 17-butyrate 0.1%
Metosyn	Fluocinonide 0.05%
Nerisone	Diflucortolone valerate 0.1%
Synalar	Fluocinolone acetonide 0.025%
Topilar	Fluclorolone acetonide 0.025%
3. Intermediate	
Alphaderm	Hydrocortisone 1%, urea 10%
Eumovate	Clobetasone butyrate 0.05%
Haelan	Flurandrenolone 0.0125%
Synandone	Fluocinolone acetonide 0.01%
Ultralanum	Fluocortolone 0.25%, fluocortolone hexanoate 0.25%, clemizole hexachlorophane 2.5%
4. Weak	
Hydrocortisone 0.1–2.5%	Hydrocortisone 0.1–2.5%
Methyl prednisolone 0.25%	Methyl prednisolone 0.25%

Fig. 13.3. Classification of topical corticosteroids – by potency

thoroughly acquainted with their use. The usual principles of steroid therapy apply in that a strong steroid preparation is used initially and with control of the disorder, the strength of steroid is reduced until eventually the weakest preparation compatible with maintenance of a normal skin is found. At this stage the steroid-sparing effect of emollients can be used to good effect. Ointments can be diluted in white soft paraffin and in this way a single steroid preparation can be used in serial dilutions at all stages of a skin disorder. This technique is particularly useful for those patients who become psychologically dependent on a strong steroid ointment. Although creams can be diluted in cetomacrogol cream BPC, the risk of bacterial contamination precludes this generally.

The efficacy of all these preparations can only be guaranteed when they are applied correctly and regularly. Although compliance may be good initially, it may rapidly decline if the condition improves, especially if the treatment is time consuming or if the topical preparations are cosmetically or socially unacceptable. Doctors often underestimate the volume of cream or ointment needed to clear a given area. 100–200 g will be needed to cover the whole body for one week and more limited areas will require 30–50 g.

On occasions rashes will require regular dressings and sometimes the skills of the district nurse or treatment-room sister in the practice may be required.

Aside from the physical aspect of treatment, this contact helps maintain the patient's motivation and affords opportunity for other problems to be voiced. Dressings in themselves serve to keep paste or ointment undisturbed and in close contact with the skin and also protect overlying clothing. Where there is associated pruritus, they protect the skin from scratching.

COMMON CHRONIC SKIN DISEASES IN GENERAL PRACTICE

Dermatitis

Dermatitis is the name given to the pattern of skin reactions evoked by damaging external stimuli. An 'eczematous' reaction is identical but is secondary to an undefined constitutional element or increased susceptibility to an otherwise mild external agent. Whatever the aetiology the clinical signs are identical, comprising initially erythema, irritation, and vesiculation. The vesicles eventually burst and weep – and later heal.

Atopic eczema

This common affliction affects between 1–3 per cent of the population and there is strong familial element in its pathogenesis. The condition often begins in the early months of life, usually with involvement of the face. As the child grows the skin becomes drier and thicker, especially at the flexures. With the passage of time there is usually continued improvement although the tendency to have a dry, itchy skin often remains throughout life.

The blemished skin of the atopic infant causes mother great distress and even with detailed explanation and reassurance, acceptance may take a long time. She may become particularly self-conscious at gatherings of mothers and young children – such as baby clinics and playgroups. The intense itching attracts mother's attention and serves to increase her anxiety – and this may be heightened still further by any concomitant asthma or hay fever developed by her offspring. As these children grow up they frequently present a well recognized blend of affection and excitability often accompanied by a reluctance to accept discipline!

Management

Before any specific treatment is instituted it is imperative that the parents understand the nature of the condition and its tendency to fluctuate between exacerbations and remissions. The sensitivity of eczematous skin must be explained and in particular its susceptibility to irritants such as soap, detergents, woollen garments, and extremes of temperature – all of which should be avoided if possible. Forewarning the family of an exacerbation of the condition during the winter months, when cold, chapping winds are in evidence, may save much needless anxiety. Supplementary counselling by the health visitor, who will be closely involved with the family at this stage, will pay enormous dividends.

The simplest therapeutic measures entail the use of emollients to soften the skin. These hydrating agents counteract the irritant dryness of eczematous skin and in addition provide some protection against external irritants. They may be used during or after bathing. Ung. emulsificans – the commonest emollient – can either be actively rubbed onto eczematous patches of skin during the bath or used as a substitute for soap. It may be helpful in the case of infants to make a solution of emulsifying ointment in hot water and add this to the bath. If this form of therapy is helpful – and its simplicity often makes it highly acceptable to children – then it can be continued once, or even twice daily with benefit. Other emollients, such as aqueous cream BP or oily cream BP trap water on skin moistened after a bath and in this way exert their action. Bath oils, such as oilatum, can be used in conjunction with emulsifying ointment or independently.

Topical corticosteroids are the mainstay of treatment, and the eczemas probably account for their greatest use in dermatology. They are suppressive in their action, rather than curative and it is essential that this is understood by the patient or relatives prior to use. Ointments are preferential in the management of dry eczematous skin, particularly as the preservatives contained in creams may exert a sensitizing action. However, creams are often prescribed because of their cosmetic acceptability and their use represents a compromise between therapeutic efficacy and patient tolerance.

The aim of the doctor is to achieve control of the eczema with the weakest steroid preparation possible. In the process one or more agents may be used – or differing dilutions of a single compound. Ultimately when the eczema has been controlled recurrence may be deferred by a mild preparation such as 10 per cent betnovate in white soft paraffin. The views of patient or parent about the efficacy or use of each particular preparation should be sought (Fig. 13.4). It is essential that compliance with the prescribed regime occurs for treatment to be successful; generally bedtime is the least harassed (and thus optimal) time of day for the application of medicaments. Parents can share the load by taking turns to supervise this ritual.

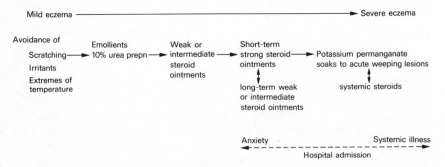

Fig. 13.4. Management of eczema.

Both practitioner and patient should be aware of the dangers of topical corticosteroids and guard appropriately against their misuse. The strongest ointment for use on the face should be 1 per cent hydrocortisone and other similarly mild preparations should be used on those areas, such as the flexures, where potency is enhanced. In very small infants the possibility of absorption and systemic toxicity with adrenal suppression must be remembered.

Pruritus can be a great problem for eczematous patients and the ensuing scratching often evokes much guilt. Simple measures are best tried first and these include keeping finger nails well manicured, encouraging the child to rub itching skin, and distracting him. Systemic antihistamines are probably effective because of their sedating effect and this can be useful at night. If there is a localized patch of eczema which is exceptionally uncomfortable, then the best therapy may be occlusion under a tar-paste bandage. This has the dual advantage of relieving the pruritus and protecting the skin from excoriation and damage. There are two types of bandage commercially available – milder ones impregnated with ichthammol and a stronger variety impregnated with coal tar. If he so desires the doctor can devise his own occlusive dressing with coal-tar paste combined with a steroid ointment. These occlusive dressings are best left *in situ* for several days.

Damaged eczematous skin is prey to infection and to counter this a wide variety of combined steroid and antibiotic preparations are available. These agents, or those containing an antiseptic such as clioquinol, are effective particularly if used in the early stages of an infection. Systemic antibiotics are rarely needed.

The benefit of all topical preparations can be enhanced by the use of a sutiable dressings. In acute weeping eczemas soaks of potassium permanganate solution followed by a dressing of light linen or cotton strips, supported by stockinette, is highly efficacious. Expandable stockinette bandages can provide supportive dressings for acute lesions on any part of the body – even to the extent of making 'mittens' for children to prevent scratching. The reassuring presence of the district nurse soothing both the patient and the rash also provides the opportunity for the patient to ask questions and glean more information about his condition. The nursing staff must thus be well briefed about the disorder, for which they are caring, and this implies close communication between doctor and nurse.

The vast majority of children with atopic eczema are managed by their family doctor. When the condition is exceptionally severe and difficult to control, or there is great parental anxiety, outpatient referral to a dermatologist will be arranged.

Admission to hospital is an uncommon event and will be sought in the rare eventuality of erythroderma developing or more commonly to give parents or child a break.

Invariably in the management of atopic eczema the question of diet and possible allergy to food will be raised. This is a difficult area with few definite guidelines. It is an almost inevitable avenue of exploration for the frustrated parent who is slowly coming to terms with his child's disorder. If parents are keen to try dietary exclusion, then it is wise to let them persist, perhaps with the caution to avoid expensive fads.

Contact dermatitis

In this condition the skin becomes senstitized to a specific substance, which is usually unreactive when applied to the skin of a normal person. In all instances the sensitizing agent must, at some time in the past, have been in contact with the patient's skin and sensitization is enhanced if the skin is damaged or injured. Stress is a much debated aetiological factor which, nevertheless, probably plays a role in exacerbations of the condition.

Although the skin changes themselves are identical with those eczematous lesions already described, the site of the lesions is related to the area of contact with the causative agent. Other areas may be later affected by secondary sensitization.

Successful treatment of contact dermatitis is dependent on the identification of the causative factor and its subsequent avoidance. This is particularly relevant when exposure to the agent has occurred during the course of the patient's occupation.

Particular attention is paid to any likely substances encountered in the 24 hours preceding the eruption. If an occupational dermatitis is suspected then any fluctuation of symptoms with time at work or home should be noted and enquiry made about dermatological problems in the rest of the workforce. The distribution of the rash often gives clues to its aetiology, for instance nickel dermatitis in the middle of the back secondary to brassiere clips and involvement of the bridge of the nose and retro-auricular folds with spectacle frame dermatitis.

The intitial management of acute dermatitis is identical with that of eczema – with the use of emollients and topical corticosteroid preparations. Occasionally resistance to treatment may necessitate the use of additional measures for short periods; severe hand dermatitis may respond more quickly if the action of topical preparations is enhanced by occlusion under polythene gloves. However, the essence of treatment is to identify the causative agent and for this patch testing is necessary.

Once the causative substance has been identified then invariably some adaptation and adjustment of life-style ensues. This is especially so in the case of an industrial dermatitis where a myriad of other factors comes into play. Any absence from work immediately imposes the added strain of a reduced income on the family. With continuing disability the feasibility of continuing in that occupation progressively diminishes. Eventually if alternative employment cannot be found within the company, then redundancy may ensue. The patient may, at this stage, be entitled to compensation, and this is another avenue that must be explored. This pathway may, of course, be exploited by the more unscrupulous individual who is dissatisfied with his position. At some stage assessment by the disablement resettlement officer may be necessary so that his advice with regard to alternative careers or re-training may be obtained.

The general practitioner's role is complex and includes managing the patient and his dermatitis, arranging certification when necessary, and supporting the family.

Neurodermatitis

This localized eczematous lesion, which is perpetuated by scratching, is commonly seen in practice. Typically the lesions are to be found in any area which is easily accessible and include the occipital area, neck, hands, and legs. Invariably the patient will freely admit to his role in the production of the lesion. In some instances the lesion reflects an underlying and unspoken anxiety and this is a possibility which should be explored; in others it seems to be a device for seeking attention and maintaining a 'sick role' with all its attendant benefits.

Treatment is the same as that for eczematous lesions with perhaps prefer ential use of occlusive dressings.

Acne vulgaris

Acne is an almost universal accompaniment to youth. Its predeliction for the face occurs at this unfortunate time when self-awareness and sensitivity are so pre-eminent and further anxiety is fostered by the media which encourages the concept of physical perfection. Against this background adolescent patients consult their general practitioners. Often they will have read copious literature in assorted magazines, watched relevant television programmes, talked with friends, and tried a variety of proprietary medicaments.

As with any pathological process, the doctor must first listen to his patient's complaints and then explain the nature of the problem in simple terms so that the basis of treatment may be better understood. Invariably he will be asked about the relative benefits of different diets, soaps, and cosmetics; but there is little evidence that modification of any of these factors influences the course of the condition. Cosmetics, however, should be lightweight and non-greasy.

The characteristic features of acne are produced by increased sebum secretion, blocking of sebaceous ducts by keratin plugs and consequent bacterial action with inflammation. Therapy is directed at reversing these abnormal changes. The patient who presents with a discrete area of acne on one part or another of the face is first offered topical therapy. There are numerous compounds available but perhaps the most widely used have benoxyl peroxide as a base. This acts by reducing the *Propionobacterium acnes* population and may be obtained in the form of creams, gels, or lotions. Whatever preparation, the principle of application is the same, treatment is started with a weak form and the strength gradually increased until benefit is found. Another line of topical attack is by the use of retinoic acid which acts by loosening the keratin plugs in the sebaceous ducts and so reducing the consequent acne. In some people it causes irritation of the skin and this side-effect can be reduced by diminishing the frequency of application. Both benoxyl peroxide and retinoic acid can be used together – benoxyl peroxide being applied in the morning and retinoic acid at night.

For widespread acneiform eruptions where administration of a topical agent is unrealistic, or those lesions which are resistant to topical therapy, supplementary tretment with systemic antibiotics may be necessary. Tetracycline in a dosage of 250 mg twice daily before meals for several months is highly successful, although treatment with erythromycin or cotrimoxazole is similarly efficacious. With all forms of therapy whether topical or systemic, prolonged treatment is essential and the patient must be warned that any response will take several weeks to become manifest and will need to be continued for at least six months. The length of treatment imposes a strain on patients' compliance and this is often a factor in unresponsive acne. There is a great temptation on the part of doctor and patient to alter treatment before it has had a chance to become established and produce any benefit.

Patients must be warned that on cessation of treatment recurrence of acne may occur and may continue to be a problem through the early years of adult life. Severe, resistant acne or a high level of anxiety on the part of the patient are often an indication for referral to a dermatologist. On occasions a patient will be referred for a specific form of therapy, for instance dermabrasion when unsightly scars predominate.

Psoriasis

Psoriasis is a common condition with an estimated one million sufferers in this country; every general practitioner has a small number of psoriatics on his list who none the less make a significant contribution to his dermatological practice. There have been many advances in the treatment of psoriasis in recent years, both in the introduction of new therapeutic measures and in the increasing sophistication and refinement of traditional remedies. It provides an excellent example of the importance of keeping up to date with new developments.

At a cellular level, psoriasis is characterized by an increased rate of turnover and this proliferation gives rise to the typical pink plaques covered by silver-grey scales. Most frequently these are found on the extensor surfaces and scalp. The condition usually appears for the first time in adolescence, although not infrequently an older patient will present with severe 'dandruff' which on closer inspection proves to be psoriasis of the scalp. Occasionally closer inspection will reveal mild psoriatic changes on other extensor surfaces or the nails. Rarely florid guttate psoriasis may present in a child after a viral infection or episode of tonsillitis.

Once the diagnosis has been made, the aetiology of the disorder and its implications for the future must be fully discussed with the patient. It is again useful to determine whether any specific stresses have precipitated the condition. Discussion may help relieve any tensions or anxieties the patient may have and also serves to strengthen the relationship between patient and doctor. The doctor must anticipate that the anger and frustration of a patient coming to terms with a chronic illness may be directed towards him.

Clearance of psoriasis involves physical treatment of one kind or another and it is imperative that the patient is fully conversant with and motivated in his task. Repeated application of one or more preparations is time consuming and calls for an obsessional approach. There is much information for the new patient to grasp and written directions on a handout sheet describing the chosen regime provides a good adjunct to verbal instructions given in the surgery.

In general practice treatment is initiated with the simplest and most cosmetically acceptable preparations. Tars have formed the basis of treatment for many years and the mildest commercially available preparation is 'Alphosyl'. which contains a 5 per cent coal-tar extract. This may be supplemented by tar baths and shampoos using a preparation such as 'Polytar Liquid'. Many of these substances are classified as borderline substances and it is important to preface any prescriptions for them with the initials ACBS. Stronger tar preparations, such as crude coal tar BPC or coal tar and salicylic acid ointment, have the advantage of greater efficacy but unfortunately their use is countered by propgressive unacceptability to the patient.

Topical corticosteroids are widely used because of their effectiveness, acceptability, and ease of preparation. Although invariably successful in the short term, a response cannot be guaranteed and often the length of remission induced is much shorter than that effected by dithranol or coal-tar preparationns. Unfortunately there is no known means of determining which patients are likely to benefit from steroid preparations. The toxicity of corticosteroids must also be borne in mind, both in the short term when large areas of the body may have to be covered, and over longer periods when powerful steroids may need to be used continuously to suppress the condition. Psoriatic skin is dry and treatment with an ointment is optimal; a useful therapeutic compromise is 10 per cent Betnovate ointment with 3 per cent liquor picis carb. in white soft paraffin.

Until recently the use of dithranol was confined to those patients in hospital or those closely supervised in the outpatient department. The traditional preparations of dithranol in lassar's paste required meticulous application, often burning normal skin and staining clothing. The introduction of new, more sophisticated formulations has allowed the general practitioner to take advantage of this powerful and highly effective form of treatment. 'Dithrolan' comprises 0.5 per cent dithranol and 0.5 per cent salicylic acid and is perfectly compatible with domiciliary usage; more recently 'Dithrocream'—containing 0.1, 0.25, and 0.5 per cent dithranol in a vanishing cream base – has been introduced. Another variation on this theme 'Psoradrate' contains 0.1 or 0.2 per cent dithranol with 17 per cent urea. Although all these preparations still share to some extent the unpleasantness of dithranol, the problems are much less and with careful guidance in a well-motivated patient, therapy can be highly successful. As with the steroids, it is best for a practitioner to select one group of dithranol preparations and then become fully conversant with their properties (Fig. 13.5).

Whilst the introduction of these more sophisticated dithranol preparations has extended the capabilities of the general practitoner, the inception of PUVA has similarly transformed the theraputic range of the dermatologist. This treatment entails taking a photosensitizing drug – 8-methoxypsoralen two hours prior to exposure to long-wave ultraviolet light (UVA) delivered by banks of special fluorescent tubes. Initially the patient receives three treatments per week until remission is induced and this usually then lasts for 4–5 months. Following remission, maintenance treatment on a weekly or fortnightly basis will serve to

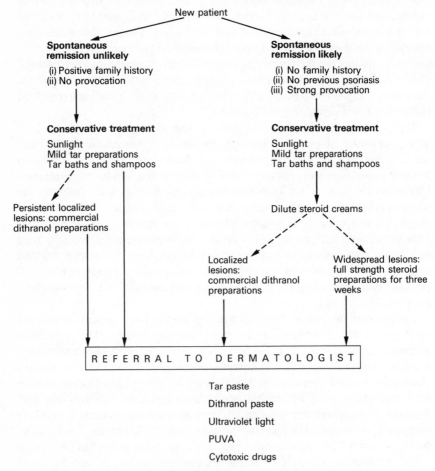

Fig. 13.5. Management of psoriasis.

keep most patients clear of psoriasis. The success rate is high with some 80–90 per cent of patients clearing completely and is highly acceptable cosmetically with the added advantage to the patient of the acquisition of a deep sun tan. Many departments of dermatology provide access to the equipment during unsocial hours so that patients need not lose time from work. Their regular visits to the dermatology department and frequent contact with other psoriatics provides the patients with much more support. PUVA enables many patients, who formerly would have required hospital admission, to be managed as out-patients.

Patients receiving PUVA incur a risk of cataract development, so appropriate goggles must be worn during treatment; there is also a risk of future development of basal cell and squamous-cell carcinomas. The dangers of these side-effects must be weighed carefully against the quality of life endured by the patient with widespread untreated psoriasis and the risks of alternative therapy with cytotoxic agents.

PUVA is now the treatment of first choice for those people over 60 years of age with at least 20 per cent of their body covered by psoriasis. In addition PUVA is partcularly effective in the treatment of pustular psoriasis of the palms and soles – a condition usually highly resistant to conventional therapy. Younger patients with severe psoriasis may also be treated with PUVA, although because of possible side-effects this is not embarked upon lightly and a stringent trial of dithranol will be tried first.

Leg ulcers

The majority of leg ulcers seen in general practice are secondary to venous insufficiency, and they form one of the most persistent and difficult dermatological problems encountered in primary care.

The raised hydrostatic pressure in the veins of the lower leg is invariably secondary to damage consequent upon a past deep-vein thrombosis; this is often aggravated by reduced muscular activity because of osteoarthritis or muscular atrophy due to age. Increased venous pressure causes blood to leak from dermal capillaries and leads eventually to infarction of the skin with subsequent ulceration.

The first aspect of management is to eliminate any reversible factors which delay healing of the lesion. Correction of anaemia, treatment of congestive cardiac failure and loss of weight will all be beneficial. The most important principle of treatment is to attempt to correct the basic venous disorder – ambulant patients should be encouraged to wear compression bandages and told to avoid standing still – or sitting for long periods with their feet down. Crêpe bandages must be applied immediately on rising in the morning or, as an alternative, medicated bandages can be used and left *in situ* for two to three weeks.

The ulcer itself is cleaned with an antiseptic such as eusol or povidone-iodine. Although ulcers are colonized by a variety of bacteria, antibiotics have a very limited role to play in their management. Systemic antibiotics rarely achieve an effective concentration at the site of the ulcer, and when topically applied exert little therapeutic influence and encourage the rapid appearance of resistant organisms. Sytemic antibodies are indicated, however, when there is an associated cellulitis around the ulcer. Swabs from uncomplicated ulcers are thus only of predictive value, indicating the most appropriate antibiotic should a cellulitis occur.

Once the ulcer has been dressed it is often appropriate to wrap the leg in a suitable medicated bandage and then apply an overlying adhesive bandage, such as elastoplast or an elastic diachylon bandage (Lestreflex). It is very common for patients with leg ulcers to become sensitized to preservatives in the preparations used with the development of an associated eczema. This may be treated initially with topical corticosteroids but patch testing will ultimately be necessary to elucidate the precise cause of the problem so that future use of the relevant agent may be avoided. Persistent ulcers which fail to respond to medical treatment may benefit from referral to a plastic surgeon for grafting.

These patients with chronic venous ulcers make a substantial contribution to the workload of the district nurse who visits them regularly in their homes over long periods. Some of the more ambulant patients may be able to make their way to the surgery and have their ulcers dressed by the practice nurse. The frustrations of managing a chronic condition such as this where progress is often slow are considerable and the district nurses, who are relatively isolated in their work, require great support and easy communication with the doctor. On rare occasions resistant ulcers necessitate admission to hospital for rest and elevation. Admission to a community hospital is particularly appropriate in these circumstances and provides a welcome respite for patient and district nurse alike.

Invariably a close relationship between nurse and patient develops. For the patient, who may well be socially isolated, the visit of the district nurse becomes a vital part of life, as she may become one of the most frequent visitors to the household. The district nurse, whilst ostensibly dressing the ulcer, will inevitably become aware of other deficiencies in that patient's life and can provide the general practitioner and health care team with valuable insight. In this way other colleagues, such as health visitors and occupational therapists, can be introduced and social supports strengthened. Free communication between the professionals involved is essential if this knowledge is to be used effectively.

At times patients use their ulcers to attract the sympathy and attention of their family and, if they are alone, the doctor and nurse.

LONG-TERM MANAGEMENT OF SKIN DISEASES

As with so many other conditions encountered in general practice, the development of a chronic skin disorder signifies the beginning of a long relationship between doctor and patient. The weeks and months after presentation of the condition are marked by great activity – the doctor will be searching for the most effective remedy for the condition and this may include referral to hospital. He will be attempting to teach the patient and his family about the disorder and aiding their adjustment to it.

Eventually a period of stability will ensue when the condition is controlled or in remission. The doctor's task in now to achieve a compromise – encouraging the patient's independence and self-reliance, but simultaneously exerting some control over the use of medication. To some extent the latter can be achieved by education, making the patient aware of the dangers associated with certain preparations; an important and practical tool, however, is the carefully managed repeat prescription. Patient and doctor must agree upon a mutually acceptable contract with the details of this appropriately recorded in the notes. It is to the advantage of all if the procedure for repeat prescriptions can be agreed between all the doctors in the partnership so that a uniform system prevails. A separate repeat prescription sheet or card in the patient's notes – stating the strength and volume of the preparation and the frequency of administration – should exist. The number of occasions on which the treatment can be repeated should be clearly detailed and known to both patient and doctor, so that no confusion need arise upon the dates for review. It is essential that those actually running the repeat prescription service, whether they be receptionists in an urban practice or dispensers in a rural one, are fully conversant with the system.

Good communications between all the relevant members of the practice team are necessary if the service is to maintain optimum efficiency and will include not only ease of access to one another but a high standard of recording in the notes. Once a contract between doctor and patient has been established, then it should be enforced; any deviation from the agreed procedure, by either party, facilitates future abuse of the system.

In the long term it is imperative that patients are reviewed at predetermined intervals, so that the progress of their disease can be monitored, any side-effects of treatment noted and their therapy reviewed in the light of new developments. This implies the presence of a 'disease index' or list of all those patients with a specific condition so that a recall system can be established.

THE GENERAL PRACTITIONER AND THE DERMATOLOGIST

The boundary between primary care and the hospital service is a variable and ill-defined one. Dermatologists only see patients on referral from their general practitioner and this is most often on an outpatient basis. Certain patients with particularly troublesome disorders will remain under the care of the outpatient department for many years but most will be referred back to their own doctor once a solution has been found to their presenting problem. A minority of patients will require admission to hospital – but as we have seen, even here new developments exert their influence – as with the psoriatics who now receive PUVA therapy.

Most patients are referred to a dermatologist because their doctor is unable to make the diagnosis or because his condition has failed to respond to the doctor's therapeutic endeavours. Many rashes are short lived and precise diagnosis is both difficult and unnecessary; inevitably the persistence of a rash excites the anxieties of the patient, his family and the doctor. Speed of referral will to some extent depend on the doctor's diagnostic and therapeutic skill, his degree of self-reliance, and his perception of that patient's need for specialized advice. The anxieties and fears of the patient and his family will greatly influence the general practitioner's management and may hasten referral. The relationship between doctor and patient and in particular the degree of confidence and trust that the doctor can inspire will have a significant effect on the course of events. Other factors tending to inhibit referral include the doctor's expertise, the distance to the hospital, and suitability of travelling arrangements.

Referral of patients to hospital fluctuates widely from doctor to doctor. In 1967 Last showed that the actual referral rate to all hospital departments varied from 5 per 1000 patients per month to 115 per 1000 patients per month, with most doctors referring 10–35 per 1000 patients per month.

Good communication between general practitioner and dermatologist is essential if maximum benefit is to be derived from the referral. The general practitioner's letter should contain a concise, but pertinent history noting in particular relevant occupational factors, details of all treatment administered and any appropriate social factors. It is valuable too to stipulate one's requirements of the referral, e.g. diagnosis, advice regarding further treatment or reassurance. Ideally the letter should be typewritten and a copy retained in the notes for reference. A similarly detailed reply is required once the patient has been assessed in the clinic; it is imperative that the family doctor is notified of any change in the treatment of those patients who regularly attend the out-patient department.

OTHER AGENCIES

In this chapter we have seen the importance of nurses and health visitors in the management of patients with skin disorders. Many sufferers have associated social or domestic problems, the stress of which exacerbates their condition. For these patients perceptive help from social workers can be of value and obviously the closer the co-operation between the primary health care team and social services, the more appropriate that help is likely to be.

Other agencies outside the National Health Service can also make a significant contribution to the welfare of these patients. The British Red Cross Society now provide a 'beauty care service' and this has been extended to the provision of camouflage clinics. The advice given at these clinics enables people with conditions as diverse as vitiligo or naevi to lead a more normal life despite their disability.

In recent years our society has witnessed the evolution of the consumer movement, and the field of dermatology has been no exception with the development of voluntary self-help organizations, some of which are listed at the end of the chapter. The first of these was the Psoriasis Association which began in 1963. Basically all such groups have common aims and they provide support for patients and their families, putting them in touch with one another and providing social contact. They help educate patients and the public on the nature and management of the relevant condition and they raise money for research. Often a regular magazine will be published by the organization in addition to leaflets and data explaining various therapeutic options that patients might be offered. As we have seen, education of the patient about his disease forms a vital part of his management and also serves to dispel a variety of 'old wives tales' that abound. Many people feel isolated and ostracized from society by their disorder and the realization that they are not alone is of great reassurance to them. Of course the benefits of these groups are not confined to the sufferers – the National Eczema Society for instance has done much to reassure and help anxious parents.

Often local meetings are held and doctors and specialists invited to participate, giving lectures, and leading discussion. Their co-operation is invaluable in the preparation of literature or in deciding on the feasibility of supporting proposed research projects. Doctors and patients can work together in this way sharing their experiences and philosophies and jointly planning improvements in dermatological services.

In many ways the management of chronic skin disease reflects the problems of general practice as a whole. Both doctor and patient must come to terms with the mutual frustration of prolonged incurable disease. The doctor must monitor the disease and its therapy whilst simultaneously helping the patient to adjust to his disability and modify his lifestyle. He must balance his medical view of the illness, where severity might be assessed by the extent of systemic complications or the toxicity of therapy, with the patients perception in which loss of social and financial status assume greater significance. A suitable equilibrium between these viewpoints must be found if the patient is to adjust to his disability and management is to be successful; this will entail the close involvement and co-operation of the patient, his family, and the practice team.

Treatment should be as practical and cosmetically acceptable as possible whilst maintaining therapeutic efficacy, and the ultimate aim of all is that the patient should return to school or work and continue to be a useful and fulfilled member of society.

PERFORMANCE REVIEW CHECK LIST

General

1. Does the practice have a policy for the management of common skin disorders?

2. Can the practice identify all patients on long-term preparations for skin disorders?

Patients on treatment

1. Is there any record of the patient's ideas or the information given to the patient?
2. Are the current drugs clearly recorded?

PATIENT ASSOCIATIONS AND SELF-HELP GROUPS

British Red Cross Society. Beauty Care and Cosmetic Camouflage.
(Contact local branches of British Red Cross.)

Dystrophic Epidermolysis Bullosa Research Association,
38 Cornwall Avenue,
Clayton,
Newcastle-under-Lyme,
Staffs.

The Lupus Group, Arthritis Care,
6 Grosvenor Crescent,
London, SW1X 7ER

Maria Scleroderma Therapy Trust,
11 Warrender Road,
Chesham,
Bucks. HP5 3NE

The National Eczema Society,
Tavistock House North,
Tavistock Square,
London, WC1H 95R

The Psoriasis Association,
7 Milton Street,
Northampton, NNZ 7JG

The Skins Disease Research Fund,
c/o St. John's Hospital for Diseases of the Skin,
5 Lisle Street,
Leicester Square,
London, WCZH 7BJ

Tuberous Sclerosis Association of Great Britain,
Church Farm House,
Church Road,
North Leigh,
Oxford OX8 6TX

PATIENT BOOKS AND LEAFLETS

Supplied by the above.

REFERENCES

Rea, J.N., Newhouse, M.L., and Halil, T. (1976): Skin disease in Lambeth, MTP, Lancaster.

Office of Population Censuses and Surveys (1974). *Morbidity statistics from general practice.* Studies on Medical and Population Subjects No. 26. HMSP.

Last, J.M. (1967). Objective measurements of quality in general practice. Suppl. to *Ann. gen. Pract.* **XII**, 2.

14 Thyroid disease

Andrew Markus

DEFINITION

Diseases of the thyroid are best considered under the headings of abnormalities of structure and of function.

Structure: Enlargement (goitre) may be diffuse or nodular, and either may be associated with normal or abnormal function. Enlargement may also be due to acute or chronic inflammation, and neoplasm.

Function: the effects on the system depend on whether there is over or under activity, and on the age at which malfunction begins.

The size of the gland is no guide to the level of function.

INCIDENCE AND PREVALENCE

In the author's practice the prevalence of all thyroid disease is 7 per 1000 patients, equally divided between over and under activity. In the last ten years there have also been two cases of Hashimoto's thyroiditis and one of thyroid carcinoma (in a total of 8500 patients) so the incidence of these conditions is very small. The sex ratio of thyrotoxicosis is female:male 30:1 and of myxoedema 15:1. The incidence of the disease over the last ten years has been 1/1000 patients/annum. This compares with an incidence of 0.2/1000 in Dr John Fry's practice (personal communication).

The 'average' GP with a list of 2500 patients may therefore expect to see 2–3 patients with thyroid disease per year, and as these conditions are eminently treatable, it is well worthwhile looking out for them – especially in female patients.

IMPACT OF THE DISEASE – PATIENT, PRACTICE, AND SOCIETY

The effect of thyroid disease on the individual varies from the minor cosmetic to the major systemic. Over and under activity of the gland may lead to serious social and medical consequences – the thyrotoxic may be labelled as a fussy neurotic complainer, and cause a lot of frustrating and unsatisfactory doctor patient contacts, whilst the undiagnosed patient with myxoedema may lose her job because of 'lack of drive', or end up in a mental hospital – lethargic, confused, or suffering from so called 'myxoedema mania'. It is therefore, important to have a high index of suspicion of malfunction of this gland, and, for patients with diagnosed disease, to have an effective system to ensure follow-up.

DIAGNOSIS AND APPROPRIATE INVESTIGATIONS

Full blown over or under activity of the thyroid gland is easy to diagnose and satisfying to treat. The confirmation of the diagnosis by biochemical means requires some knowledge of basic thyroid physiology.

The function of the thyroid gland is to synthesize and store thyroxine (T_4) and trio-idio thyronine (T_3), and to liberate these hormones into the system in appropriate amounts. Iodine is required for synthesis, and the trapping of this by the thyroid gland is enhanced by thyroid stimulating hormone (TSH) and opposed by thiocyanates and perchlorates. The iodine is linked with tyrosine to form T_3 and T_4 and this step is inhibited by thiouracil and carbimazole. The liberation of the thyroid hormones (stored in the gland in combination with glycoproteins) into the bloodstream is activated by TSH.

In the blood the majority of hormonal iodine is in the form of thyroxine, in balance with a much smaller quantity of T_3 (though some people are T_3 rather than T_4 secretors, and in them there is a larger amount of T_3 circulating). Only about 0.03 per cent of the circulating T_4 is 'free', the rest being protein bound, mainly to thyroxine-binding globulin (TBG), with which it is in equilibrium. This free thyroxine (and T_3) would be the best indicator of thyroid function, as it is not dependent on the absolute levels of serum proteins, but its estimation is only now beginning to be offered as a service by specialised laboratories. The T_3 and T_4 levels estimated by most laboratories give the *total* T_3 and T_4 level in the blood, which, as explained above, is mostly protein bound. The level of free T_4 in the blood is controlled through a feedback mechanism by TSH – a fall in the level of thyroid hormones in the blood causes a rise in TSH secretion (see Fig. 14.1).

Thyroid hormones influence cellular metabolism in all tissues. The maturation of the body – skeletal, sexual, and mental, depends on normal function. Thyroid hormones increase oxidation and carbohydrate breakdown in the liver and peripheral tissues, as well as protein catabolism. The serum cholesterol level is in part controlled by these hormones, rising in thyroid deficiency, though not falling in overactivity.

The rational use of tests of thyroid function depends on the understanding of the above facts, because, as stated before, the size of the gland is no guide to its level of function.

Physiological tests

Serum thyroxine
The *total* level (bound and unbound) of T_4 or T_3 may be measured by radio-immunoassay – the free amount of these hormones is too small to be measured

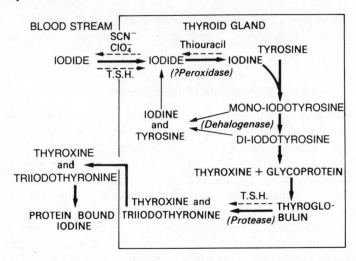

Fig. 14.1. Diagrammatic summary of the sequences in the biosynthesis of thyroxine and tri-iodothyronine in the thyroid gland. Broken arrows indicate agents which accelerate or retard the formation of thyroid hormones. (From *Price's textbook of the practice of medicine* (ed. Sir Ronald Bodley Scott) Clarendon Press, Oxford (1978).)

in routine circumstances – and therefore both these levels are affected by the level of thyroid-binding proteins. This is raised in pregnancy and in women taking oestrogens, including the contraceptive pill, but allowances can be made by determining the 'free thyroxine index' (FTI) (see below).

T_3 resin uptake

This rather confusingly named test does *not* measure the serum T_3, but the proportion of circulating thyroxine-binding protein *not* bound with thyroid hormone. Radioactive T_3 is added *in vitro* to the patient's serum. Those binding sites not already saturated take up T_3, and the remainder is absorbed onto a resin and measured. In thyrotoxicosis a large proportion of thyroid-binding protein is occupied, and there is less room for the radioactive T_3 – a larger proportion of this will therefore be left to be absorbed onto the resin. The reverse holds in myxoedema. The reason for the usefulness of this test is that with alterations of the thyroid-binding protein levels, the movement of the T_3 resin test result is in the opposite direction to the level of the serum hormones.

'Free thyroxine index' (FTI)

Multiplication of the serum T_4 level by the result of the T_3 resin test gives a result independent of the level of thyroid-binding protein, and is by convention called the 'free thyroxine index'. *This figure is the single most reliable indicator of thyroid function.*

Other tests: ^{131}I test

A dose of radioactive iodine is given to the patient and its 'trapping' by the thyroid gland is measured after a delay of a few hours. It is a test which tends to be used only under special rare circumstances, such as when viral thyroiditis is suspected, as there may then be a tranisent high uptake.

TSH level

Because of the 'feedback' effect, a raised TSH level is found in primary myxoedema and is a useful diagnostic test. It is also (see below) the single most important index of the satisfactory treatment of myxoedema with substitution therapy. The test is *not* helpful in thyrotoxicosis as the TSH levels are frequently normal in this condition.

TRH (thyroid releasing hormone) test

TSH levels are tested before and after the injection of TRH. This test is useful in distinguishing primary hypothyroidism from that secondary to pituitary failure, or for borderline hyperthyroidism.

Aetiological tests

Thyroid antibodies

Various tests are available, of which the most sensitive is a complement fixing test which is positive in 98 per cent of patients with Hashimoto's thyroiditis. As it is also positive in 83 per cent of patients with primary myxoedema, and in about 65 per cent of those with thyrotoxicosis, the diagnostic value of this test is not great. However, it has some predictive value in patients with treated thyrotoxicosis, as those with high pre-treatment antibody levels are more likely to develop myxoedema subsequently.

Thyroid scan

This test helps to distinguish hyperthyroidism due to general overactivity of the gland from that due to autonomous toxic nodules – so called 'hot nodules'.

'Best buy' in thyroid tests

In suspected hyperthyroidism: serum T_3 level (some people are T_3 secretors, and as in normal T_3 and T_4 are in balance, measurement of T_3 covers all eventualities).

In suspected hypothyroidism: serum T_4 level (there is less T_3 present than T_4 normally and in the lower ranges measuring T_3 becomes inaccurate), and serum TSH.

In complicated situations: e.g. with concurrent disease or drug therapy – free thyroxine index.

BUT, it is well to remember that, especially in older patients, the diagnosis of myxoedema should be made on clinical grounds, and clinical impressions should not be over-ruled by normal function tests.

MANAGEMENT

Simple goitre

By definition this includes all non-malignant enlargement of the thyroid gland, which is not accompanied by abnormal function. By common usage autoimmune diseases of the thyroid such as Hashimoto's thyroiditis are excluded from this category.

Enlargement of the gland due to goitrogens will reduce if these are withdrawn, though that due to iodine deficiency may not subside of iodine is given, especially if the deficiency has long been standing. Surgery is the only other treatment available, and may be indicated on grounds of appearance, pressure on surrounding structures, or possibility of malignancy.

Follow up after surgery is important, especially if thyroid antibody levels were raised pre-operatively, as under these circumstances the development of hypothyroidism is more likely (see before).

Hyperthyroidism

This state may be caused by generalized overactivity of the gland, such as in Graves' disease (which accounts for 99 per cent of cases) or by overactivity of localized areas. Graves' disease is not associated with increased TSH concentrations in the blood, but is probably due to the effect of IgG immunoglobulins (of which the best recognized is LATS, long-acting thyroid stimulator) on the thyroid gland.

Before treatment, confirmation of the diagnosis should be sought by using one of the tests previously described, otherwise confusion with an anxiety state may result in wrong treatment.

Graves' disease may be treated by antithyroid drugs, radioactive iodine, or surgery. The method chosen depends on the size of the gland, the age and wishes of the patient, and the availability of radiotherapy and surgical services. A beta-adrenergic blocking drug may be used initially to give symtomatic relief of excessive sweating and increased heart rate, but this is emphatically not definitive treatment. If an unselective beta-blocker such as propranolol is used, 40 mg three times a day is a reasonable dose, but should be avoided in patients with asthma. Heart failure may be precipitated by this treatment and will need the concurrent use of digitalis and/or diuretics.

Antithyroid drugs are usually the treatment of first choice in young to middle-aged adults. The initial dose of carbimazole is 10 mg three times a day and of propyl-thiouracil 100 mg three times a day. Either treatment may cause rashes, gastrointestinal upsets and drug fever, and also agranulocytosis. All patients should be told to report sore throats at once. Regular white cell counts, formerly advised, are probably not very helpful as the onset of marrow supression is liable to be sudden. The object of treatment by many experts nowadays is virtual ablation of the gland for the period of treatment, maintaining the initial drug dose throughout, rather than trying to 'titrate' it against the patient's clinical condition. If this approach is used, it is best to give thyroxine 0.1 mg daily throughout treatment – this helps maintain the euthyroid state and possibly helps to stop the gland enlarging during treatment. 18–24 months treatment is usually advised, and some 40 per cent of patients relapse after therapy.

Radioactive iodine treatment is usually reserved for patients aged over 40, and is the treatment of choice in younger patients with recurring problems. The treatment takes up to three months to achieve maximum effect, and during this time a beta-blocker can be used to reduce symptoms. The main problem with this form of treatment is that in the ten years following it, 40 per cent of patients become hypothyroid, and subsequently even more. Adequate follow up, which needs to be maintained long after discharge from hospital clinics, is therefore vital (see below).

Surgical treatment is indicated when the gland is large, either in the neck or retrosternally, and causing symptoms; in young patients with recurrent problems; in those contemplating pregnancy, and in those patients who do not wish for prolonged surveillance. Having said that, the development of hypothyroidism occurs in around 20 per cent of patients within six years of surgery and there is a 5 per cent recurrence rate for thyrotoxicosis. Surgical treatment is also advised for patients with toxic nodular goitres in whom cardiovascular symptoms may predominate.

It will be seen from the above that the likelihood of hypothyroidism after *any* form of treatment is very high and increases over the post treatment years. Adequate follow up is therefore vital.

Hypothyroidism

The clinical picture of hypothyroidism depends on the age at which thyroid deficiency first affects the body. Congenital and childhood deficiency result in cretinism and dwarfism respectively, which are both very rare conditions, and outside the scope of this book. Adult hypothyroidism is most commonly due to primary deficiency in the function of the thyroid gland, though it may, much more rarely, be secondary to pituitary malfunction. It is more common in women than men, and is especially prevalent in the 30–50 age group. The serum of the majority of patients contains thyroid antibodies, so the cause is likely to be due to an auto-immune process in most patients. The most obvious manifestation of this kind of activity is the hypothyroidism following Hashimoto's thyroiditis, a chronic inflammatory disease of the thyroid gland, caused by thyroid antibodies, commonly resulting in myxoedema.

From the general practice point of view the main problem with the diagnosis of hypothyroidism is its frequently insidious onset, with the consequent difficulty in picking up symptoms and signs, especially in patients one sees often. It is a diagnosis liable to be made by a partner or locum who has never seen the patient before, whilst the patient's own doctor is away on holiday. Symptoms of lethargy, muscular pains, cold intolerance, and perhaps tingling in the hands (due to a 'carpal tunnel' syndrome) should alert the doctor. Full-blown confusional states may also occur. The appearance and the voice of the patient may be pathognomonic, and it should be remembered that, paradoxically, hypertension is common in myxoedema, and may be resistant to treatment with hypotensives – just as the treatment of auricular fibrillation in undiagnosed thyrotoxic patients is resistant to treatment with digitalis.

An attempt has been made by Gillewicz *et al.* (1969) to apply statistical methods to the clinical diagnosis of hypothyroidism. Table 14.1 is reproduced for interest, but has not been found helpful by the present author.

Table 14.1. *Hypothyroid diagnostic index*

Symptoms	Present	Absent	Signs	Present	Absent
Diminished sweating	+6	−2	Slow movement	+11	−3
Dry skin	+3	−6	Coarse skin	+7	−7
Cold intolerance	+4	−5	Cold skin	+3	−2
Weight increase	+1	−1	Per orbital		
Constipation	+2	−1	puffiness	+4	−6
Hoarseness	+5	−6	Slow ankle jerk	+15	−6
Paraesthesiae	+5	−4	Slow pulse	+4	−4
Deafness	+2	0			
		Euthyroid	− 30 or less		
		Doubtful	− 29 to + 19		
		Hypothyroid + 20 or more			

It must be emphasized that although the diagnosis of hypothyroidism is best confirmed by serum T_4 estimations, mild cases may only have a raised TSH level, or normal blood findings altogether. Such patients deserve a trial of treatment on clinical grounds alone.

The treatment of hypothyroidism is usually straightforward and is by the use of thyroxine in a single daily dose of 0.1–0.2 mg. The best index of adequate therapy (apart from the condition of the patient) is a fall in the TSH level to normal. In elderly patients, especially those with heart disease, such as angina pectoris, it is wise to start with a lower dose, such as 0.025 mg daily, rising in weekly stages to standard levels.

PRACTICE ORGANIZATION

Whatever abnormality of the thyroid is, or has been, present in a patient, it is very helpful to have the names listed, either as part of a general disease index, or otherwise. Some method has to be devised whereby patients who miss follow-up appointments come to notice. A simple way is for the names of patients to be written on a small card index card, and for these to be filed in a 'tickler' system, by months when the patient should return. Anyone defaulting can then be contacted. This is the kind of information which a computer could effectively be used to supply.

AUDIT

The effectiveness of management may be checked by extracting the records of patients via the disease index, and seeing to what extent the euthyroid state has been achieved and maintained. This state will need to be defined in biochemical and/or clinical terms. There are no generally accepted guidelines as to how often patients should be seen, or blood tests be performed – though *a priori* one would expect more frequent examinations to be necessary if treatment has been recent. The setting of guidelines could be one of the products of audit activity – by, say, performing annual tests and examinations, it would be possible to show whether, from a long-term point of view, these are too frequent, or not frequent enough, to predict the maintenance of the euthyroid state satisfactorily. Criteria (guidelines) can then be worked out to represent good practice, and the achievement of these criteria can be reviewed by, say, annual reaudit. This kind of activity could be organized on an area basis at postgraduate meetings. To the author's knowledge this has not been done, though individual workers (such as Mourin 1976) have published results from their own practice, and Howie and Butt (1982) have described a trainee group project.

INDICATIONS FOR REFERRAL

Patients with straightforward thyrotoxicosis or myxoedema need not be referred to hospital if the diagnosis can be confirmed by biochemical tests and the best treatment is medical. The more complicated patient, perhaps with concurrent disease such as diabetes, may benefit from a consultant opinion. Treatment by surgery or ^{131}I will of course entail specialist involvement but in every case long-term GP follow up is mandatory and the responsibility for this must be clearly defined, otherwise the patient falls between the two stools of hospital and general practice.

PERFORMANCE REVIEW CHECK LIST

General
1. Can the practice identify all its patients on thyroid replacement?
2. Is there a mechanism for following up all patients who have had thyroid surgery and thyrotoxicosis?

Patients on treatment

1. Is there a clear indication in the records of why the patient was started on thyroid replacement?
2. Is there a record of thyroid function tests at subsequent assessments?
3. Is there any record of the patient's ideas or the information given to the patient?
4. Are the current drugs and dosage clearly recorded?

REFERENCES

Billewicz, W.Z., Chapman, R.S., Crooks, J., Day, M.E., Gossage, J., Wayne, E. and Young, J.A. (1969). Statistical methods applied to the diagnosis of hypothyroidism. *Q. Jl med.* **38**, 255–66.

Howie, J.G.R. and Butt, A.J.M. (1982). Managing thyroid illness: a trainee group project. *Br. med. J.* **285**, 1541–2.

Mourin, K.A. (1976). Auditing and evaluation in general practice. *J. R. Coll. gen. Practrs* **26**, 726–33.

15 Conclusions

John Hasler and Theo Schofield

In this book we have argued that an increasing proportion of medical time will need to be spent in the management of chronic disease in the future. We have highlighted the size of the problem and emphasized that some of the most important aspects of management are not clinical in the accepted sense of the word. Many of the features of effective practice organization have been described.

We have demonstrated that the management of common chronic diseases is, for the most part, well within the competence of the general practitioner. But we have gone further: we have declared our belief that most patients are more logically, effectively, and economically managed in general practice. Further, not only should this be better for patients, but it should ensure that the general practitioner remains a broadly based clinician, thereby freeing the specialist to concentrate on the more difficult problems.

If, on the other hand, general practitioners choose to opt out and expect the hospital outpatient department to supervise the increasing number of routine long-term problems, then the consequences of that decision should be obvious. The hospital specialist's time becomes increasingly burdened with patients who do not require his particular expertise, and the time he has available to deal with the more complex problems, legitimately his concern, becomes progressively limited. At the same time, the scarce financial resources of an ever-increasing hospital budget are diluted still further.

But the implications are greater still for general practice. Many would question the right of the general practitioner to continue to enjoy his central position in the National Health Service if a major part of everyday clinical medicine is handed over.

In any civilised country such as ours, with its long and great tradition of general practice, people have a right to receive the best possible care for those diseases which cannot be prevented or cured. We hope that this book will, in some small measure, motivate, and help general practitioners to provide a substantial part of that care.

Index